STATINS TOXIC SIDE EFFECTS

Evidence From 500 Scientific Papers

by

David Evans

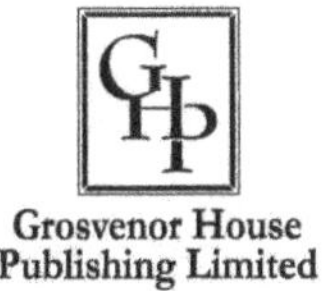

Grosvenor House
Publishing Limited

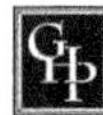

This book is published by
Grosvenor House Publishing Ltd
28-30 High Street, Guildford, Surrey, GU1 3EL.
www.grosvenorhousepublishing.co.uk

A CIP record for this book
is available from the British Library

ISBN 978-1-78148-390-9

This book is dedicated to my wonderful wife Julie for her patience, support and love

Also by David Evans

Cholesterol and Saturated Fat Prevent Heart Disease: Evidence From 101 Scientific Papers

Low Cholesterol Leads To An Early Death: Evidence From 101 Scientific Papers

Medical/liability disclaimer

This book is intended solely for informational and educational purposes and not as medical advice, nor to replace the advice of a doctor or other health care professionals. Anyone wishing to embark on any dietary or lifestyle change must first consult with their health care professional.

The decision to use any information in this book is entirely the decision of the reader, who assumes full responsibility for any and all consequences arising from such a decision. Neither the author nor the publisher shall be held liable for any consequences resulting or allegedly resulting from use of information in this book.

About the author

David is a qualified nutritional adviser. He runs a website called *Healthy Diets and Science* (www.dietsandscience.com) which is devoted to examining the scientific evidence regarding the effects of diet, pharmaceutical drugs and lifestyle on health. David has previously written books examining the influence of dietary cholesterol and saturated fat on heart disease and the impact of cholesterol levels on health. He is married to Julie, has four children, two step-children – ages 17 to 31 – and six grandchildren.

Foreword

by
Tom Naughton
Health writer, researcher and filmmaker

Judging by the constant parade of TV advertisements for statins, you'd think they're the greatest drugs ever developed. *Lowers "bad" cholesterol! Reduces heart attacks by 33 percent! A low risk of side-effects!* Well, heck, what's not to like? Perhaps we should all be taking statins along with our daily vitamin pills, just to on the safe side.

If you're a speed-reader and happen to watch TV through binoculars, you might just catch one of the disclaimers that appear briefly in tiny print. Using the freeze-frame option on my remote, I saw one disclaimer that the statin being advertised has not actually been shown to reduce heart attacks. (This fact didn't prevent the woman in the ad from dancing a happy little jig to celebrate her lower cholesterol.) Another disclaimer stated that a reduction in heart attacks was only demonstrated in a particular "high risk" group. Given that statins are handed out like candy on Halloween, that "high risk" group must be the biggest minority on the planet.

If you take a peek at the actual research (which I have), you'll quickly find that the supposed benefits of statins aren't nearly as impressive or ubiquitous as we've been led to believe. Yes, one brand of statin may have reduced the rate of heart attacks by 33 percent – in one particular "high risk" group, anyway – but you have to understand how that number is calculated: among high-risk men enrolled in the years-long study, three out of every 100 who took a placebo had a heart attack; while in the statin-taking group, two out of every 100 had a heart attack. Two is a 33% reduction from three ... but in real terms, it means years of taking a statin apparently prevented one heart attack for every 100 high-risk men. Oh, and by the way, there was no reduction in the overall death rate.

You might be thinking to yourself, "Okay, so perhaps statins don't actually prevent all that many fatal heart attacks. But they do lower cholesterol, so why not take them? What can it hurt?"

The answer is: plenty.

To begin with, statins can literally make you hurt. One of the most common side-effects is pain in the muscles and joints. Soon after my mother began taking a statin, she ended up taking a daily pain-killer as well. (Her doctor, like so many doctors, never attributed the onset of aches and pains to the statin.)

Even if your muscles don't ache, they not may function as well. A study of professional athletes showed that most who are prescribed statins stop taking them. You and I may not notice if we become a bit weaker and slower, but professional athletes certainly do – after all, losing a bit of strength and speed can cost them their careers.

But muscle pains are just the tip of the iceberg. Despite the manufacturers' claims of *a low incidence of side-effects*, independent research is concluding that side-effects are quite common with statins ... including everything from diabetes to liver damage to memory loss.

But you don't have to take my word for it. In this book, David Evans presents summaries of 500 scientific papers – yes, 500 – in which the researchers concluded that statins caused or were at least associated with very negative health effects. These are the studies your doctor probably hasn't seen and which the statins manufacturers would like to pretend don't exist.

But they do exist. For your sake, and for the sake of any loved ones who are taking statins, I'd urge you to give these studies a look.

I don't believe you'll find them so effectively gathered and summarized anywhere else.

Table of contents

Introduction

Are you fearful of high cholesterol? Are you taking, or have you been advised to start taking cholesterol lowering statin drugs? It is essential you have the knowledge of statins debilitating and toxic side effects. This book, based on the evidence of 500 peer-reviewed scientific papers, provides you with that knowledge.

People of an ever decreasing age are been urged, almost mandated, to have their cholesterol numbers checked, and an ever increasing percentage of them are then advised by a member of the medical profession to take a statin drug to lower their "dangerously high" levels.

Consider the above paragraph with the following data.

Figures drawn from 192 countries by the World Health Organisation reveal the following:

- Women with cholesterol levels of 177 mg/dL (4.6 mmol/L) and under have a 250% higher death rate than women with cholesterol levels of 212 mg/dL (5.5 mmol/L) and over.
- Men with cholesterol levels of 177 mg/dL (4.6 mmol/L) and under have a 138% higher death rate than men with cholesterol levels of 212 mg/dL (5.5 mmol/L) and over.

Statin drugs generate annual sales of $34 billion and now exceed a quarter of a trillion dollars since they were first marketed around two and a half decades ago. The total sales of atorvastatin (Lipitor) have been worth more than $140 billion to the pharmaceutical giant Pfizer.

Statin drugs are purported to prevent cardiovascular disease by cutting cholesterol levels.

However, again, data collected by the World Health Organiszation from 192 countries shows a surprising story:

- Women with cholesterol levels of 177 mg/dL (4.6 mmol/L) and under have a 93% higher death rate from cardiovascular diseases than women with cholesterol levels of 212 mg/dL (5.5 mmol/L) and over.
- Men with cholesterol levels of 177 mg/dL (4.6 mmol/L) and under have a 27% higher death rate from cardiovascular diseases than men with cholesterol levels of 212 mg/dL (5.5 mmol/L) and over.

So, worldwide data reveals that higher cholesterol levels are associated with a longer lifespan and a reduced risk of cardiovascular disease, and figures show that cholesterol lowering drugs (statins) sales are in the tens of billions of dollars annually.

Why then, do virtually all the medical profession, the media, our friends and family think it is a wise decision to lower cholesterol levels with a statin drug? And why are they wrong? This book will provide answers.

As mentioned above, this book uses evidence from 500 scientific papers drawn from peer-reviewed scientific journals. These 500 papers reveal that statin drugs do not save lives. The evidence shows that statin drugs do not add one day to your lifespan, but they do have a plethora of toxic side effects that adversely impact the quality of life of millions of people.

Using the data from the 500 scientific papers, the book will show you some of statins toxic side effects:

- The disturbing effects of statins on death rates, heart disease, stroke, diabetes and cancer.
- Statins are a health disaster for those with an underactive thyroid.
- How statins cause muscle disease, kidney disease, liver disease, pancreatitis and multiorgan failure.
- The dire consequences of statin use on the nervous system.
- Autoimmune diseases, arthritis and skin infections may result from statin use.
- Evidence is presented that reveal statins are deleterious for those that have asthma and lung diseases.
- Exercise performance is severely restricted by the use of the drug.
- People taking statins are found to have a 'foggy' brain, depression and an increased risk of violence and suicidal thoughts.
- Statins can damage your eyes and give you headaches.
- They can make men impotent, damage sperm quality and cause birth defects.
- Bowel problems, urinary tract infections and other general infections are exacerbated with statin use.
- Bone structure may be compromised and tendon rupture is more common when using the drug.

Again using the scientific papers, this book examines how statins deplete us of vital nutrients, and the mechanisms of how statins poison us are explained.

You may be wondering who issues the guidelines for cholesterol lowering and statin use. A chapter is devoted to this subject. This chapter shows that the advice given by the authorities to continually lower cholesterol levels bears no relationship to the actual evidence the authorities presented.

You will discover that statin manufacturers pay for the trials that are used as evidence to increase the use of statin drugs. You will learn that statin manufacturers pay out millions of dollars to doctors, professors and scientists who design, carry out and convey the results of these studies. You will be shown the close links between high-level health policy makers and statin manufacturers. You will find out that doctors are almost mandated to prescribe you statin drugs.

However, there is a chink of light at the end of the tunnel. Not all in the medical profession have been bedazzled by the cholesterol lowering statin colossus. Observations and wisdom is gathered from independently minded eminent professors and doctors. These medical professionals provide thoughtful and compelling evidence that statin drugs are overhyped, overused, are not safe and should not be used.

How to use this book

This book contains 500 scientific papers which have virtually all been published in peer-reviewed scientific journals.

The format of the book has been designed so you can analyse each paper independently, although you could read the whole book through, or pick a chapter where you need particular knowledge.

Every paper has a heading that gives the essence of its findings. Each paper also contains the name of the author, the title of the paper, and where and when it was published.

I then try and describe the findings of the paper in a concise, easy to read manner. However, some unfamiliar words are in the text, which are explained in the Glossary.

For an example of the layout, Paper 17 is shown below:

Paper 17:
Statin use increases the size of brain haemorrhage
Ricard G et al Statins may increase intracerebral hemorrhage volume. *Canadian Journal of Neurological Sciences* 2010 Nov;37(6):791-6

The paper heading is "Statin use increases the size of brain haemorrhage".

G Ricard was the author. (et al means "with others"). So other people also contributed to the paper.

The title of the paper is "Statins may increase intracerebral hemorrhage volume".

It was published in the *Canadian Journal of Neurological Sciences.*

The date, volume and page numbers etc. of this paper is 2010 Nov;37(6):791-6

You may be wondering what peer-reviewed scientific journals are.

Peer review is a process that journals use to ensure the articles they publish represent the best scholarship currently available. When an article is submitted to a peer-reviewed journal, the editors send it out to other scholars in the same field (the author's peers) to get their opinion on the quality of the scholarship, its relevance to the field, its appropriateness for the journal, etc. If these "peers" find the proposed article does not meet these rigorous standards then the article is rejected. This process is in stark contrast to the articles written in newspapers which are based on circulation figures and personal opinions. It may be argued that the peer review process is not without its faults. Many studies conducted on the efficacy of drugs are sponsored by the pharmaceutical company manufacturing the drug, and bias, personal opinion, and the design of the study to ensure it will find answers that will please the sponsor, may creep into the process. This is reflected in titles of some papers bearing little resemblance to the findings of the study and the habit of many researchers to maximize any trivial benefits of a drug whilst at the same time minimalizing any toxic effects. However, in most scientific papers the results of the investigations can be found, sometimes buried very deeply, and rigorous and thorough reading of the whole papers rather than just the headlines will reveal the facts.

Chapter 1

Statins don't save lives

Statins, or to give them their full title: 3-hydroxy-3-methylglutaryl-coenzyme (HMG-CoA) reductase inhibitors, are among the biggest-selling medicines in the world, generating billions in revenue for pharmaceutical companies.

Statins medications include: Atorvastatin (lipitor), Fluvastatin (lescol), lovastatin (mevacor), pitavastatin (livalo), pravastatin (pravachol), rosuvastatin (crestor) and simvastatin (zocor). Some statins may be known by different brand names, and some are combined with other drugs such as the ezetimibe/simvastatin combination (vytorin).

Statin drugs are used to lower cholesterol levels. Propaganda emanating from the statin pharmaceutical goliaths alleges that high cholesterol is unhealthy, thereby statins are wonder drugs and "save thousands of lives every year".

However, is this true?

Do statins save lives?

The following 32 papers investigate the effect of statins on mortality rates in a variety of people, from those who are healthy with (normal or "high" cholesterol levels), to those who have heart disease, stroke, cancer, diabetes and other life-threatening conditions.

Paper 1:
Statins increase the risk of serious adverse cardiovascular events

Crouse JR 3rd et al Effect of rosuvastatin on progression of carotid intima-media thickness in low-risk individuals with subclinical atherosclerosis: the METEOR Trial. *Journal of the American Medical Association* 2007 Mar 28;297(12):1344-53

This study (Measuring Effect on Intima-Media Thickness: an Evaluation of Rosuvastatin, METEOR) investigated the effects of statins in participants with a low risk of heart disease. The two-year study, based at Wake Forest University, was a randomised, double-blind, placebo-controlled trial of 984 individuals, average age 57 years. The participants received either a daily 40-mg dose of rosuvastatin or placebo.

The study found:

- Cholesterol levels reduced by 33% in the statin users and remained the same in those on placebo.
- Low density lipoprotein (LDL) cholesterol levels reduced by 49% in the statin users and remained the same in those on placebo.
- Statin users had a 21% increased risk of death compared to placebo.
- Statin users had a 423% increased risk of a serious adverse cardiovascular event compared to placebo.
- Statin users had a 5% increased risk of developing cancer compared to placebo.
- Statin users had a 5% increased risk of muscle pain compared to placebo.
- Statin users had a 121% increased risk of elevated liver enzymes compared to placebo.
- Statin users had a 56% increased risk of developing arthritis compared to placebo.
- Statin users had a 42% increased risk of joint pain compared to placebo.
- Statin users had a 20% increased risk of headaches compared to placebo.
- Statin users had a 43% increased risk of dizziness compared to placebo.

Paper 2:
Simvastatin is associated with higher death rates, higher cardiac death rates and increased risk of cancer

Teo KK et al Long-term effects of cholesterol lowering and angiotensin-converting enzyme inhibition on coronary atherosclerosis: The Simvastatin/Enalapril Coronary Atherosclerosis Trial (SCAT). *Circulation* 2000 Oct 10;102(15):1748-54

One of the aims of this long-term, multicentre randomized, double-blind, placebo-controlled trial was to evaluate the effects of simvastatin in patients with normal cholesterol levels and with detectable plaque build up in at least three major coronary artery segments. The study, headed by Professor Koon Teo – an expert in clinical trials and epidemiology studies on cardiovascular diseases – lasted for four years, and included a total of 460 patients: 230 received simvastatin and 230, a placebo.

Professor Teo found:

- The patients receiving simvastatin had a 117% increased risk of death compared to the patients receiving placebo.
- The patients receiving simvastatin had a 76% increased risk of cardiac death compared to the patients receiving placebo.
- The patients receiving simvastatin had a 225% increased risk of non-cardiac death compared to the patients receiving placebo.
- The patients receiving simvastatin had a 9% increased risk of a heart attack compared to the patients receiving placebo.
- The patients receiving simvastatin had a 78% increased risk of cancer compared to the patients receiving placebo.

Paper 3: Scientists raise fears of cancer link to statin used by thousands

Rossebo AB et al Intensive lipid lowering with simvastatin and ezetimibe in aortic stenosis. *New England Journal of Medicine* September 25, 2008; 359(13): 1343-56

This trial (Simvastatin and Ezetimibe in Aortic Stenosis, SEAS) observed the effects of the drug Inegy (a combination of simvastatin and ezetimibe). The trial was a randomised, double-blind trial involving 1,873 patients with mild-to-moderate, asymptomatic aortic stenosis (obstruction of blood flow across the aortic valve). The patients received either 40 mg of simvastatin plus 10 mg of ezetimibe or placebo daily and were followed for 52 months.

The study revealed:

- Those taking the simvastatin/ezetimibe combination had a 4% increased risk of death compared to those taking placebo.
- Those taking the simvastatin/ezetimibe combination had a 21% increased risk of death from heart failure compared to those taking placebo.

- Those taking the simvastatin/ezetimibe combination had a 67% increased risk of death from cancer compared to those taking placebo.
- Those taking the simvastatin/ezetimibe combination had a 195% increased risk of death from violence or accidents compared to those taking placebo.

Professor Heinz Drexel, of the University of Innsbruck in Austria and spokesman for the European Society of Cardiology, said: *"I am not sure that the efficacy is proven and I am not sure that the safety is proven. I wouldn't take the drug myself"*.

In Britain, about 300,000 NHS prescriptions were dispensed for Inegy in 2006 – 2008.

Paper 4:
Lovastatin increases the death rate by 150-300%

Bradford RH et al Expanded Clinical Evaluation of Lovastatin (EXCEL) Study Results: 1. Efficacy in Modifying Plasma Lipoproteins and Adverse Event Profile in 8245 Patients With Moderate Hypercholesterolemia *Archives of Internal Medicine* 1991; 151 (1): 43-49

This double-blind, diet and placebo controlled study investigated the relationship between statins and death rates. In the study, 8,245 'patients', aged 18 to 70, with cholesterol levels between 232mg/dL (6.0 mmol/l) and 300mg/dL (7.8 mmol/l) received one of four different doses of lovastatin (Mevacor) or a placebo.

The study found after one year:

- Higher transaminase levels (which may be an indicator of liver damage) were found in the subjects taking statins.
- Higher incidences of clinical adverse experiences requiring patients to discontinue the 'treatment' were found in the subjects taking statins.
- 16% more patients taking 20 mg/day statins discontinued their treatment compared to patients taking placebo.
- 50% more patients taking 80 mg/day statins discontinued their treatment compared to patients taking placebo.
- Higher levels of muscle damage were detected in the subjects taking statins.
- The four groups taking lovastatin lowered their low density lipoprotein (LDL) cholesterol levels by 24%-40%.

- The four groups taking lovastatin lowered their cholesterol levels by 17%-29%.
- The death rate of the four groups taking various doses of lovastatin was 150-300% higher than the placebo group.

Paper 5: Statin use is associated with an increased risk of adverse events and death in patients undergoing coronary artery bypass surgery for unstable angina

Ali IS et al Preoperative statin use and in-hospital outcomes following heart surgery in patients with unstable angina. *European Journal of Cardiothoracic Surgery* 2005 Jun;27(6):1051-6

Unstable angina happens when blood flow to the heart is suddenly slowed by narrowed vessels or small blood clots that form in the coronary arteries. Unstable angina is a warning sign that a heart attack may soon occur. It is an emergency. It may happen at rest or with light activity.

This Canadian study investigated the effects of preoperative statin use in patients with unstable angina undergoing coronary artery bypass graft/valve surgery. The study matched 534 patients taking statins with 534 patients not on statins from 1,706 patients classified with Canadian Cardiovascular Society Angina Grading IV (the most severe grade of angina). In this study, composite outcome refers to adverse events namely: dying in hospital, needing intra-aortic balloon pump use, heart attack, needing use of a ventilator and stroke.

The Canadian researchers found:

- Patients taking statins had a 10% increased risk of death whilst in hospital compared to patients not taking statins.
- Patients taking statins had a 14% increased risk of composite outcomes compared to patients not taking statins.

Paper 6: Cardiac surgery patients taking statins have a 24% increased risk of death

Mohamed R et al Preoperative statin use and infection after cardiac surgery: a cohort study. *Clinical Infectious Diseases* 2009 Apr 1;48(7):e66-72

This study, led by Dr Rachid Mohamed at the University of Alberta, explored the effects of preoperative statin use in adults who had undergone cardiac surgery. The study included 7,733 non-transplant cardiac surgery patients who were followed for 30 days.

Dr Mohamed's investigations revealed:

- Patients taking statins had a 24% increased risk of death compared to patients not taking statins.
- Patients taking statins had an 11% increased risk of death due to infection compared to patients not taking statins.
- Patients taking statins had an 8% increased risk of any infection compared to patients not taking statins.

Paper 7: Statin taking cardiac surgery patients have a 42% increased risk of death

Hinz J et al Hemodynamic effects of peri-operative statin therapy in on-pump cardiac surgery patients. *Journal of Cardiothoracic Surgery* 2012 Jul 13;7:39

German researchers examined the effect of statin therapy on patients undergoing cardiac surgery with cardiopulmonary bypass. (Cardiopulmonary bypass is a technique that temporarily takes over the function of the heart and lungs during surgery, maintaining the circulation of blood and the oxygen content of the body.) The study included 478 patients who stayed in hospital for an average of 25 days. They were divided into (i) statin taking group, and (ii) non statin group.

The researchers found:

- Patients taking statins had a 42% increased risk of death whilst in hospital compared to patients not taking statins.
- The statin taking group had a significant 16% lower Systemic Vascular Resistance Index compared to the non statin group. (A decrease of Systemic Vascular Resistance Index is evidence for systemic inflammation.)

Paper 8: Statins increase the risk of hospital acquired thrombocytopenia in heart attack patients

Nikolsky E et al Impact of in-hospital acquired thrombocytopenia in patients undergoing primary angioplasty for acute myocardial infarction. *American Journal of Cardiology* 2005 Aug 15;96(4):474-81

Thrombocytopenia is the term for a reduced platelet (thrombocyte) count. Platelets are tiny cells that circulate in the blood and whose function is to take part in the clotting process. Platelets are essential in the formation of blood clots to prevent haemorrhage – bleeding from a ruptured blood vessel. An adequate number of normally functioning platelets is also needed to prevent leakage of red blood cells from apparently uninjured vessels.

Percutaneous coronary intervention is a coronary revascularisation technique used in the treatment of ischemic heart disease. Percutaneous coronary intervention involves non-surgical widening of the coronary artery, using a balloon catheter to dilate the artery from within. A metallic stent is usually placed in the artery after dilatation.

Dr Eugenia Nikolsky, a Professor of Medicine in Cardiology, explored the influence of statins on the incidence and prognostic significance of hospital acquired thrombocytopenia, in patients with a heart attack who underwent percutaneous coronary intervention. The study included 1,975 patients who received balloon angioplasty.

Dr Nikolsky reported:

- Those who used statins had a 228% increased risk of developing hospital acquired thrombocytopenia compared to those who did not use statins.
- Those who developed hospital acquired thrombocytopenia had a 270% higher in-hospital rates of major hemorrhagic complications.
- Those who developed hospital acquired thrombocytopenia had a 156% greater requirement for blood transfusions.
- Those who developed hospital acquired thrombocytopenia had a 33% longer hospital stay.
- Those who developed hospital acquired thrombocytopenia had a 400% increased risk of death after 30 days.
- Those who developed hospital acquired thrombocytopenia had a 156% increased risk of death after one year.

Paper 9:
Statin use increases the risk of death and major cardiovascular events in abdominal aortic aneurysm patients

Sun T et al A two-year follow-up for Chinese patients with abdominal aortic aneurysm undergoing open/endovascular repair. *Chinese Medical Journal (England)* 2014 Feb;127(3):457-61

This study evaluated the independent predictors of mortality and morbidity in abdominal aortic aneurysm patients undergoing elective surgical treatment. (An abdominal aortic aneurysm is a dilation (ballooning) of part of the aorta that is within the abdomen. An abdominal aortic aneurysm usually causes no symptoms unless it ruptures (bursts). A ruptured abdominal aortic aneurysm is often fatal.)

The study lasted for two years and included 386 abdominal aortic aneurysm patients, average age 70.6 years.

Regarding statin use, the study found:

- Patients using statins had a 92% increased risk of death compared to patients not taking statins.
- Patients using statins had a 194% increased risk of a major cardiovascular event (congestive heart failure, angina, stroke and non-fatal heart attack etc.) compared to patients not taking statins.

Paper 10:
Lovastatin treatment is associated with a higher death rate and a higher risk of heart attack in angioplasty patients

Weintraub WS et al Lack of effect of lovastatin on restenosis after coronary angioplasty. Lovastatin Restenosis Trial Study Group. *New England Journal of Medicine* 1994 Nov 17;331(20):1331-7

This six-month, randomised, double-blind trial (Lovastatin Restenosis Trial LRT) evaluated the effects of lovastatin in 404 patients who had undergone angioplasty. (Angioplasty is the technique of mechanically widening narrowed or obstructed arteries.) The patients received either lovastatin (40 mg orally twice daily) or placebo.

The trial revealed:

- Patients receiving lovastatin had a 200% increased risk of death compared to the patients receiving placebo.
- Patients receiving lovastatin had a 177% increased risk of a heart attack compared to the patients receiving placebo.

Paper 11: Pravastatin treatment increases the risk of death by 301% after balloon angioplasty

Bertrand ME et al Effect of pravastatin on angiographic restenosis after coronary balloon angioplasty. The PREDICT Trial Investigators. Prevention of Restenosis by Elisor after Transluminal Coronary Angioplasty. *Journal of the American College of Cardiology* 1997 Oct;30(4):863-9

This French based study investigated the effects of pravastatin treatment after coronary balloon angioplasty. In a multicentre, randomised, double-blind trial, 695 patients received either pravastatin (40 mg/day) or placebo for six months after successful balloon angioplasty.

- The study found that the patients on statin treatment had a 301% increased risk of death compared to the patients receiving placebo.

Paper 12: Statins should not be given to patients with heart failure

Tavazzi L et al Effect of rosuvastatin in patients with chronic heart failure (the GISSI-HF trial): a randomised, double-blind, placebo-controlled trial. *Lancet* 2008 Oct 4;372(9645):1231-9

The study (Gruppo Italiano Per Lo Studio Della Sopravvivenza Nell'Infarto Miocardico–Heart Failure: Rosuvastatin GISSI-HF) investigated the effects of rosuvastatin in patients with heart failure. The study, led by Dr Luigi Tavazzi, Professor of Cardiology at the University of Pavia, included 4,574 patients aged 18 years or older with chronic heart failure who were assigned to either rosuvastatin 10 mg daily (2,285) or placebo (2,289) and followed up for 3.9 years.

The trial identified:

- Statin users had a 4% decreased risk of death from cardiovascular reasons compared to placebo.
- Statin users had a 12% increased risk of sudden cardiac death compared to placebo.
- Statin users had a 23% increased risk of fatal and non fatal stroke compared to placebo.
- Statin users had a 2.5% increased risk of death compared to placebo.

Dr Tavazzi said: *"In conclusion, results from the GISSI-HF trial might help physicians in taking the following decisions. First, not prescribing statins to patients with heart failure of non-ischaemic cause. Second, stopping statins in patients with heart failure of ischaemic cause".*

Paper 13: Statins are independently and significantly associated with a higher risk of death in elderly patients with heart failure

Charach G et al Low levels of low-density lipoprotein cholesterol: a negative predictor of survival in elderly patients with advanced heart failure. *Cardiology* 2014;127(1):45-50

This Tel Aviv University study aimed to examine the impact of statins and low-density lipoprotein (LDL) cholesterol levels on survival rates in elderly patients with moderate and severe heart failure. The study included 212 patients, average age 77 years, who were followed for 3.7 years. The patients were divided into three groups according to LDL cholesterol levels:

- Group one had LDL cholesterol levels less than 90 mg/dL (2.32 mmol/l).
- Group two had LDL cholesterol levels between 90-115 mg/dL (2.32-3.00 mmol/l).
- Group three had LDL cholesterol levels above 115 mg/dL (3.00 mmol/l).

The Israeli researchers unearthed:

- The total cholesterol level of group one patients was 31% lower than group three patients.
- Group one patients were over twice as likely to be on statins as group three patients.
- Only 34% of group one patients survived longer than 50 months, whereas 58% of group three patients survived longer than 50 months.

The leader of the study, Dr Gideon Charach, concluded: *"Low LDL cholesterol levels are associated with a reduced survival in elderly patients with clinically controlled moderate and severe heart failure. Statins were independently and significantly associated with a higher risk of mortality".*

Paper 14: Statins double the risk of death in patients with coronary artery disease

Blankenhorn DH et al Coronary angiographic changes with lovastatin therapy. The Monitored Atherosclerosis Regression Study (MARS). *Annals of Internal Medicine* 1993 Nov 15;119(10):969-76

This randomised, double-blind, placebo-controlled, multicenter study assessed the effects of lovastatin in patients with coronary artery disease. The trial included 270 patients, 37 to 67 years old, who received either 80 mg/day of lovastatin, or placebo.

- The study found that the patients receiving lovastatin had a 104% increased risk of death.

Paper 15: Stroke victims taking statins have a 140% increased risk of infection

Montaner J et al Simvastatin in the acute phase of ischemic stroke: a safety and efficacy pilot trial. *European Journal of Neurology* 2008 Jan; 15(1):82-90

This Spanish based study was a double-blind, randomised, multicentre clinical trial to study the effects of simvastatin in patients during the first 90 days after a cortical stroke. The study included 60 patients with cortical strokes (a cortical stroke occurs when the blood supply to the outside, or cortex, of the brain is reduced or blocked, which results in brain damage) who were given either simvastatin or placebo at three to 12 hours from symptom onset.

The trial ascertained:

- More patients taking simvastatin died compared to patients taking placebo.
- Patients taking simvastatin had a 140% increased risk of infection compared to patients taking placebo.

Paper 16: The adverse effects of statins on stoke patients

Amarenco P et al High-dose atorvastatin after stroke or transient ischemic attack. *New England Journal of Medicine* 2006 Aug 10;355(6):549-59

This study was called the Stroke Prevention by Aggressive Reduction in Cholesterol Levels trial (SPARCL). It investigated the effect of statins on patients on patients who had recently had a stroke or transient ischemic attack. The study included 4,731 patients who had had a stroke or transient ischemic attack within one to six months before the start of the study. In the study, which lasted for seven years, a group of 2,365 patients received 80 mg of atorvastatin per day and a group of 2,366 patients received placebo.

SPARCL revealed:

- There were five more deaths in the group of patients receiving statins compared to the placebo group.
- There was one more death from cardiac causes in the group of patients receiving statins compared to the placebo group.
- There were four more deaths from cancer in the group of patients receiving statins compared to the placebo group.
- There were six more deaths from infections in the group of patients receiving statins compared to the placebo group.
- There were five more deaths from accidents or violence in the group of patients receiving statins compared to the placebo group.
- The patients in the statin group suffered 43 more adverse events (such as accidental injury, back pain, diarrhoea, headache etc.) compared to the placebo group.
- 73 more patients in the statin group had to discontinue study treatment because of an adverse event compared to the placebo group.
- The patients in the statin group had a 363% increased risk of elevated levels of the liver enzymes alanine aminotransferase and aspartate aminotransferase compared to the placebo group. (High levels of alanine aminotransferase and aspartate aminotransferase may indicate the presence of liver disease.)

Paper 17:
Statin use increases the size of brain haemorrhage

Ricard G et al Statins may increase intracerebral hemorrhage volume. *Canadian Journal of Neurological Sciences* 2010 Nov;37(6):791-6

This study investigated the association of statins with the initial size of intracerebral (brain) haemorrhage and the subsequent increase in area of the haemorrhage. The study included 303 patients, aged 18 years and over, who had the size of the haemorrhage measured when they were first admitted to hospital and again within a 72-hour period.

The head researcher of the study Dr Geneviève Ricard from the University of Sherbrooke reported:

- The size of the brain haemorrhage was 95% larger in the patients taking statins compared to patients not taking statins.
- The size of the brain haemorrhage increased by an extra 1100% in the patients taking statins compared to patients not taking statins.
- During hospitalisation the patients taking statins had an 18% increased risk of death compared to patients not taking statins.

Dr Ricard concluded: *"Our results suggest that statin use prior to intracerebral haemorrhage is associated with higher hematoma volume and may contribute to haemorrhage volume progression"*.

Paper 18: Stroke patients taking statins have a 32% increased risk of death

Rocco A et al Impact of statin use and lipid profile on symptomatic intracerebral haemorrhage, outcome and mortality after intravenous thrombolysis in acute stroke. *Cerebrovascular Diseases* 2012;33(4):362-8

The aim of this German study was to assess the impact of statin use and cholesterol levels on brain haemorrhage, outcome and death rates following thrombolysis in ischaemic stroke. (Thrombolysis is a pharmacological treatment to dissolve dangerous clots in blood vessels, improve blood flow and prevent damage to tissues and organs, and is often used as an emergency treatment to dissolve blood clots that form in arteries feeding the heart and brain.) The study included 1,066 patients with ischaemic stroke, who were followed for three months.

A favourable outcome was classed as modified Rankin scale 0-1. (Modified Rankin scale measures the degree of disability in people that have suffered a stroke and runs from 0-6 where 0 is perfect health without symptoms and 6 is death.)

The study identified the following:

- Patients taking statins had a 5% increased risk of brain haemorrhage compared to nonusers.
- Patients taking statins had a 32% increased risk of death compared to nonusers.
- Patients taking statins had an 11% decreased chance of a favourable outcome compared to nonusers.
- Patients with high levels of low density lipoprotein (LDL) cholesterol had a 4% reduced risk of brain haemorrhage.
- Patients with low levels of high density lipoprotein (HDL) cholesterol had a 78% increased risk of brain haemorrhage.

Paper 19:
Statin use is associated with a 68% increased risk of death in patients with stroke-associated infection

Yeh PS et al Effect of statin treatment on three-month outcomes in patients with stroke-associated infection: a prospective cohort study. *European Journal of Neurology* 2012 May;19(5):689-95

The purpose of this study was to examine the influence of statin treatment on death rates in patients with stroke-associated infection. The study lasted for three months and included 514 patients with acute ischaemic stroke or transient ischaemic attack (average age, 74 years) with infection occurring in the first seven days after admission to hospital. All patients had not received statin treatment prior to admission, and 121 patients received statins within three days of admission.

- The study found that statin use was associated with a 68% increased risk of death in patients with stroke-associated infection.

Paper 20:
Statin use associated with increased risk of brain hemorrhage after stroke treatment

Meier N et al Prior statin use, intracranial hemorrhage, and outcome after intra-arterial thrombolysis for acute ischemic stroke. *Stroke* 2009 May;40(5):1729-37

This study was headed by Dr Niklaus Meier, a senior physician at the University Hospital Bern. The study evaluated the influence of statin pretreatment and cholesterol levels on the incidence of intracranial hemorrhage in 311 patients with acute ischemic stroke receiving intra-arterial thrombolysis treatment.

The investigations of Dr Meier and his colleagues revealed:

- The cholesterol levels of patients who had an intracranial hemorrhage were 2.5% lower than patients who did not have an intracranial hemorrhage.
- Statin users had a 210% increased risk of an intracranial hemorrhage compared to nonusers.
- Three months after their stroke, statin users had a 59% increased risk of death compared to nonusers.

Paper 21:
Atorvastatin increases the death rate in diabetic patients

Knopp RH et al Efficacy and safety of atorvastatin in the prevention of cardiovascular end points in subjects with type 2 diabetes: the Atorvastatin Study for Prevention of Coronary Heart Disease Endpoints in non-insulin-dependent diabetes mellitus (ASPEN). *Diabetes Care* 2006 Jul;29(7):1478-85

The purpose of this randomised, double-blind, parallel-group trial was to assess the effect of 10 mg of atorvastatin versus placebo in subjects with type 2 diabetes and low LDL cholesterol levels. The study lasted four years and included 2,410 subjects who were assigned to receive 10 mg of atorvastatin or placebo.

The study found:

- Those who were assigned atorvastatin had a 1.7% increased risk of death compared to those who were assigned placebo.
- Those who were assigned atorvastatin had a 1.7% increased risk of a cardiovascular death compared to those who were assigned placebo.
- Those who were assigned atorvastatin had a 7% increased risk of adverse events compared to those who were assigned placebo.
- Those who were assigned atorvastatin had a 91% increased risk of cancer compared to those who were assigned placebo.

- Those who were assigned atorvastatin had a 91% increased risk of muscle pain compared to those who were assigned placebo.
- Those who were assigned atorvastatin had a 17% increased risk of elevated liver enzymes compared to those who were assigned placebo.
- Those who were assigned atorvastatin had a 197% increased risk of renal disorder compared to those who were assigned placebo.

Paper 22:
Statin treatment increases cardiovascular diseases in diabetics by 31%

Bruno G et al C-reactive protein and five-year survival in type 2 diabetes: the Casale Monferrato Study. Diabetes 2009 Apr;58(4):926-33 *Diabetes* 2009 Apr;58(4):926-33

The objective of this University of Torino study was to determine to what extent various diabetic risk factors and diabetic treatments influence five-year cardiovascular death rates and total death rates in type two diabetic individuals. The study lasted for five years, with 11,717 years of observation on 2,381 subjects with type two diabetes.

- Regarding statins, the study observed those who were taking statins had an increase of 2% in total death rates and an increase of 31% in death from cardiovascular diseases.

Paper 23:
Statins increase the risk of death by 21% in women with breast cancer

Nickels S et al Mortality and Recurrence Risk in Relation to the Use of Lipid-Lowering Drugs in a Prospective Breast Cancer Patient Cohort. *PLoS One* 2013 Sep 25;8(9):e75088

This study investigated the effects of cholesterol lowering drugs (the vast majority (85%) were taking statins) on women diagnosed with breast cancer. Dr Stefan Nickels and his colleagues from the German Cancer Research Centre analyzed data from the German Mammacarcinoma risk factor investigation *plus* (MARIEplus) study. They looked at 3,189 women, aged 50 and older, for 5.3 years.

Dr Nickel's research revealed:

- Women taking statins had a 21% increased risk of death compared to women not taking statins.
- Women taking statins had a 4% increased risk of death from breast cancer compared to women not taking statins.
- Women taking statins had a 49% increased risk of death from causes other than breast cancer compared to women not taking statins.

Paper 24:
The link between statins and bladder cancer

Crivelli JJ et al Effect of statin use on outcomes of non-muscle-invasive bladder cancer. *BJU International* 2013 Jul;112(2):E4-E12

Non-muscle-invasive bladder cancer (or superficial bladder cancer) may be treated by removal of the tumor, whereas invasive bladder cancer generally requires surgery to remove the bladder and the surrounding organs.

Transurethral resection of the bladder is a surgical procedure that is used both to diagnose bladder cancer and to remove cancerous tissue from the bladder.

The objective of the study was to assess the impact of statin use on outcomes of patients with non-muscle-invasive bladder cancer. The study included 1,117 patients who had undergone transurethral resection of the bladder treatment for non-muscle-invasive bladder cancer. The 1,117 patients included 931 with a first-time diagnosis of non-muscle-invasive bladder cancer.

The findings of the study identified:

- In all 1,117 patients, those who used statins had a 23% increased risk of death from bladder cancer and a 14% increased risk of death from any cause compared to those who did not use statins.
- In the 931 patients with a first-time diagnosis of non-muscle-invasive bladder cancer, those who used statins had a 27% increased risk of death from bladder cancer and a 15% increased risk of death from any cause compared to those who did not use statins.

Paper 25: Statins increase the risk of death in four year trial

Asselbergs FW et al Effects of fosinopril and pravastatin on cardiovascular events in subjects with microalbuminuria. *Circulation* 2004 Nov 2;110(18):2809-16

Microalbuminuria is when excess amounts of a protein called albumin pass through the kidneys and into the urine. This can be a sign of underlying conditions such as kidney disease or cardiovascular disease.

One of the aims of this Dutch study (Prevention of Renal and Vascular Endstage Disease Intervention Trial PREVEND IT) was to investigate the effect of statins on people aged 28 to 75 years old with microalbuminuria. This section of the study, which lasted nearly four years, included 217 people who were given statins and 216 people who were given a placebo.

- This double-blind, randomised, placebo controlled trial found that those given statins had a 6% increased risk of death compared to those given a placebo.

Paper 26: 2% increased risk of death for patients with kidney disease who take statins

Baigent C et al The effects of lowering LDL cholesterol with simvastatin plus ezetimibe in patients with chronic kidney disease (Study of Heart and Renal Protection): a randomised placebo-controlled trial. *Lancet* 2011 Jun 25;377(9784):2181-92

This study, (Study of Heart and Renal Protection SHARP), investigated the effect of a daily dose of simvastatin 20 mg plus ezetimibe 10 mg in patients with chronic kidney disease. This randomised double-blind trial included 9,270 patients with chronic kidney disease (3,023 on dialysis and 6,247 not) with no known history of myocardial infarction or coronary revascularisation. The trial lasted for 4.9 years and 4,650 patients were assigned to receive simvastatin plus ezetimibe and 4,620 to placebo.

- The SHARP study found that patients who received simvastatin plus ezetimibe had a 2% increased risk of death compared to the patients who received placebo.

Paper 27:
Fluvastatin increases the risk of death in kidney transplant patients

Holdaas H et al Effect of fluvastatin on cardiac outcomes in renal transplant recipients: a multicentre, randomised, placebo-controlled trial. *Lancet* 2003 Jun 14;361(9374):2024-31

This study (Assessment of LEscol in Renal Transplantation ALERT) investigated the effects of fluvastatin on kidney transplant patients. The study was a randomised, double-blind, placebo-controlled trial and included 2,012 renal transplant recipients. The patients were assigned either fluvastatin or placebo and were followed for 5.1 years.

The ALERT study ascertained:

- The low density lipoprotein (LDL) cholesterol of those in the fluvastatin group was lowered by 32% compared to the placebo group.
- Those in the fluvastatin group had a 2% increased risk of death compared to those in the placebo group.

Paper 28:
Review of 14 studies finds that statins increase the risk of death by 30% in kidney transplant patients

Navaneethan SD et al HMG CoA reductase inhibitors (statins) for kidney transplant recipients. *Cochrane Database of Systemic Reviews* 2009 Apr 15;(2):CD005019

This paper assessed the effects of statin therapy on kidney transplant recipients. The paper analysed the results of 14 studies with 3,045 participants that compared death rates of patients.

- The analysis found that kidney transplant patients that received statins had a 30% increased risk of death compared to patients who did not take statins.

Paper 29:
Statin treatment leads to worse outcome for patients in an intensive care unit

Terblanche MJ et al Statins do not prevent acute organ failure in ventilated ICU patients: single-centre retrospective cohort study. *Critical Care* 2011;15(1):R74

This 15-day study analysed the effects of statins on ventilated intensive care unit patients. The study included 1,397 mechanically ventilated patients without nonrespiratory organ failure within 24 hours after admission. The overall lengths of intensive care unit and hospital stays were five and 15 days, respectively. Patients receiving statins stayed longer in the intensive care unit by three days.

The study revealed:

- Patients taking statins had a 22% increased risk of organ failure compared to patients not taking statins.
- Patients taking statins had a 25% increased risk of liver failure compared to patients not taking statins.
- Patients taking statins had an 8% increased risk of liver impairment compared to patients not taking statins.
- In the intensive care unit setting, patients taking statins had a 0.7% increased risk of death compared to patients not taking statins.
- In the hospital setting, patients taking statins had a 19% increased risk of death compared to patients not taking statins.

Paper 30:
Statins increase the risk of death by 45% in patients with ventilator-associated pneumonia

Papazian L et al Effect of Statin Therapy on Mortality in Patients With Ventilator-Associated Pneumonia: A Randomized Clinical Trial. *Journal of the American Medical Association* 2013 Oct 23;310(16):1692-700

Ventilator-associated pneumonia is the most common infection in the intensive care unit and is associated with substantial death rates.

The objective of the study, headed by Professor Laurent Papazian head of the intensive care unit North Hospital Marseille, was to determine the effects of statins on 28-day death rates in patients with ventilator-associated pneumonia. This randomised, placebo-controlled, double-blind, parallel-group, multicenter trial (named the Statin-VAP study) performed in 26 intensive care units in France included 300 patients who took either simvastatin or placebo.

- The study found that patients taking statins had a 45% increased risk of death in 28 days compared to patients not taking statins.

The trial was due to analyse 1,002 patients but was stopped early because of the excess deaths in the patients taking simvastatin. Professor Papazian commented: *"It would have been ethically unacceptable to continue the trial after the interim analysis, which showed higher day-28 mortality in the simvastatin group"*.

Paper 31:
Statins increase the death rate by 53% in intensive care unit patients

Fernandez R et al Statin therapy prior to ICU admission: protection against infection or a severity marker? *Intensive Care Medicine* 2006 Jan;32(1):160-4

This Barcelona based study examined the impact of statin therapy on hospital death rates in patients at a high risk of acquiring infections while in an intensive care unit. Data was analysed from 438 patients at high risk of intensive care unit acquired infections, i.e., those receiving mechanical ventilation for more than 96 hours.

- The study found that patients who were taking statins had a 53% increased risk of death in hospital compared to patients not on statins.

Paper 32:
Stopping statins lowers the risk of death in patients hospitalised with acute infections

Kruger PS et al Continuation of statin therapy in patients with presumed infection: a randomized controlled trial. *American Journal of Respiratory and Critical Care Medicine* 2011 Mar 15;183(6):774-81

Researchers from The Princess Alexandra Hospital in Australia explored the effect of discontinuing statins in patients hospitalised for acute infections. They designed a randomised double-blind placebo-controlled trial that contained 150 patients, average age 68 years, who were on pre-existing statin therapy requiring hospitalisation for infection. In the 28-day trial 75 patients continued to take statins and 75 patients discontinued their statins and took placebo.

The Australian researchers discovered:

- The cholesterol levels of patients continuing to take statins remained similar at the end of the study, whereas the cholesterol levels of those discontinuing statins rose by 1.60 mmol/L (50 mg/dL).

- The low density lipoprotein (LDL) cholesterol levels of patients continuing to take statins remained similar at the end of the study, whereas the levels of those discontinuing statins rose by 1.09 mmol/L (42 mg/dL).
- The patients continuing to take statins had a 50% increased risk of death compared to those discontinuing statins.

This scientific evidence in this chapter has revealed that statin drugs are not the wonder drugs that "save thousands of lives every year". In fact the studies in Chapter 1 show that statins may increase the death rate in healthy people and in those with a variety of health issues.

- These studies have reported more deaths in statin takers in people with no health problems and those with "high" cholesterol.
- Patients with plaque build up in their arteries or unstable angina, are shown to die earlier if they take statins.
- In those with cardiovascular problems such as coronary heart disease, heart failure and stroke, and those who have surgery to help these conditions, a higher death rate has been reported in the patients prescribed statins.
- The data reveals people with diabetes, cancer and kidney disease may die quicker with statins.
- The evidence suggests that patients in hospital for kidney transplants or intensive care have less chance of survival if they are given statins.

However, statins main claim to fame is that they prevent heart attacks and stroke. The next chapter investigates that claim.

Chapter 2

Epidemic of heart failure

Your doctor will probably tell you to "take a statin drug to reduce your risk of having a heart attack or stroke". You may naturally assume by this statement that statins must somehow strengthen the heart and brain to prevent any damage occurring.

This chapter will examine the claim that statins are beneficial for heart function and stroke prevention.

Paper 33: Statins are associated with decreased myocardial function

Rubinstein J et al Statin therapy decreases myocardial function as evaluated via strain imaging. *Clinical Cardiology* 2009 Dec;32(12):684-9

The myocardium is the heart's muscular wall. It contracts to pump blood out of the heart then relaxes as the heart refills with returning blood. This vital function pumps blood to the cells and tissues of the body. A decrease in myocardial function is associated with angina and a chronic impairment of blood flow is associated with heart failure.

An echocardiogram is a test that uses sound waves to create pictures of the heart. The picture is more detailed than a standard X-ray image.

This study, based at The Michigan State University, sought to identify changes in myocardial function associated with statin use in 28 patients without heart disease. The myocardial function of 12 patients that were on statin therapy were compared with 16 controls who were not taking statins. The Michigan researchers, headed by cardiologist Dr Jack Rubinstein used the echocardiography techniques, Tissue Doppler Imaging and Strain Imaging.

The findings from the echocardiogram revealed:

- There was statistically significant worsening of diastolic function parameters in the statin group as measured via Tissue Doppler Imaging in the lateral wall of the heart.
- There was a larger and more significant decrease in heart function in the statin group when evaluated with Strain Imaging.

Dr Rubinstein concluded: "*Statin therapy is associated with decreased myocardial function*".

Paper 34:
Atorvastatin worsens heart function in 71% of patients

Silver MA et al Effect of atorvastatin on left ventricular diastolic function and ability of coenzyme Q10 to reverse that dysfunction. *American Journal of Cardiology* 2004 Nov 15;94(10):1306-10

Cardiologist Dr Marc Silver and his team evaluated left ventricular diastolic function before and after statin therapy. The study included 14 patients (who met the National Cholesterol Education Program's recommendations for initiating pharmacologic therapy), aged 51-79 years, who completed three to six months on atorvastatin.

- The evaluation found that 71% of the patients had worsening of left ventricular diastolic function after taking statins.

Dr Silver concluded: "*For more than a decade, there has been a suggestion of impairment of diastolic function after the administration of statins, and our findings suggest that this may be a common event and potentially a precursor to symptoms associated with ventricular dysfunction*".

Paper 35:
Simvastatin treatment lowers the energy producing nutrient coenzyme Q10

Watts GF et al Plasma coenzyme Q (ubiquinone) concentrations in patients treated with simvastatin. *Journal of Clinical Pathology* 1993 Nov;46(11):1055-7

The author of the study, Dr Gerald Watts a senior consultant physician, specialising in cardiometabolic medicine, notes that coenzyme Q10 is essential for mitochondrial function (energy production) and antioxidant activity.

This study assessed the effects of statin treatment on coenzyme Q10 levels. The study included:

- 20 patients with "high" cholesterol treated with a low-fat diet and simvastatin.
- 22 patients with "high" cholesterol treated with a low-fat diet alone.
- 20 normal controls. (Normal diet.)

The study identified:

- Patients treated with simvastatin had a significantly lower coenzyme Q10 levels than either patients receiving diet alone or normal controls.
- The higher the dose of simvastatin, the lower the coenzyme Q10 levels.

Dr Watts concludes: "*We suggest that a reduction in plasma coenzyme Q10 may underpin some of the severe side-effects of statins… a reduction in coenzyme Q10 may also compromise the course of coronary atherosclerosis… we recommend that consideration be given to measuring plasma coenzyme Q10 in patients receiving statins and particularly in those with clinically important cardiac disease*".

Paper 36:
Statin treatment may lead to heart failure

Langsjoen PH et al The clinical use of HMG CoA-reductase inhibitors and the associated depletion of coenzyme Q10. A review of animal and human publications. *Biofactors* 2003;18(1-4):101-11

The author of this paper, Dr Peter Langsjoen, is a specialist in Coenzyme Q10 and cardiology. Dr Langsjoen has authored many papers outlining Coenzyme Q10 deficiency as a factor in heart disease. Dr Langsjoen's papers have demonstrated the association of advanced congestive heart failure with low blood levels of Coenzyme Q10 and shown, unequivocally, that replenishing Coenzyme Q10 dramatically helps the failing heart.

In this review of the scientific literature, Dr Langsjoen found:

- The depletion of the essential nutrient Coenzyme Q10 by the increasingly popular cholesterol lowering drugs, statins, has grown from a level of concern to one of alarm.
- With ever higher statin potencies and dosages, and with steadily shrinking target levels of low density lipoprotein (LDL) cholesterol, the prevalence and severity of Coenzyme Q10 deficiency is increasing noticeably.
- Statin-induced Coenzyme Q10 depletion is well documented in animal and human studies with detrimental cardiac consequences in both animal models and human trials.
- This drug-induced nutrient deficiency is dose related and more notable in settings of pre-existing Coenzyme Q10 deficiency such as in the elderly and in heart failure.

Dr Langsjoen concludes: "*We are currently in the midst of a congestive heart failure epidemic in the United States… As physicians, it is our duty to be absolutely certain that we are not inadvertently doing harm to our patients by creating a wide-spread deficiency of a nutrient critically important for normal heart function*".

Paper 37: People treated with lovastatin may be subjected to a possible increased impairment of health and even to a life-threatening status

Folkers K et al Lovastatin decreases coenzyme Q levels in humans. *Proceedings of the National Academy of Sciences of the United States of America* 1990 Nov;87(22):8931-4

This study, (headed by Dr. Karl Folkers, of the University of Texas at Austin, considered to be the "father" of Coenzyme Q10 in the United States), investigated the effect of statin therapy on coenzyme Q10 levels and heart disease risk. The study included five hospitalized cardiac patients, 43-72 years old, and one volunteer aged 43.

The New York Heart Association Functional Classification provides a simple way of classifying the extent of heart failure. It places patients in one of four categories based on how much they are limited during physical activity. Class I is mild cardiac disease, whilst class IV is very severe cardiac disease.

Ejection fraction is a measurement of the percentage of blood leaving your heart each time it contracts. A normal heart's ejection fraction may be between 55% and 70%. A measurement under 40% may be evidence of heart failure or heart muscle disease. An ejection fraction between 40% and 55% indicates damage.

Patient 1

- A 55-year-old man with a weak heart, class III New York Heart Association, (coenzyme Q10 level was 0.67 ug/ml, ejection fraction 60%) was treated with 100 mg of coenzyme Q10 daily in May 1984.
- One month later (June 1984), the coenzyme Q10 level had increased to 1.73 pg/ml and the ejection fraction had increased to 74%.
- From July 1984 to September 1987, administration of coenzyme Q10 maintained a level of coenzyme Q10 of 1.73-2.78 ug/ml and an ejection fraction of 64-70%. During these three years of therapy with coenzyme Q10, the heart failure decreased from class III to class II and the quality of life significantly improved.
- Beginning in September 1987, the patient was treated with 40 mg of lovastatin daily and by March 1988, the patient had steadily deteriorated from a liveable class II to near class IV, known to be life threatening.
- His blood coenzyme Q10 level was 2.52 Mg/ml in September 1987 when treatment with lovastatin was initiated. About six months later (March 1988), his blood coenzyme Q10 level had diminished to 1.15 pg/ml, and by August 1988, it had decreased to the very low level of 0.64 g/ml and the ejection fraction had diminished to 54%. He required surgery and could not be treated with coenzyme Q10.
- Coenzyme Q10 was resumed at 166 mg/day in August 1988. The blood coenzyme Q10 increased to 1.39 ug/ml in one month and was stabilized at 1.55 ug/ml in November 1988 and 1.66 ug/ml in April 1989.
- The increase in the dosage of coenzyme Q10 to 166 mg allowed cardiac stabilization with acceptable blood levels of coenzyme Q10 and ejection fractions.

Dr Folkers notes that it is clear the administration of lovastatin to the patient over time significantly reduced blood levels of coenzyme Q10 and reduced the pumping of blood by the heart as monitored by the lowering of the ejection fraction.

Patient 2

- A 46-year-old man with a weak heart, class III New York Heart Association, (coenzyme Q10 level was 0.78 ug/ml, ejection fraction 62%) was treated with 100 mg of coenzyme Q10 daily in October 1984.
- During the next two years his coenzyme Q10 levels increased to 1.79-2.31 ug/ml and his ejection fraction increased to 68-71%.
- Also during this 24-month period, his cardiac function and his quality of life improved from class III to class I.
- Beginning in April 1987 he was given 20 mg of lovastatin daily.
- Six-18 months later, his blood coenzyme Q10 levels steadily declined from 2.29 to 1.82 to 1.50 to 1.12 ug/ml and his cardiac function deteriorated from class I to class II.
- In October 1988 the administration of lovastatin was terminated, and by March 1989, his blood coenzyme Q10 level had increased to 1.87 ug/ml and his cardiac status improved from class II to class I.

In this patient, levels of coenzyme Q10 decreased over time from the administration of lovastatin, whilst levels of coenzyme Q10 increased when the administration of lovastatin was terminated.

Patient 3

- A woman of age 43 years had a weak heart severe class IV New York Heart Association when treatment with coenzyme Q10 (100 mg per day) was initiated.
- Between March 1986 and September 1987, her coenzyme Q10 levels improved up to 4.5 ug/ml and her ejection fraction up to 60%. Her clinical status improved to class III.
- Treatment with 20 mg of lovastatin was initiated in September 1987, and by March 1988, her coenzyme Q10 levels had dropped to 2.5 ug/ml, her cardiac condition had significantly deteriorated to a severe class IV, and she was referred for a heart transplant.

This patient had a severe deterioration in her heart condition after statin therapy and she was referred for a heart transplant.

Patient 4

- A 72-year-old woman with a weak heart, class III New York Heart Association (coenzyme Q10 level was 0.79 ug/ml, her ejection fraction 58%) was treated with 100 mg of coenzyme Q10 daily in March 1986.
- After three months, her coenzyme Q10 level improved to 1.21 ug/ml but the ejection fraction remained at 58%.
- In September 1986, the coenzyme Q10 dosage was increased to 133 mg daily and during March to September 1987 her coenzyme Q10 levels improved up to 2.23 ug/ml and ejection fraction up to 64%.
- In September 1987, the administration of lovastatin was initiated at 20 mg daily.
- By March 1988, the blood CoQ1O level had decreased to 0.99 ug/ml and the ejection fraction decreased to 61%.

On administration of lovastatin the levels of coenzyme Q10 significantly diminished in this patient and she had deterioration in her clinical status.

Patient 5

- A 66-year-old man with a weak heart, class I New York Heart Association (ejection fraction 85%) was given lovastatin therapy in January 1988.
- One year later, his coenzyme Q10 level was 0.61 ug/ml, his ejection fraction had decreased to 52% and he had deteriorated to a class III.

Statin therapy caused a definite worsening in heart function in this patient.

Volunteer

- A 43-year-old man was given lovastatin.
- His levels of coenzyme Q10 decreased and was accompanied by a measurable decrease in cardiac function.

Dr Folkers concludes: *"Administration of lovastatin does indeed lower tissue levels of coenzyme Q10 which may decrease cardiac function to variable degrees... some of the side effects from lovastatin, particularly liver disease, may be caused by the depression of body levels of coenzyme Q10... people treated with lovastatin may be subjected to a possible increased impairment of health and even to a life-threatening status".*

Paper 38:
Atrial fibrillation induced by simvastatin

Akahane T et al Atrial fibrillation induced by simvastatin treatment in a 61-year-old man. *Heart and Vessels* 2003 Jul;18(3):157-9

This paper describes the case of a man who developed atrial fibrillation after starting statin therapy. Atrial fibrillation is a heart condition that causes an irregular and often abnormally fast heart rate.

- A 61-year-old man started simvastatin treatment (5 mg once daily).
- Two weeks later, he developed palpitation.
- He visited hospital because the palpitation was persistent for two days.
- An electrocardiogram revealed atrial fibrillation.
- Simvastatin was withdrawn and his heart rate returned to normal after three days.
- The patient was followed for 19 months after the withdrawal of simvastatin and has not complained of palpitation while also maintaining a normal heart rhythm.

Paper 39:
Statin users have an 82% higher risk of microalbuminuria

van der Tol A et al Statin use and the presence of microalbuminuria. Results from the ERICABEL trial: a non-interventional epidemiological cohort study. *PLoS One* 2012;7(2):e31639

Microalbuminuria occurs when very small amounts of a protein called albumin pass through the kidneys and into the urine. This can be a sign of underlying conditions such as kidney disease or cardiovascular disease.

This Belgium study, the Early Renal Impairment and Cardiovascular Assessment in BELgium, (ERICABEL), evaluated the association between statins and microalbuminuria. The study included 1,076 patients, aged 40 to 70 years, with high blood pressure, who were followed for five years.

- The study found that statin users had an 82% higher risk of microalbuminuria compared to nonusers.

Paper 40:
Abdominal aortic aneurysms expand more with statin use

Ferguson CD et al Association of statin prescription with small abdominal aortic aneurysm progression. *American Heart Journal* 2010 Feb;159(2):307-13

Abdominal aortic aneurysm is recognized as an important cause of death in older men. An abdominal aortic aneurysm is when the large blood vessel (aorta) that supplies blood to the abdomen, pelvis, and legs becomes abnormally large or balloons outward. The larger the aneurysm, the more likely it is to rupture and break open.

This study, based at James Cook University Australia, assessed the association of statin treatment (and other medications) and with abdominal aortic aneurysms expansion. The study, which lasted for six years, included 652 patients undergoing surveillance of small abdominal aortic aneurysms.

- Regarding statins, the study revealed those taking statins had a 23% increased risk of their abdominal aortic aneurysm expanding more than average compared to those not taking statins.

Paper 41:
Simvastatin/ezetimibe use associated with vasculitis

Sen D et al ANCA-positive vasculitis associated with simvastatin/ezetimibe: expanding the spectrum of statin-induced autoimmunity? *International Journal of Rheumatic Diseases* 2010 Aug;13(3):e29-31

Vasculitis is inflammation of the blood vessels. If a blood vessel is inflamed it can narrow or close off. This limits or prevents blood flow through the vessel. Antineutrophil cytoplasmic antibodies are autoantibodies (where the body harms itself) and are associated with vasculitis.

- A patient developed vasculitis after simvastatin/ezetimibe use.
- The patient was found to be antineutrophil cytoplasmic antibody-positive.
- Investigations revealed the disease was statin induced.
- The patient demonstrated complete resolution of symptoms simply by withdrawing the drug.

Paper 42:
Statins increase calcium deposits in the arteries by 7%

Houslay ES et al Progressive coronary calcification despite intensive lipid-lowering treatment: a randomised controlled trial. *Heart* 2006 Sep;92(9):1207-12

A coronary artery calcium scan is a test that looks for specks of calcium in the walls of the coronary (heart) arteries. The amount of calcium detected in the coronary arteries is converted to a calcium score. A high coronary artery calcium score is an independent predictor of coronary heart disease events.

Calcific aortic stenosis is where calcium deposits narrow the aortic valve of the heart and decreases blood flow from the heart.

The objective of this Scottish study, named the Scottish Aortic Stenosis and Lipid Lowering Therapy, Impact on Regression (SALTIRE), was to evaluate the effect of statins on coronary artery calcification in patients with calcific aortic stenosis. The study was a double-blind randomised controlled trial, and included 102 patients (who were followed for at least two years) who were randomly assigned to receive either atorvastatin 80 mg daily or placebo.

- The Scottish researchers identified that patients assigned to statins had a 7% higher increase in coronary artery calcification compared to placebo patients.

Paper 43:
Statin use is associated with increased amounts of coronary artery plaque

Nakazato R et al Statins use and coronary artery plaque composition: Results from the International Multicenter CONFIRM Registry. *Atherosclerosis* 2012 Nov;225(1):148-53

The study, based at The Cedars-Sinai Medical Center in Los Angeles, examined the relationship between statin use and the presence of coronary artery plaque. The study included 6,673 individuals, average age 59 years, who had their coronary artery plaque assessed.

The plaque was graded as:

- Non-calcified
- Mixed
- Calcified

The results from the study unearthed:

- Compared to the individuals not taking statins, those taking statins had an 11% increased presence of non-calcified plaque.
- Compared to the individuals not taking statins, those taking statins had a 46% increased presence of mixed plaque.
- Compared to the individuals not taking statins, those taking statins had a 54% increased presence of calcified plaque.

Paper 44:
Statins can damage the lining of blood vessels

Dick M et al Statin Therapy Influences Endothelial Cell Morphology and F-Actin Cytoskeleton Structure When Exposed to Static and Laminar Shear Stress Conditions. *Life Sciences* 2013 May 2;92(14-16):859-65

The aim of the study was to determine how statin drugs affect endothelial cell shape and F-actin cytoskeleton arrangement. (Endothelial cells are the thin layer of cells that line the interior surface of blood vessels and lymphatic vessels, and F-actin cytoskeleton is part of the cells scaffolding or skeleton.) In the study, human endothelial cells were cultured in the laboratory and were then treated with statins.

The findings of the study revealed:

- After been treated with statins the endothelial cells became rounded, which is associated with unhealthy cells in arteries prone to developing a build up of plaque.
- After been treated with statins the F-actin cytoskeleton structure was disorganized and fragmented, which can lead to cell death.

The significance of the results of the study is that endothelial cells and F-actin cytoskeleton arrangement are adversely impacted by statin treatment, which may increase the risk of arterial plaque and cell death.

Paper 45: Statin users at risk of deep vein thrombosis

Freeman DJ et al Incident venous thromboembolic events in the Prospective Study of Pravastatin in the Elderly at Risk (PROSPER). *BMC Geriatricts* 2011 Feb 22;11:8

Thromboembolism is the formation in a blood vessel of a clot (thrombus) that breaks loose and is carried by the blood stream to plug another vessel.

The study, led by Dr Dilys Freeman (an expert in cardiovascular disease), aimed to determine the effect of pravastatin on venous thromboembolic events (deep venous thrombosis and pulmonary embolism) in older people. The study included 5.699 men and women aged 70-82 who were followed for an average of 3.2 years.

- Dr Freeman and her team observed that statin users had a 42% increased risk of venous thromboembolic events compared to those who did not use statins.

Paper 46: Cardiac surgery patients on statins have a 10% increased risk of delirium

Burkhart CS et al Modifiable and nonmodifiable risk factors for postoperative delirium after cardiac surgery with cardiopulmonary bypass. *Journal of Cardiothoracic and Vascular Anesthesia* 2010 Aug;24(4):555-9

Delirium may manifest as severe confusion and disorientation, developing with relatively rapid onset. Postoperative delirium after cardiac surgery is associated with increased death rates.

The study sought to identify risk factors associated with the development of postoperative delirium in elderly patients after elective cardiac surgery. The study included 113 patients aged 65 or older undergoing elective cardiac surgery with cardiopulmonary bypass.

- Regarding statins, the study found that patients taking statins had a 10% increased risk of delirium compared to patients not taking statins.

Paper 47: Statins increase the risk of delirium by 52% after cardiac operations

Mariscalco G et al Preoperative statin therapy is not associated with a decrease in the incidence of delirium after cardiac operations. *Annals of Thoracic Surgery* 2012 May;93(5):1439-47

The first author of this study, Dr Giovanni Mariscalco, is a consultant in cardiac surgery at Cardiac Surgery Unit of Varese University Hospital. The study investigated the association between preoperative statins with the incidence of postoperative delirium in patients undergoing coronary artery bypass grafting. The study included 1,577 patients receiving preoperative statins who were matched with a control group of 1,577 not receiving statins.

- The study found patients receiving preoperative statins had a 52% increased risk of postoperative delirium compared to patients not taking statins.

Paper 48: Statins increase heart attack risk by 6.25% in balloon angioplasty patients

Veselka J et al Effect of two-day atorvastatin pretreatment on the incidence of periprocedural myocardial infarction following elective percutaneous coronary intervention: a single-center, prospective, and randomized study. *American Journal of Cardiology* 2009 Sep 1;104(5):630-3

The purpose of this randomised study, based in the Czech Republic, was to investigate the link between two-day atorvastatin therapy and the incidence of heart attacks (around the time of intervention) in patients with stable angina pectoris undergoing balloon angioplasty (percutaneous coronary intervention). (Percutaneous coronary intervention involves non-surgical widening of the coronary artery, using a balloon catheter to dilate the artery from within. A metallic stent is usually placed in the artery after dilatation to allow blood to flow more freely through it.) The study included 200 patients with stable angina pectoris who were not taking statins and who had been referred for percutaneous coronary intervention. Before undergoing the percutaneous coronary intervention the patients received a two-day pretreatment regimen with either atorvastatin 80 mg per day or no statin treatment.

- The results of the study revealed that patients with stable angina pectoris undergoing percutaneous coronary intervention taking atorvastatin had a 6.25% increased risk of heart attack compared to those not taking statins.

Paper 49: Statins increase the risk of angina by 15% in patients receiving angioplasty treatment

Zbinden S et al Effect of statin treatment on coronary collateral flow in patients with coronary artery disease. *Heart* 2004 Apr;90(4):448-9

Collateral blood vessels are small capillary-like branches of an artery that form over time in response to narrowed coronary arteries. The collaterals "bypass" the area of narrowing and help to restore blood flow.

A balloon occlusion test is a way to see whether one artery can be temporarily or permanently blocked without significantly affecting the level of blood in your brain. The procedure utilizes an X-ray and a special dye to create detailed images of your arteries and a small balloon, which when inflated will temporarily block your artery.

This study, headed by Dr Stephan Zbinden a Senior Physician in non-invasive Cardiology, investigated the influence of statins on the formation of collateral arteries in patients with coronary artery disease undergoing coronary angioplasty. The study included 500 patients who had their collateral blood vessels assessed whilst undergoing angioplasty.

Dr Zbinden reported:

- Measurement by electrocardiogram revealed patients taking statins had a 14% increased risk of insufficient collateral arteries compared to patients not taking statins.
- Patients taking statins had a 15% increased risk of suffering angina during a balloon occlusion test compared to patients not taking statins.

Paper 50:
Statins increase the risk of acute stent thrombosis

Shen J et al Impact of statins on clopidogrel platelet inhibition in patients with acute coronary syndrome or stable angina. *Zhonghua Xin Xue Guan Bing Za Zhi* 2008 Sep;36(9):807-11

Acute stent thrombosis is when a previously placed stent in a heart artery (coronary artery) suddenly becomes blocked by a blood clot. This can result in a heart attack or even death.

This study investigated the impact of statins (pravastatin, fluvastatin, atorvastatin) on patients with acute coronary syndrome or stable angina who had just undergone a coronary angiography/ percutaneous coronary intervention (the procedure that widens the artery and a stent (tube) is placed in the artery to keep it open). The study included 1,015 patients who were allocated into groups and received either:

- Pravastatin
- Fluvastatin
- Atorvastatin
- Placebo

The study identified:

- Patients taking Pravastatin had a 12% increased risk of acute stent thrombosis compared to patients taking placebo.
- Patients taking Fluvastatin had a 37% increased risk of acute stent thrombosis compared to patients taking placebo.
- Patients taking Atorvastatin had a 25% increased risk of acute stent thrombosis compared to patients taking placebo.

Paper 51: In patients undergoing major vascular surgery, statins are associated with an increased risk of cardiac death or nonfatal heart attack

Boersma E et al Predictors of cardiac events after major vascular surgery: Role of clinical characteristics, dobutamine echocardiography, and beta-blocker therapy. *Journal of the American Medical Association* 2001 Apr 11;285(14):1865-73

The object of the study (Dutch Echocardiographic Cardiac Risk Evaluation Applying Stress Echocardiography DECREASE) was to examine the relationship between various therapies and cardiac events in patients undergoing major vascular surgery. The study included 1,351 patients who were followed for 30 days.

- Regarding statins, DECREASE ascertained that patients taking statins had a 10% increased risk of cardiac death or nonfatal heart attack compared to patients not taking statins.

Paper 52:
Statins associated with increased bleeding in the brain in patients with intracerebral hemorrhage

Haussen DC et al Statin Use and Microbleeds in Patients With Spontaneous Intracerebral Hemorrhage. *Stroke* 2012 Oct;43(10):2677-81

Microbleeds (or microhaemorrhages) are pinpoint drops of blood that leak from blood vessels in the brain that may increase the risk of stroke and cognitive dysfunction.

The cortico-subcortical region of the brain is the outer layers and the area beneath the outer layers.

The study, based at the prestigious Harvard Medical School, examined the effects that statin use had on microbleeds in patients with intracerebral (brain) hemorrhage. The study included 163 patients with intracerebral hemorrhage.

The Harvard researchers discovered:

- Statin users had significantly lower cholesterol and low-density lipoprotein (LDL) cholesterol levels compared to nonusers.
- Statins users had a 172% increase in microbleeds compared to nonusers.
- Statins users had a 315% increase in cortico-subcortical microbleeds compared to nonusers.

Paper 53:
Statin use associated with an increased risk of post stroke infection

Becker K et al Early statin use is associated with increased risk of infection after stroke. *Journal of Stroke and Cerebrovascular Diseases* 2013 Jan;22(1):66-71

This study assessed the impact of early statin use on the risk of infection in stroke patients. The study included 112 patients admitted to hospital with ischemic stroke, average age 57.

The lead author of the study, Dr Kyra Becker, is a University of Washington Professor of Neurology and of Neurological Surgery. Her clinical interests include stroke prevention and treatment.

- Professor Becker and her team found that patients taking statins prior to admission to hospital, or who had started statin therapy by day three after the stroke had a 749% increased risk of infection in the first 15 days after stroke compared to patients not on statins or who started on statins later than three days after stroke onset.

Professor Becker notes that: *"Statins can interfere with initiation of the innate immune response"* and concludes: *"Our data suggest that early statin use appears to be associated with an increased risk of post stroke infection"*.

Paper 54:
Statin users have a higher risk for subarachnoid hemorrhage-related vasospasm

Singhal AB et al SSRI and statin use increases the risk for vasospasm after subarachnoid haemorrhage. *Neurology* 2005 Mar 22;64(6):1008-13

Vasospasm refers to a condition in which a blood vessel's spasm leads to a narrowing of the blood vessels resulting from contraction of the muscular wall of the vessels. This can lead to tissue to a restriction in blood supply to tissues causing tissue death. Vasospasm is a major contributor to post-operative stroke and death especially after aneurysmal subarachnoid haemorrhage (where a blood vessel bursts in or around the brain). Vasospasm typically appears four to ten days after subarachnoid haemorrhage.

This study, led by Dr Aneesh Singhal an Associate Professor of Neurology at The Harvard Medical School, investigated the effects of various pharmaceutical drugs on the risk for vasospasm in patients who had suffered an aneurysmal subarachnoid haemorrhage. The study included 514 patients who were evaluated for vasospasm between days four and 14.

Regarding statins, the study observed:

- The proportion of patients taking statins increased significantly across three worsening categories (none, asymptomatic, symptomatic) of vasospasm.
- Patients taking statins had a 175% increased risk of vasospasm compared to patients not taking statins.

Dr Singhal concluded: *"Statin users have a higher risk for subarachnoid hemorrhage-related vasospasm"*.

Paper 55:
Statins, stroke victims and the risk of intracranial haemorrhage

Engelter ST et al IV thrombolysis and statins. *Neurology* 2011 Aug 30;77(9):888-95

Intravenous thrombolysis involves the use of thrombolytic drugs, which break down and dissolve blood clots. Intravenous thrombolysis may be used for the treatment of ischaemic strokes (when blood clots block the flow of blood to the brain).

This Swiss study explored the effect of statin use in stroke patients receiving intravenous thrombolysis. The study included 4,012 intravenous thrombolysis treated patients.

The study found:

- Statin users had an 11% less chance of reaching an excellent three-month outcome compared to nonusers.
- Statins users had a 15% increased risk of intracranial (brain) haemorrhage compared to nonusers.

Paper 56:
Statins increase the risk of hemorrhagic stroke by 73%

Vergouwen MD et al Statin Treatment and the Occurrence of Hemorrhagic Stroke in Patients With a History of Cerebrovascular Disease. *Stroke* 2008;39:497

The purpose of this review was to analyse the effect of statin treatment on the occurrence of ischemic and hemorrhagic strokes in patients with a history of cerebrovascular disease. The Dutch investigators searched the scientific literature and found four studies for analysis. The four studies included 8,832 patients with a history of cerebrovascular disease (stroke).

The review identified that:

- Statins decreased the risk of ischemic stroke by 20%.
- Statins increased the risk of hemorrhagic stroke by 73%.

Paper 57:
Patients taking atorvastatin after a stroke have a 68% increased risk of suffering another stroke

Goldstein LB et al Hemorrhagic stroke in the Stroke

Prevention by Aggressive Reduction in Cholesterol Levels study. *Neurology* June 10, 2008 vol. 70 no. 24 Part 2 2364-2370

This paper analysed the association between statins and hemorrhagic stroke in patients who had suffered a recent stroke. The study was a double-blind, randomized, placebo-controlled trial and included 4,731 patients, aged 18 years and over, who were followed for 4.9 years. The patients received either:

- Atorvastatin 80 mg per day.
- Placebo.

Dr Larry Goldstein from Duke University Medical Centre headed the study which revealed:

- Patients who received the statin had a 68% increased risk of fatal and non-fatal hemorrhagic stroke compared to those who received placebo.
- Patients who received the statin had a 140% increased risk of non-fatal hemorrhagic stroke compared to those who received placebo.

Dr Goldstein concluded: "*Hemorrhagic stroke was more frequent in those treated with atorvastatin*".

The papers in this chapter reveal that statins severely compromise heart function and increase the risk of brain haemorrhage.

- Echocardiograph and other techniques have found that statin users have a significant decrease in heart function.
- Statins deplete the essential enzyme coenzyme Q10. Coenzyme Q10 deficiency is a well-known factor in heart disease.
- Patients taking statins may suffer more damage and inflammation to the arteries.
- Studies have shown that increased arterial plaque and calcium deposits are associated with statin use.
- Cardiac surgery patients using statins could have elevated risks of delirium, thrombosis, angina and heart attack.
- Brain haemorrhage risk is heightened with people taking statins.
- Stroke patients on statins may have more bleeding and an increased risk of infection.

Dr Duane Graveline, a family doctor and a former astronaut, aerospace medical research scientist and flight surgeon, sums up the result of statins effects on coenzyme Q10 levels and its effects on the heart: "*Coenzyme Q10 is an anti-oxidant that is also critical for cell wall integrity and for the production of adenosine triphosphate (ATP), our cellular fuel. Coenzyme Q10 inhibition will contribute to mitochondrial DNA mutation and ATP insufficiency. It was known that the present epidemic of congestive heart failure would inevitably follow the use of statins for coronary artery disease control. When the coenzyme Q10, vital for heart cell function, is inhibited by statins, it is not difficult to predict heart failure as a result*".

Chapter 3

It's official: Statins increase the risk of diabetes

In 2012, the American Food and Drug Administration (FDA) announced that people being treated with statins may have an increased risk of raised blood sugar levels and the development of Type two diabetes. The FDA said they will be changing the drug labels of statin products to reflect these new concerns. (These labels are not the sticker attached to a prescription drug bottle, but the package insert with details about a prescription medication, including side effects.)

The following 25 papers explore the research to see how the FDA reached the conclusion that statins increase the risk of diabetes.

Paper 58: Statin use is associated with accelerated artery calcification in type two diabetes

Saremi A et al Progression of Vascular Calcification Is Increased With Statin Use in the Veterans Affairs Diabetes Trial (VADT). *Diabetes Care* Nov 2012; 35(11): 2390–2392

The objective of the study, led by diabetes expert Dr Aramesh Saremi, was to determine the effect of statin use on progression of calcification in the arteries of type two diabetics. (The higher the calcification, the higher the risk of a cardiac event.) The study included 197 participants with type two diabetes.

The study determined:

- Coronary artery calcification was significantly higher in more frequent statin users than in less frequent users.
- Aortic artery calcification was higher in more frequent statin users than in less frequent users.

- In participants initially not receiving statins, progression of both coronary artery calcification and aortic artery calcification was significantly increased in frequent statin users.

Paper 59: Atorvastatin increases the risk of diabetes

Koh KK et al Atorvastatin causes insulin resistance and increases ambient glycemia in hypercholesterolemic patients. *Journal of the American College of Cardiology* 2010 Mar 23;55(12):1209-16

Elevated levels of fasting insulin is the single greatest marker to assess a person's risk for cardiovascular disease and diabetes.

The term HbA1c refers to glycated haemoglobin. It develops when haemoglobin, a protein within red blood cells that carries oxygen throughout your body, joins with glucose in the blood, becoming 'glycated'. By measuring glycated haemoglobin (HbA1c), clinicians are able to get an overall picture of what our average blood sugar levels have been over a period of weeks/months. For people with diabetes this is important as the higher the HbA1c, the greater the risk of developing diabetes-related complications.

Insulin sensitivity describes how sensitive the body is to the effects of insulin. Someone said to be insulin sensitive will require smaller amounts of insulin to lower blood glucose levels than someone who has low sensitivity. Low insulin sensitivity can lead to a variety of health problems. The body will try to compensate for having a low sensitivity to insulin by producing more insulin. However, a high level of circulating insulin (hyperinsulinemia) is associated with damage to blood vessels, high blood pressure, heart disease and heart failure, diabetes, obesity, osteoporosis and even cancer.

This study investigated the association between statins and diabetes risk. The study was a randomized, single-blind, placebo-controlled parallel study that was conducted in 44 patients taking placebo and in 42, 44, 43, and 40 patients given daily atorvastatin 10, 20, 40, and 80 mg, respectively, during a two-month treatment period.

The study ascertained:

- Atorvastatin at 10, 20, 40, and 80 mg daily significantly increased fasting insulin levels by 25%, 42%, 31%, and 45%, respectively.

- Atorvastatin at 10, 20, 40, and 80 mg daily significantly increased glycated hemoglobin levels (HbA1c levels) by 2%, 5%, 5%, and 5%, respectively.
- Atorvastatin at 10, 20, 40, and 80 mg daily decreased insulin sensitivity by 1%, 3%, 3%, and 4%, respectively.

Stain treatment increased fasting insulin levels, increased glycated hemoglobin levels and decreased insulin sensitivity, which all indicate an increased risk of diabetes.

Paper 60:
Rosuvastatin is associated with a dose-dependent increase in insulin resistance

Kostapanos MS et al Rosuvastatin treatment is associated with an increase in insulin resistance in hyperlipidaemic patients with impaired fasting glucose. *International Journal of Clinical Practice* 2009 Sep;63(9):1308-13

Insulin resistance is a condition in which the body produces insulin but does not use it effectively. When people have insulin resistance, glucose builds up in the blood instead of being absorbed by the cells, leading to type two diabetes or prediabetes.

Impaired fasting glucose, more commonly known as prediabetes refers to a condition in which the fasting blood glucose level is consistently elevated above what is considered normal levels; however, it is not high enough to be diagnosed as diabetes. This prediabetic state is associated with insulin resistance and increased risk of cardiovascular disease.

HOmeostasis Model Assessment (HOMA-IR) has been widely utilized as insulin resistance index in clinical and epidemiological studies. Low HOMA values indicate high insulin sensitivity, whereas high HOMA values indicate insulin resistance.

Elevated insulin is associated with insulin resistance, diabetes, heart disease and numerous other health conditions.

This study assessed the effect of rosuvastatin treatment on patients with impaired fasting glucose, who are at high risk to develop diabetes. The medical records of 72 patients with impaired fasting glucose on varying doses of rosuvastatin (10, 20 and 40 mg per day) were analysed over a 12-week period.

The study brought to light:

- Rosuvastatin treatment was associated with a dose-dependent significant increase in HOMA-IR values by 25.4%, 32.3% and 44.8% at the dose of 10, 20 and 40 mg per day respectively.
- Rosuvastatin treatment was associated with a dose-dependent significant increase in insulin levels by 21.7%, 25.7% and 46.2% at the dose of 10, 20 and 40 mg per day respectively.

The data from the study reveals that in patients with impaired fasting glucose, rosuvastatin treatment was associated with a dose-dependent increase in insulin resistance.

Paper 61:
Atorvastatin therapy worsens insulin sensitivity in women with polycystic ovary syndrome

Puurunen J et al Statin Therapy Worsens Insulin Sensitivity in Women With Polycystic Ovary Syndrome (PCOS): A Prospective, Randomized, Double-Blind, Placebo-Controlled Study. *Journal of Clinical Endocrinology and Metabolism* 2013 Dec;98(12):4798-807

Dr Johanna Puurunen headed a team from The Helsinki University Central Hospital for this study. Dr Puurunen notes that women with polycystic ovary syndrome have an increased risk of developing type two diabetes.

The objective of the study was to explore the effects of atorvastatin in women with polycystic ovary syndrome. In this six-month, randomised, double-blind, placebo-controlled study, women with polycystic ovary syndrome were either treated with atorvastatin 20 mg per day, (15 women) or placebo (13 women).

Dr Puurunen's research revealed:

- Insulin levels significantly increased in the atorvastatin group.
- Insulin sensitivity decreased in the atorvastatin group.

The study results show that statins worsen insulin sensitivity in women with polycystic ovary syndrome and increases their risk of type two diabetes.

Paper 62:
Statins are associated with adverse effects on insulin resistance

Moutzouri E et al Comparison of the effects of simvastatin vs. rosuvastatin vs. simvastatin/ezetimibe on parameters of insulin resistance. *International Journal of Clinical Practice* 2011 Nov;65(11):1141-8

The aim of this study (lead author Dr Elisavet Moutzouri from The University of Ioannina) was to compare the effects of three different regimens of cholesterol-lowering drugs on insulin resistance. The study included 153 patients who received either: (i) simvastatin 40 mg (ii) rosuvastatin 10 mg (iii) simvastatin 10 mg/ezetimibe10 mg combination for 12 weeks.

- The study found all three treatment regimens were associated with significant increases in HOMA-IR and fasting insulin levels. (Elevated HOMA-IR and fasting insulin levels are linked to increased insulin resistance.)

Dr Moutzouri concludes: *"Simvastatin 40 mg, rosuvastatin 10 mg and simvastatin/ezetimibe 10/10 mg are associated with similar adverse effects on insulin resistance"*.

Paper 63:
Use of statins is associated with increased insulin resistance in patients undergoing coronary artery bypass grafting

Sato H et al Statin intake is associated with decreased insulin sensitivity during cardiac surgery. *Diabetes Care* 2012 Oct;35(10):2095-9

This study, published in the prestigious *Diabetes Care* journal, investigated the association between preoperative statin therapy and insulin sensitivity during surgery in 120 nondiabetic patients undergoing coronary artery bypass grafting.

High blood sugar levels and a greater oscillation (greater variation) of blood sugar levels lead to damaged blood vessels and diabetes and may cause a multitude of complications such as: Kidney disease or kidney failure requiring dialysis, strokes, heart attacks, visual loss or blindness, immune system suppression with increased risk for infections, erectile dysfunction, nerve damage causing tingling, pain or decreased sensation in the feet, legs, and hands, and poor circulation to the legs and feet, with poor wound healing. In extreme cases, because of the poor wound healing, amputation is required.

The findings of the study detected:

- Insulin sensitivity was ~20% lower in those taking statins compared to those not taking statins.
- Blood sugar levels were 9% higher in those taking statins compared to those not taking statins.
- The oscillation of blood sugar levels was larger in those taking statins compared to those not taking statins.

The study results show that preoperative use of statins is associated with increased insulin resistance in nondiabetic patients undergoing coronary artery bypass grafting.

Paper 64: Statins associated with insulin resistance during major non-cardiac surgery

Turan A et al Effect of statins on insulin requirements during non-cardiac surgery. *Anaesthesia and Intensive Care* 2014 May;42(3):350-5

This study, based at The Cleveland Clinic, (which is regarded as one of the top four hospitals in the United States), examined the impact of statin use on glucose concentrations and insulin requirements during surgery. The study of 173 adults having major non-cardiac surgery, compared statin and non-statin users on total amount of intraoperative insulin to maintain plasma glucose concentration within 4.4 to 6.1 mmol/l.

The Cleveland researchers unearthed:

- Statin users needed 45% more insulin to maintain normal glucose levels compared to non-statin users.
- There was a trend toward insulin resistance intraoperatively among statin users during the major non-cardiac surgery.

Paper 65: Statin use is associated with a rise of fasting blood glucose levels in patients with and without diabetes

Sukhija R et al Effect of statins on fasting plasma glucose in diabetic and nondiabetic patients. *Journal of Investigative Medicine* 2009 Mar;57(3):495-9

Cardiologist Dr Rishi Sukhija and his colleagues from the University of Arkansas looked at the effects of statins on fasting blood sugar levels. The study included diabetics and non-diabetics, statin users and nonusers, and analysed the change in fasting blood sugar levels in 345,417 patients, average age 61, over a two year period.

Dr Sukhija found:

- Fasting blood sugar levels increased by an extra 29% in non-diabetic statin users compared to non-diabetic nonusers.
- Fasting blood sugar levels increased by an extra 18% in diabetic statin users compared to diabetic nonusers.

Dr Sukhija concluded: "*Statin use is associated with a rise of fasting blood glucose levels in patients with and without diabetes*".

Paper 66:
Statin usage leads to elevated levels of glucose in the blood in patients with type two diabetes

Simsek S et al Effects of rosuvastatin and atorvastatin on glycaemic control in Type 2 diabetes – the CORALL study. *Diabetes Medicine* 2012 May;29(5):628-31

This study was given the title; COmpare the effect of Rosuvastatin with Atorvastatin on apoB/apoA-1 ratio in patients with Type 2 diabetes meLLitus and dyslipidaemia study (CORALL). The aim of the study, (headed by Dr Suat Simsek from the Department of Internal Medicine/Diabetes Centre, Medical Centre Alkmaar), was to examine whether high-dose statin therapy in patients with Type two diabetes influenced variables of glycaemic control. (*Glycaemic control* is a medical term referring to the typical levels of blood sugar (glucose) in a person with diabetes. Many of the long-term complications of diabetes result from many years of elevated levels of glucose in the blood.) The study lasted for 24 weeks and included 263 patients, average age 60 years, who had type two diabetes and were given either atorvastatin or rosuvastatin.

The study discovered:

- The HbA(1C) levels of patients given 80 mg atorvastatin daily increased by 7%.
- The HbA(1C) levels of patients given 40 mg rosuvastatin daily increased by 5%.

- The fasting glucose levels of patients given 80 mg atorvastatin daily increased by 3.4%.
- The fasting glucose levels of patients given 40 mg rosuvastatin daily increased by 3.2%.

Dr Simsek concludes: "*Glycaemic control deteriorated in patients with diabetes following high-dose statin therapy*".

Paper 67:
Statin use is associated with increased HbA1c levels in patients with high blood pressure

Liew SM et al Statins use is associated with poorer glycaemic control in a cohort of hypertensive patients with diabetes and without diabetes. *Diabetology and Metabolic Syndrome* 2014 Apr 23;6:53

Associate Professor Su May Liew and her researchers from the University of Malaya, sought to determine the association between the use of statins and glycaemic control in patients with high blood pressure. The study included 1,060 patients.

The Malaysian study reported:

- Analysis of the whole group found that statin users had 29% higher HbA1c levels than statin nonusers.
- Analysis of those with diabetes found that statin users had 20.8% higher HbA1c levels than statin nonusers.

Professor Liew concluded: "*Statins use is associated with increased HbA1c levels among hypertensive patients and hypertensive patients with diabetes*".

Paper 68:
Statins may trigger the onset and worsening of diabetes

Ohmura C et al Acute onset and worsening of diabetes concurrent with administration of statins. *Endocrine Journal* 2005 Jun;52(3):369-72

This paper reports a patient in whom the administration of statins might have triggered the onset and worsening of diabetes. The patient was a 48-year-old man who underwent annual medical examination but had never been told of high blood sugar.

The paper found:

- Four months after the commencement of atorvastatin (10 mg/day) treatment, a diagnosis of diabetes was made from his symptoms of high blood sugar.
- His after-meal glucose level had risen to 29.8 mmol/l (536 mg/dL). Normal levels are below 8.1 mmol/L (8.1 mmol/L).
- His HbA1c levels (a measurement of average blood sugar levels over the previous three months) had risen to 11.5%. Normal levels are below 5.6%.
- Three months after the cessation of atorvastatin, almost complete resolution of diabetes was observed.
- During the subsequent three months, diet therapy alone was sufficient to control blood sugar levels.
- Pravastatin (20 mg/day) was then prescribed and during the next three months his HbA1c levels gradually increased.
- After discontinuation of pravastatin, his HbA1c levels gradually decreased.

This case shows that statins may trigger the onset and worsening of diabetes.

Paper 69:
Statin use is associated with weight gain and a large increase in diabetes

Sugiyama T et al Different Time Trends of Caloric and Fat Intake Between Statin Users and Nonusers Among US Adults: Gluttony in the Time of Statins? *Journal of the American Medical Association International Medicine* 2014 Jul;174(7):1038-45

This Japanese study examined the effects of statins on caloric intake, weight gain and diabetes. The study lasted eleven years and included 27,886 adults, 20 years or older, who completed a 24-hour dietary recall.

The study found over an 11-year period:

- The caloric intake of statin users increased by 9.6%.
- The caloric intake of nonusers DECREASED by 1.9%.
- The BMI of statin users increased by 1.3.
- The BMI of nonusers increased by 0.5.

- Diabetes increased by 7.8% in statin users.
- Diabetes DECREASED by 0.4% in nonusers.

This study shows statin use is associated with weight gain and a large increase in diabetes.

Paper 70: The risk of diabetes rises as adherence with statin therapy increases

Corrao G et al Statins and the Risk of Diabetes: Evidence From a Large Population-Based Cohort Study. *Diabetes Care* 2014 Aug;37(8):2225-32

This study was conducted by Professor Giovanni Corrao and his associates from the University of Milano-Bicocca. The objective of the study was to investigate the relationship between adherence with statin therapy and the risk of developing diabetes. The seven-year study included 115,709 patients who were newly treated with statins. Adherence was measured by the proportion of days covered with statins.

The Italian study determined:

- Compared with patients with very low adherence (proportion of days covered less than 25%), those with low adherence (proportion of days covered 26-50%) had a 12% increased risk of developing diabetes.
- Compared with patients with very low adherence (proportion of days covered less than 25%), those with intermediate adherence (proportion of days covered 51-75%) had a 22% increased risk of developing diabetes.
- Compared with patients with very low adherence (proportion of days covered less than 25%) those with high adherence (proportion of days covered more than 75%) had a 32% increased risk of developing diabetes.

Professor Corrao concluded: *"In a real-world setting, the risk of new-onset diabetes rises as adherence with statin therapy increases"*.

Paper 71: Medical records show that statins are associated with a 14% increased risk of type two diabetes

Danaei G et al Statins and Risk of Diabetes: An analysis of electronic medical records to evaluate possible bias due to differential survival. *Diabetes Care* 2013 May;36(5):1236-40

This Harvard study analysed the relationship between statins and type two diabetes. Data was drawn from the medical records of 285,864 men and women aged 50-84 years who were followed for ten years.

- The study found that statin therapy was associated with a 14% increased risk of type two diabetes.

Paper 72:
Statins hamper the beneficial effects of lifestyle intervention in people at high risk of type two diabetes

Rautio N et al Do statins interfere with lifestyle intervention in the prevention of diabetes in primary healthcare? One-year follow-up of the FIN-D2D project. *British Medical Journal* 2012 Sep 13;2(5)

The objective of the study, (conducted by Dr Nina Rautio and colleagues from the Pirkanmaa Hospital, Tampere, Finland) was to examine whether the use of statins is associated with the incidence of type two diabetes among individuals at high risk for type two diabetes participating in one-year lifestyle intervention study. The study included 2,798 non-diabetic individuals, aged 18–87 years, who had elevated fasting glucose levels.

Lifestyle counselling was performed either in group sessions or individually. Advice was given on diet, weight control, meal frequency and quality, physical activity, smoking, alcohol use and diabetes as a disease in general. Group sessions were mainly weight maintenance or exercise groups and lectures concerning diabetes and lifestyle changes.

The Finnish researchers observed:

- Statin users had a 17% increased risk of developing type two diabetes compared to non-statin users.
- Fasting glucose levels increased by 0.08 mmol/L (1.44 mg/dL) in statin users, but remained unchanged in nonusers.

Dr Rautio concluded: "*The finding that fasting glucose slightly increased in statin users in spite of lifestyle interventions suggests the view that the use of statins might have unfavourable effects on glucose metabolism and that statins might hamper beneficial effects of lifestyle intervention in people at high risk of type two diabetes*".

Paper 73:
A significant association is found between new onset treated diabetes in those treated with statins

Zaharan NL et al Statins and risk of treated incident diabetes in a primary care population. *British Journal of Clinical Pharmacology* 2013 Apr;75(4):1118-24

The aims of this study were to:

- Examine the incidence of new onset diabetes in patients treated with different types of statins.
- Examine the relationship between the duration and dose of statins and the subsequent development of new onset diabetes.

The study (lead author Dr Nur Lisa Zaharan a senior lecturer at the University of Malaysia) included 1,235,671 individuals who were followed for eight years.

Dr Zaharan's findings revealed:

- Statin use was associated with a 20% increased risk of new onset diabetes.
- There was a statistically significant overall dose and duration effect increase in new onset diabetes for all statins, excepting fluvastatin, which only demonstrated a duration effect.

Dr Zaharan finished: "*In conclusion, we found a significant association between new onset treated diabetes in those treated with statin therapy. This was associated with increased duration and dose of treatment suggesting a possible biologically plausible effect*".

Paper 74:
Statins increase risk of diabetes by 32% in patients with impaired glucose tolerance

Shen L et al Role of diuretics, β blockers, and statins in increasing the risk of diabetes in patients with impaired glucose tolerance: reanalysis of data from the NAVIGATOR study *British Medical Journal* 9 December 2013;347:f6745

The objective of this study, published in the prestigious *British Medical Journal,* was to examine the association of various drugs in patients with impaired glucose tolerance with new onset diabetes. The study lasted five years and included 9,306 patients. (If you have impaired glucose tolerance, your blood glucose is raised beyond the normal range but it is not so high that you have diabetes. However, if you have impaired glucose tolerance you are at risk of developing diabetes.)

- Regarding statins, the study found that statin use was associated with a 32% increased risk of new onset diabetes.

Paper 75: Men with prostate cancer taking statins have an increased risk of developing diabetes

Lage MJ et al Association between androgen-deprivation therapy and incidence of diabetes among males with prostate cancer. *Urology* 2007 Dec;70(6):1104-8

This study investigated various factors that may be involved in the development of diabetes in men diagnosed with prostate cancer. The study included 8,481 men with prostate cancer.

- Regarding statins the study found that men taking statins had a 35% increased risk of diabetes compared to men not taking statins.

Paper 76: In postmenopausal women using statins the risk of diabetes increases by 48%

Culver AL et al Statin Use and Risk of Diabetes Mellitus in Postmenopausal Women in the Women's Health Initiative. *Archives of Internal Medicine* 2012 Jan 23;172(2):144-52

This study, based at the world-renowned Mayo Clinic, investigated whether the incidence of diabetes is associated with statin use among postmenopausal women. The trial included 161,808 postmenopausal women aged 50 to 79 who were followed for three years, which amounted to 1,004,466 person years of follow up.

- The study identified that statin use was associated with a 48% increase in diabetes.

Paper 77:
Statin use is associated with an increased risk of diabetes, which increases with longer duration of use

Macedo AF et al Statins and the risk of type 2 diabetes mellitus: cohort study using the UK clinical practice research datalink. *BMC Cardiovascular Disorders* 2014 Jul 15;14(1):85

This study, headed by Assistant Professor Ana Filipa Macedo, aimed to assess the effect of statins on type two diabetes development. The study comprised of 2,016,094 individuals, including 430,890 people who received a statin, matched to 1,585,204 people not prescribed a statin.

The study ascertained:

- Statin users had a 57% increased risk of developing diabetes compared to nonusers.
- The risk of developing diabetes increased with longer duration of statin use:
    - o Statin users who were followed for one to three years had a 22% increased risk of diabetes.
    - o Statin users who were followed for 15 to 20 years had a 263% increased risk of diabetes.

Professor Macedo concluded: *"Statin use is associated with an increased risk of T2DM (type two diabetes), which increases with longer duration of use"*.

Paper 78:
Elderly people taking statins have a 124% higher risk of diabetes

Dybicz SB et al Prevalence of diabetes and the burden of comorbid conditions among elderly nursing home residents. *American Journal of Geriatric Pharmacotherapy* 2011 Aug;9(4):212-23

The aim of the study, published in *The American Journal of Geriatric Pharmacotherapy,* was to estimate the prevalence of diabetes (and factors associated with diabetes) in the elderly living in nursing homes. The study lasted for 12 months and included 2,317 residents from 23 nursing homes, aged 65 and over.

- Regarding statins, the study revealed that those taking statins had a 124% increased risk of having diabetes compared to those not taking statins.

Paper 79:
Statins associated with a significantly increased risk of new onset diabetes in liver transplant recipients

Cho Y et al Statin therapy is associated with development of new onset diabetes after transplantation (NODAT) in liver recipients with high fasting plasma glucose. *Liver Transplantation* 2014 May;20(5):557-63

The aim of this study, carried out in the Department of Internal Medicine at the Yonsei University College of Medicine, was to investigate the association between statin therapy and the development of new onset diabetes after transplantation in liver transplant recipients. The study, which lasted for about 42 months, included 364 liver transplant recipients who underwent transplantation between the ages of 20 and 75 years without a previous history of diabetes.

- The researchers observed that statin use was significantly associated with a 132% increased risk of new onset diabetes after transplantation.

Paper 80:
Statins increase the risk of diabetes by 185% in patients with high blood pressure

Izzo R et al Primary prevention with statins and incident diabetes in hypertensive patients at high cardiovascular risk. *Nutrition, Metabolism and Cardiovascular Diseases* 2013 Nov;23(11):1101-6

This study evaluated the risk of type two diabetes in relation to statin prescription in non-diabetic outpatients' patients with high blood pressure but free of cardiovascular disease. The study included 4,750 patients, average age 58 years, who were followed for at least 12 months.

- At the end of the study the prevalence of diabetes was 185% higher in those taking statins compared to those not taking statins.

Paper 81:
Statins increase the risk of diabetes by 199%

Giudice R et al Does Therapy With Statins Increase Risk Of Diabetes? *Circulation* 2010; 122: A14293

The study was led by Dr Renata Giudice from Federico University in Naples. The study evaluated the risk of diabetes in relation to statin therapy in patients free of diabetes at the start of the study. The study included 1,760 non-diabetic participants, (average age 52 years), who were followed for 3.5 years.

- By the end of the follow-up period Dr Giudice found that the prevalence of new diabetes was 199% higher in patients on statins compared to those not taking statins.

Paper 82:
Statins increase the risk of diabetes in kidney transplant patients

Choe EY et al HMG CoA Reductase Inhibitor Treatment Induces Dysglycemia in Renal Allograft Recipients. *Transplantation* 2014 Feb 27;97(4):419-25

The aim of this Korean study was to evaluate the influence of statins on the development of dysglycemia in kidney transplant patients. (Dysglycemia is defined as diabetes and/or impaired fasting glucose.) The study included 394 patients without previously known diabetes or impaired fasting glucose who had undertaken kidney transplantation. Patients were grouped into the two groups according if they used statins (245 statin users and 149 nonusers).

The research unearthed:

- Statin users had a 208% increased risk of dysglycemia compared to nonusers.
- The time to development of dysglycemia after transplantation was shorter in the statin group (38.8 months) than in the control group (47.2 months).

The scientific evidence shows the FDA were correct in their findings that statins may exacerbate the risk of diabetes.

- Calcium deposits accumulate more in the arteries of diabetics taking statins.
- Insulin levels and insulin resistance is increased in statin users, whereas insulin sensitivity is decreased. Blood glucose levels are more likely to be elevated when prescribed statins. (Increased insulin and glucose levels lead to diabetes.)
- Patients undergoing surgery who injest statins have a higher risk of diabetes.
- The papers in this chapter show that statins make both apparently healthy people, and patients with various conditions, susceptible to the dangers of diabetes.
- People at heightened risk of diabetes with statin intake include: The elderly, those with high blood pressure, women with polycystic ovary syndrome, postmenopausal women, men with prostate cancer, and patients undergoing liver or kidney transplants.
- The scientific literature shows that those who take more statins and those that have a longer duration of use of statins have an increased risk of type two diabetes.

Dr Stephen Sinatra, a cardiologist and Assistant Clinical Professor of Medicine at the Univesity of Connecticut School of medicine, comments: "*Statins have the potential to contribute to type two diabetes to a degree that in 2012 the FDA mandated statin manufacturers to place a diabetes warning on their labels. Moreover, there is evidence that these drugs can produce arterial calcification in diabetic men*".

Chapter 4

Statins and cancer: Cause for concern

Headlines in the media offer spectacularly different viewpoints on the subject of statins and cancer risk. In the UK for instance on the 4th July the *Daily Mail* reported: "*Taking statins could help prevent breast cancer*" yet, a couple of weeks later, on the 20th July 2014, the *Daily Express* headline read: "*New research suggests statins drug can double breast cancer risk*".

Drs Thomas Newman and Stephen Hulley from the University of California analysed all the studies with stain-treated laboratory animals and found that in every study statins have caused cancer. Of course results should not be automatically extrapolated to humans from animal studies.

Therefore in this chapter, 43 scientific papers are reviewed to ascertain if there is any correlation between statin use and cancer risk in humans.

Paper 83:
Statins and the risk of developing cancer
Vinogradova Y et al Exposure to statins and risk of common cancers: a series of nested case-control studies. *BMC Cancer* 2011 Sep 26;11:409

This UK study investigated the association between statins and cancer. The study included 88,125 patients diagnosed with cancer who were compared with 362,254 participants free from cancer.

The study found:

- Those taking statins for less than 12 months had a 1% increased risk of developing cancer than those not taking statins.
- Those taking statins for more than 49 months had a 4% increased risk of developing cancer than those not taking statins.

Paper 84:
Pravastatin increases the risk of cancer by 6%

Bonovas S et al Does pravastatin promote cancer in elderly patients? A meta-analysis. *Canadian Medical Association Journal* 2007 Feb 27;176(5):649-54

The aim of the study, conducted by Dr Stefanos Bonovas from the Department of Pharmacology at the University of Athens, was to assess the effect of pravastatin therapy on cancer risk. The study analysed the results of 12 pravastatin trials which included 42,902 men and women, (21,454 patients in pravastatin groups and 21,448 in control groups).

This Greek study found:

- Pravastatin users had a 6% increased risk of cancer compared to non-statin users.
- Pravastatin therapy was associated with an increasing risk of cancer as the patient age increased. E.g. the oldest pravastatin users – aged over 75 – had a 22% increased risk of cancer compared to nonusers.

Dr Bonovas concluded: "*This analysis showed that pravastatin therapy was associated with an increasing risk of cancer as age increased*".

Paper 85:
In patients undergoing treatment for bladder cancer, statins are significantly associated with an increased risk of tumor progression

Hoffmann P et al Use of statins and outcome of BCG treatment for bladder cancer. *New England Journal of Medicine* 2006 Dec 21;355(25):2705-7

This study was led by Dr Paul Hoffman of the Jules Bordet Institute in Brussels. The study investigated the association between statins and bladder cancer. The study, which lasted for 46 months, analyzed the clinical outcomes of 84 patients who had received the bacille Calmette–Guérin vaccine for the treatment of non–muscle-invasive bladder cancer.

The investigations revealed:

- In 53% of the patients who took statins, the tumor became more aggressive, whereas this change occurred in only 18% of the patients who did not take statins.

- 42% of the patients in the statin group had to undergo radical cystectomy, (radical cystectomy is the removal of the entire bladder, nearby lymph nodes, part of the urethra, and nearby organs that may contain cancer cells), as compared with only 14% of the patients who did not take statins.

Dr Hoffmann concluded: "*The use of statins was significantly associated with an increased risk of tumor progression and a subsequent need for radical cystectomy*".

Paper 86:
Long-term statin users have a 21% increased risk of bladder cancer compared to nonusers

Zhang XL et al Statin use and risk of bladder cancer: a meta-analysis. *Cancer Causes and Control* 2013 Apr;24(4):769-76

This paper analysed the scientific data between January 1966 and October 2012 to quantify the association between statin use and risk of bladder cancer. A total of 13 studies contributed to the analysis.

The analysis found:

- Statin users had a 7% increased risk of bladder cancer compared to nonusers.
- Long-term statin users had a 21% increased risk of bladder cancer compared to nonusers.

Paper 87:
Simvastatin may be harmful rather than beneficial for multiple myeloma patients

Sondergaard TE et al A phase II clinical trial does not show that high dose simvastatin has beneficial effect on markers of bone turnover in multiple myeloma. *Hematological Oncology* 2009 Mar;27(1):17-22

Multiple myeloma is a type of bone marrow cancer. The cancer affects the plasma cells inside the bone marrow, which are an important part of the immune system.

Osteoclasts are a type of cell that destroys bone and osteoblasts are cells that help to build bone. Normally, the activity of the osteoclasts and osteoblasts is well balanced – the osteoclasts clear out the old bone and the osteoblasts begin the rebuilding of new bone. In patients with multiple myeloma, osteoclasts activity is increased and bone destruction ensues.

Collagen is a major constituent of bone and provides the bone with strength and flexibility. When the urinary level of collagen is high, this indicates that bone is being destroyed faster than it is replaced. This indicates osteoporosis in the making.

Lead researcher Teis Esben Sondergaard and his team from the University of Southern Denmark investigated the effect of high dose simvastatin on biochemical markers of bone turnover and disease activity in six patients (age 62-83 years) with multiple myeloma. The patients were treated with simvastatin (15 mg per kg per day) for seven days followed by a rest period of 21 days in two four-week cycles.

The study observed:

- Osteoclast activity in serum and levels of collagen fragments in urine increased for all patients temporarily during the seven days of treatment with high dose simvastatin indicating that osteoclasts may have been stimulated rather than inhibited.
- All six patients experienced gastrointestinal symptoms.
- Three patients had nausea or vomiting, two patients had constipation, one had abdominal pain and there was one incidence of diarrhoea.
- Myalgia (muscle pain) and other muscular symptoms were reported by five patients.
- There was one incident of deep venous thrombosis and one of Achilles tendonitis.
- One patient suffered from fatigue and depression.
- One patient had neutropenia (low levels of white blood cells).
- Two patients died of pneumonia.

Sondergaard concluded: "*This sign of a transient stimulation of osteoclast activity suggests that high dose simvastatin may be harmful rather than beneficial for multiple myeloma patients. For this reason and because of gastro-intestinal side effects the study was stopped prematurely*".

Paper 88:
Women using statins for more than five years have a 27% increased risk of breast cancer

Boudreau DM et al Statin use and breast cancer risk in a large population-based setting. *Cancer Epidemiology Biomarkers and Prevention* 2007 Mar;16(3):416-21

The objective of this Seattle based study was to evaluate the relationship between statin use and breast cancer risk. The study included 92,788 women, aged 45 to 89, who were followed for 6.4 years.

The study reported:

- Statin users had a 7.4% increased risk of breast cancer compared to nonusers.
- A longer duration of statin use led to an increased risk of breast cancer:
    - o Statin use of three to 4.9 years was associated with a 4% increased risked of breast cancer.
    - o Statin use of over five years was associated with a 27% increased risked of breast cancer.

Paper 89:
Women using statins have a 9% increased risk of breast cancer

Beck P et al Statin use and the risk of breast cancer. *Journal of Clinical Epidemiology* 2003 Mar;56(3):280-5

Canadian researchers examined the association of statin use and breast cancer. The study included 13,592 statin users and 53,880 nonexposed subjects who were followed for up to 8.5 years.

- The researchers identified that women using statins had a 9% increased risk of breast cancer compared to women not exposed to statins.

Paper 90:
Statin users have a 13% increased risk of breast cancer

Chan TF et al Statin use and the risk of breast cancer: a population-based case-control study. *Expert Opinion on Drug Safety* 2014 Mar;13(3):287-93

The aim of this Taiwanese study was to investigate whether the use of statins was associated with breast cancer risk. The study included 565 breast cancer cases, aged 50 years and older, and 2,260 matched controls.

- The study observed that those who used statins had a 13% increased risk of breast cancer compared to those with no use of statins.

Paper 91:
Increased risk of breast cancer related to statin use

Eaton M et al Statins and breast cancer in postmenopausal women without hormone therapy. *Anticancer Research* 2009 Dec;29(12):5143-8

This study, led by Dr Mark Eaton from the University of North Dakota School of Medicine and Health Sciences, investigated the association between statin use and risk of breast cancer among overweight or obese postmenopausal women who have never used hormone therapy. The study included 95 women with breast cancer and 94 controls. The women were aged from 55 to 81 years old and had a body mass index over 25.0 kg/m2.

Dr Eaton and his colleagues discovered:

- Women who used statins had a 30% increased risk of breast cancer compared to women not using statins.
- Women who used lovastatin, simvastatin, fluvastatin, or atorvastatin type statins had a 310% increased risk of breast cancer.

Paper 92:
Statin use increases the risk of breast and prostate cancer

Coogan PF et al Statin use and the risk of breast and prostate cancer. *Epidemiology* 2002 May;13(3):262-7

This study, from the Boston University School of Medicine, assessed the relationship of statin use to the risk of breast and prostate cancer. The study included 1,132 women with breast cancer and 1,009 men with prostate cancer who were compared with 1,331 women and 1,387 men without breast or prostate cancer.

The study ascertained:

- Women using statins had a 50% increased risk of breast cancer compared to women not using statins.
- Men using statins had a 20% increased risk of prostate cancer compared to men not using statins.

Paper 93:
Women who take statins may be at increased risk for the development of breast cancer

Mortimer JE et al Effect of statins on breast cancer incidence: Findings from the Sentara Health Plan. *American Society of Clinical Oncology* 22: 2003 (abstr 373)

The study was set up to determine if the use of statins had an impact on breast cancer incidence in women. The study included 66,843 women aged over 35.

- The study shows that women who take statins have a 54% increased risk for the development of breast cancer compared with women not taking statins.

Paper 94:
Long-term use of statins increases the risk of breast cancer
McDougall JA et al Long-term statin use and risk of ductal and lobular breast cancer among women 55-74 years of age. *Cancer Epidemiology, Biomarkers and Prevention* 2013 Sep;22(9):1529-37

Invasive ductal carcinoma refers to cancer that has broken through the wall of the milk duct and begun to invade the tissues of the breast.

Invasive lobular carcinoma. This means that the cancer started in the cells that line the lobules of the breast and has spread into the surrounding breast tissue.

This study, authored by Jean McDougall a Postdoctoral Fellow from the Fred Hutchinson Cancer Research Centre, investigated the relationship between long-term statin use and the risk of breast cancer. The study included 916 women with invasive ductal carcinoma breast cancer and 1,068 women with invasive lobular carcinoma breast cancer who were compared with 902 women free of breast cancer. The women were aged between 55-74 years.

The study found:

- Current users of statins for ten years or longer had a 83% increased risk of invasive ductal carcinoma breast cancer compared to women who had never used statins.
- Current users of statins for ten years or longer had a 97% increased risk of invasive lobular carcinoma breast cancer compared to women who had never used statins.

McDougall concluded: *"All statins inhibit HMG-CoA reductase at the rate-limiting step of the mevalonate pathway, an intricate biochemical pathway required for the production of cholesterol, isoprenoids, dolichol, ubiquinone, and isopentenyladine. Laboratory studies have investigated how disrupting the melavonate pathway may lead to carcinogenesis. Our finding of an increased risk only among current long-term statin users suggests that the chronic dysregulation of the mevalonate pathway and/or long-term lowering of serum cholesterol may contribute to breast carcinogenesis".*

Paper 95:
Statin use increases the risk of multiple colorectal adenomas by 25%

Wei JT et al Reported use of 3-hydroxy-3-methylglutaryl coenzyme A reductase inhibitors was not associated with reduced recurrence of colorectal adenomas. *Cancer Epidemiology, Biomarkers and Prevention* 2005 Apr;14(4):1026-7

This study investigated the association of statins with the risk of recurrent colorectal adenomas. (An adenoma (a type of polyp) is a benign tumour. Colorectal adenomas are removed because of their tendency to become malignant and to lead to colon cancer.) The study analysed data from three randomised trials (Polyp Prevention Study, Calcium Polyp Prevention Study and Aspirin/Folate Polyp Prevention Study) regarding the recurrence of colorectal adenomas in patients with a history of adenomas. The trials included 2,638 patients.

The analysis revealed:

- Statin users had a 3% increased risk of any adenoma compared to statin never-users.
- Statin users had a 13% increased risk of any advanced adenoma compared to statin never-users.
- Statin users had a 25% increased risk of multiple adenoma compared to statin never-users.

Paper 96:
Increase in colorectal cancer cases in statin users

Cheng MH et al Statin use and the risk of colorectal cancer: a population-based case-control study. *World Journal of Gastroenterology* 2011 Dec 21;17(47):5197-202

The aim of the study was to investigate whether the use of statins is associated with colorectal cancer risk. The study included 1,156 colorectal cancer cases that were aged 50 years and older and had a first-time diagnosis of colorectal cancer and 4,624 matched controls.

The results of the study revealed:

- Statins users had a 9% increased risk of colorectal cancer compared to those who did not take statins.
- Statin users with the highest cumulative statin use had a 30% increased risk of colorectal cancer compared to those who did not take statins.

Paper 97:
Statin users of ten years have a 30% increased risk of colorectal cancer

Yang YX et al Chronic statin therapy and the risk of colorectal cancer. *Pharmacoepidemiology and Drug Safety* 2008 Sep;17(9):869-76

The study sought to clarify the association between long-term statin therapy and the risk of colorectal cancer. This study was conducted among patients aged 50 years or more and with five or more years of colorectal cancer-free initial follow-up. The study, based at the University of Pennsylvania, included 4,432 colorectal cancer patients and 44,292 control subjects.

The study identified:

- Those who had been taking statins for five or more years had a 10% increased risk of colorectal cancer compared to nonusers of statins.
- Those who had been taking statins for ten years had a 30% increased risk of colorectal cancer compared to nonusers of statins.

Paper 98:
Statins increase the risk of recurrent adenomatous polyps by 36%

Parker-Ray N et al Statin use does not prevent recurrent adenomatous polyp formation in a VA population. *Indian Journal of Gastroenterology* 2010 Jun;29(3):106-11

The lead author of the study, Dr Nikki Parker-Ray, specialises in gastroenterology. The aim of the study was to evaluate whether statin use was associated with recurrent adenomatous polyps. The study included 197 patients, (average age 63 years), who had undergone polypectomy (removal of a polyp) between January 1, 1999 and December 31, 2001 and surveillance colonoscopy by December 2006. (Colonoscopy is a test that allows your doctor to look at the inner lining of your large intestine. During a colonoscopy, tissue samples can be collected (biopsy) and abnormal growths can be taken out.)

- Dr Parker-Ray found that statin users had a 36% increased risk of recurrent adenomatous polyps compared to nonusers.

Paper 99:
Statins increase the risk of developing colorectal adenomas

Bertagnolli MM et al Statin use and colorectal adenoma risk: results from the adenoma prevention with celecoxib trial. *Cancer Prevention Research* (Philadelphia, Pa) 2010 May;3(5):588-96

This study, headed by Dr Monica Bertagnolli from the Brigham and Women's Hospital, investigated the relationship between statin use and colorectal adenoma risk in patients with a high risk of recurrent colorectal adenomas. The study analysed data from 2,035 adenoma patients from a previous adenoma prevention trial (Adenoma Prevention with Celecoxib, APC trial) in which patients received celecoxib (drug to prevent cancer) or placebo.

After three years, the study found:

- Statin users of over three years who received placebo had a 47% increased risk of recurrent colorectal adenomas compared to statin nonusers.
- Statin users of over three years who received celecoxib 200 mg twice daily had a 3% increased risk of recurrent colorectal adenomas compared to statin nonusers.
- Statin users of over three years who received celecoxib 400 mg twice daily had a 16% increased risk of recurrent colorectal adenomas compared to statin nonusers.
- Statin users who received placebo had a 214% increased risk of a cardiovascular adverse event compared to statin nonusers.

- Statin users who received celecoxib 200 mg twice daily had 45% increased risk of a cardiovascular adverse event compared to statin nonusers.
- Statin users who received celecoxib 400 mg twice daily had 27% increased risk of a cardiovascular adverse event compared to statin nonusers.

Dr Bertagnolli concludes: *"For patients at high risk of colorectal cancer, statins do not protect against colorectal neoplasm's and may even increase the risk of developing colorectal adenomas"*.

Paper 100:
Statins increase the risk of colon adenomas by 54%

Eddi R et al Association of Type 2 Diabetes and Colon Adenomas. *Journal of gastrointestinal cancer* 2012 Mar;43(1):87-92

This three-year study, based at Seton Hall University School of Health and Medical Sciences, of 783 people (of which 261 had adenomas) sought to determine (i) the association between type two diabetes and colon adenomas and (ii) factors that increase the risk of adenomas.

The study detected:

- Those who had diabetes had a 45% increased risk of developing colon adenomas.
- Use of statins increased the risk of adenoma by 54%.

Paper 101:
Statin users have a 37% increase in gastric cancer risk

Shimoyama S Statins and gastric cancer risk. *Hepato-gastroenterology* 2011 May-Jun;58(107-108):1057-61

Dr Shouji Shimoyama, whose research interests include oesophageal and gastric oncology and upper gastrointestinal endoscopy, reviewed the scientific literature concerning the effect of statins on gastric cancer incidence published between 1993 and 2008. He found six eligible publications, three were for gastric cancer risk and three were for upper gastrointestinal cancer risk.

Dr Shimoyama found:

- Statin users had a 37% increase in gastric cancer risk.
- Statin users had a 20% increase in upper gastrointestinal cancer.

Paper 102:
Trend of increased kidney cancer risk with statins

Chiu HF et al Statin use and the risk of kidney cancer: a population-based case-control study. *Expert Opinion on Drug Safety* 2012 Jul;11(4):543-9

The objective of the study was to investigate whether the use of statins was associated with kidney cancer risk. The study included 177 kidney cancer cases and 708 controls aged 50 or over.

The findings of the study revealed:

- Those who were prescribed statins had an 8% increased risk of kidney cancer compared to those that did not take statins.
- Those with the highest use of statins had a 28% increased risk of kidney cancer compared to those that did not take statins.

The author of the paper, Professor Hui-Fen Chiu, advises: "*There is a trend of increased kidney cancer risk with higher cumulative (statin) defined daily doses, and consequently that it is prudent to continue monitoring cancer incidence among long-standing statin users*".

Paper 103:
Statins increase the risk of renal cell carcinoma

Chéry L et al NSAID and statin use and risk of renal cell carcinoma. *American Urological Association Annual Meeting*; May 19-23, 2012; Atlanta, GA. Abstract 575

This study was authored by Dr Lisly Chéry, a urology resident at the University of Washington School of Medicine in Seattle. Dr Chéry notes that renal cell carcinoma, the most common type of kidney cancer, is the sixth most common cancer in men and the eighth most common cancer in women.

This study set out to determine the effect of various pharmaceutical drugs on the risk of renal cell carcinoma. The study included 77,048 individuals aged 50 to 76 years.

- Regarding statins, the study found those who were taking statins had a 10% increased risk of developing renal cell carcinoma.

Paper 104:
Rosuvastatin (Crestor) is associated with a 2.8-fold increased risk of lung cancer

Lai SW et al Statins use and female lung cancer risk in Taiwan. *Libyan Journal of Medicine* 2012 Dec 27;7(0):1-3

The mission of this study was to clarify the association between statins use and female lung cancer risk. The study included 1,117 women with newly diagnosed lung cancer, average age 66.5 years, who were compared to 4,468 age-matched women without lung cancer.

The results of the study ascertained:

- Statin use was associated with a 7% increased risk of lung cancer.
- Rosuvastatin (Crestor) use of over 12 months' duration was associated with a 2.8-fold increased risk of lung cancer.

Paper 105:
Statins increase lymphoid malignancy rates by 124%

Iwata H et al Use of hydroxy-methyl-glutaryl coenzyme A reductase inhibitors is associated with risk of lymphoid malignancies. *Cancer Science* 2006 Feb;97(2):133-8

Lymphoid malignancies include lymphoma and myeloma. Lymphoma is cancer that starts in the lymph glands or other organs of the lymphatic system. Myeloma, also known as multiple myeloma, is a cancer arising from plasma cells, a type of white blood cell which is made in the bone marrow.

The study examined the association between statin use and development of lymphoid malignancies. Statin use of 221 cases with proven lymphoid malignancies (lymphoma and myeloma), from Toranomon Hospital (Tokyo, Japan) was compared with statin use of 879 patients without malignancies from the same hospital.

- The observations from the study identified there was a 124% higher frequency of statin use among patients with lymphoid malignancies in comparison with the other patients.

Paper 106:
Statin use is associated with increased blood loss during prostate surgery

Truesdale MD et al Impact of HMG-CoA reductase inhibitor (statin) use on blood loss during robot-assisted and open radical prostatectomy. *Journal of Endourology* 2011 Sep;25(9):1427-33

Blood loss is a major surgical complication and death rates may be up to 20% in the presence of severe bleeding.

A radical prostatectomy is an operation to remove the prostate gland and some of the tissue around it. It is done to remove prostate cancer.

Hematocrit is a blood test that measures the percentage of the volume of whole blood that is made up of red blood cells. This measurement depends on the number of red blood cells and the size of red blood cells.

Urologist Dr Matthew Truesdale and his colleagues from the Columbia University Medical Centre looked at the impact of statin use on blood loss during open radical prostatectomy and robot-assisted radical prostatectomy (where the surgeon moves the robotic arm while sitting at a computer monitor near the operating table). Blood loss was defined as % hematocrit change presurgery vs. postsurgery. The hematocrit levels were measured in 3,578 patients who had undergone prostatectomy for prostate cancer. Average patient age was 60.2 years.

Dr Truesdale reported:

- For open radical prostatectomy, hematocrit levels decreased by an extra 11.2% in statin users compared to nonusers.
- For robot-assisted radical prostatectomy, hematocrit levels decreased by an extra 0.8% in statin users compared to nonusers.

Dr Truesdale concluded: "*Statin use is associated with increased blood loss during radical prostatectomy*".

Paper 107:
Cholesterol-lowering drugs and prostate cancer incidence

Jacobs EJ et al Cholesterol-lowering drugs and advanced prostate cancer incidence in a large U.S. cohort. *Cancer Epidemiology, Biomarkers and Prevention* 2007 Nov;16(11):2213-7

The purpose of this large Atlanta based study was to examine the association between use of cholesterol-lowering drugs and prostate cancer incidence. The study included 55,454 men who were followed for six years. (Of the men using cholesterol-lowering drugs 86% were on statins.)

The observations from the study indicated:

- Men using cholesterol-lowering drugs for less than five years had a 2% increased risk of prostate cancer compared to men not using cholesterol-lowering drugs.
- Men using cholesterol-lowering drugs for more than five years had a 6% increased risk of prostate cancer compared to men not using cholesterol-lowering drugs.

Paper 108:
Men taking statins have an 11% increased risk of high-grade prostate cancer

Freedland SJ et al Statin use and risk of prostate cancer and high-grade prostate cancer: results from the REDUCE study. *Prostate Cancer and Prostatic Diseases* 2013 Sep;16(3):254-9

This study examined the association between statins and prostate cancer and low-grade and high-grade prostate cancer. The study included 6,729 men aged 50-75 years, who were followed for four years. (Low-grade cancer is likely to develop more slowly than high-grade cancer.)

The investigations revealed:

- Men taking statins had a 5% increased risk of prostate cancer compared to men not taking statins.
- Men taking statins had a 3% increased risk of low-grade prostate cancer compared to men not taking statins.
- Men taking statins had an 11% increased risk of high-grade prostate cancer compared to men not taking statins.

Paper 109:
The association between statins and prostate cancer

Murtola TJ et al Cholesterol-lowering drugs and prostate cancer risk: a population-based case-control study. *Cancer Epidemiology, Biomarkers and Prevention* 2007 Nov;16(11):2226-32

Researchers from the University of Tampere evaluated the association between cholesterol-lowering medication use and prostate cancer risk.

The study included all newly diagnosed prostate cancer cases in Finland during 1995 to 2002 and matched controls (24,723 case control pairs).

The Finnish researchers found:

- Those taking statins had a 7% increased risk of prostate cancer compared to those not taking statins.
- Those taking fibrates had a 5% increased risk of prostate cancer compared to those not taking fibrates.
- Those taking other cholesterol-lowering medications (resins and acipimox) had a 16% increased risk of prostate cancer compared to those not taking cholesterol-lowering medications.
- Those with 14-167 cumulative daily doses of statins had a 6% increased risk of prostate cancer compared to those not taking statins.
- Those with 915-6,781 cumulative daily doses of statins had a 13% increased risk of prostate cancer compared to those not taking statins.

Paper 110:
Statins and non-steroidal anti-inflammatory drugs increase the risk of prostate cancer by 10%

Coogan PF et al Statin and NSAID use and prostate cancer risk. *Pharmacoepidemiology and Drug Safety* 2010 Jul;19(7):752-5

The aim of this Boston University study was to investigate the association of statins and non-steroidal anti-inflammatory drugs with the risk of prostate cancer. The study included 1,367 men, (aged 40-79) with prostate cancer and 2,007 men without prostate cancer.

The results of the study determined:

- Men taking statins had a 10% increased risk of prostate cancer compared to men not taking statins.
- Men with joint use of statins and non-steroidal anti-inflammatory drugs had a 10% increased risk of prostate cancer compared to men not taking statins or non-steroidal anti-inflammatory drugs.
- Men taking statins for over ten years had a 40% increased risk of prostate cancer compared to men not taking statins.

Paper 111:
Statins raise prostate cancer risk of obese men

Agalliu I et al Statin Use and Risk of Prostate Cancer: Results from a Population-based Epidemiologic Study. *American Journal of Epidemiology*2008;168(3):250-260

Assistant Professor Dr Ilir Agalliu, and his Seattle based team, conducted a study of 1,001 prostate cancer cases, aged 35-74 years, and 942 age-matched controls to evaluate the risk of prostate cancer associated with statin use.

The Seattle study reported:

- Those who had used statins for more than ten years had an 11% increased risk of prostate cancer compared to nonusers.
- In obese men, current use of a statin was associated with a 50% increased risk of prostate cancer compared to nonusers.
- In obese men, use of a statin for five or more years was associated with a 80% increased risk of prostate cancer compared to nonusers.

Dr Agalliu Concluded: "*Obese men who use statin medications, particularly for longer durations, have an increased risk of prostate cancer relative to obese nonusers*".

Paper 112:
Statin users have a 15% increased risk of prostate cancer recurrence

Mass AY et al Preoperative statin therapy is not associated with biochemical recurrence after radical prostatectomy: our experience and meta-analysis. *Journal of Urology* 2012 Sep;188(3):786-91

The purpose of this New York University School of Medicine study was to investigate whether statins were associated with prostate cancer recurrence in men after radical prostatectomy. The study included 1,446 patients, who were followed for 57 months, who underwent radical prostatectomy.

- In the study, the New York University researchers found that statin users had a 15% increased risk of prostate cancer recurrence compared to nonusers.

Paper 113:
Statin use increases the risk of recurrence of prostate cancer

Rioja J et al Impact of statin use on pathologic features in men treated with radical prostatectomy. *Journal of Urology* 2010;183(4):e51

This study, led by Dr Jorge Rioja, evaluated the effect of statin use on prostate cancer. The study included 3,748 prostate cancer patients who had a radical prostatectomy.

Dr Rioja observed:

- Statin users had a 15% increased risk of recurrence of prostate cancer compared to nonusers.
- Statin users had a 33% larger tumour size than nonusers.

Paper 114:
Statin users have an 18% increased risk of recurrence of prostate cancer

Ku JH et al Relationship of statins to clinical presentation and biochemical outcomes after radical prostatectomy in Korean patients. *Prostate Cancer and Prostatic Diseases* 2011 Mar;14(1):63-8

In this study, urologist Dr Ja Hyeon Ku set out to determine whether or not statins influence biochemical recurrence in patients undergoing surgical treatment for prostate cancer. The study reviewed data from 687 men who had undergone radical retropubic prostatectomy. (Radical retropubic prostatectomy is a surgical procedure in which the prostate gland is removed through an incision in the abdomen. It is most often used to treat individuals who have early prostate cancer.)

- Dr Ku found that patients taking statins had an 18% increased risk of recurrence of prostate cancer compared to patients not taking statins.

Paper 115:
Statins increase the risk of prostate cancer

Wuermli L et al Hypertriglyceridemia as a possible risk factor for prostate cancer. *Prostate Cancer and Prostatic Diseases* 2005;8(4):316-20

This Swiss study assessed various factors in patients with prostate cancer and compared them with patients with benign prostatic hyperplasia. (Benign prostatic hyperplasia is an increase in size of the prostate gland without malignancy present and it is so common as to be normal with advancing age.) The study included 504 patients diagnosed with prostate cancer and 565 age-matched patients with benign prostatic hyperplasia.

- Regarding statins, the study found that statin usage was 23% higher in the patients that had developed prostate cancer compared to the patients with an enlarged prostate.

Paper 116:
Statin users are at an increased risk for recurrence of prostate cancer following removal of the prostate

Ritch CR et al Effect of statin use on biochemical outcome following radical prostatectomy. *British Journal of Urology international* 2011 Oct;108(8 Pt 2):E211-6

The first author of the study, Dr Chad R. Ritch, is a fellowship-trained urologist with expertise in Urologic Oncology. He specializes in the treatment of prostate, bladder, kidney and testicular cancer. The objective of the study was to determine the relationship between statin use and cancer recurring (biochemical recurrence) following radical prostatectomy. 1261 patients were analysed of which 281 were statin users.

Dr Ritch's research ascertained:

- Statin users had a 54% increased risk of prostate cancer recurring compared to non-statin users.
- Statin users had a lower five-year survival compared with non-statin users.

Dr Ritch concluded: "*Statin users are at an increased risk for biochemical recurrence following radical prostatectomy*".

Paper 117:
Statins increase the risk of prostate cancer by 55%

Chang CC et al Statins increase the risk of prostate cancer: A population-based case-control study. *The Prostate* 2011 Dec;71(16):1818-24

The aim of the study was to investigate whether the use of statins was associated with prostate cancer risk. The study examined 388 prostate cancer cases and 1,552 controls.

The study results revealed:

- Those who used statins had a significant 55% increase in prostate cancer risk compared to those with no use of statins.
- Those who had the lowest statin dose had a 17% increase in prostate cancer risk compared to those with no use of statins.
- Those who had the highest statin dose had an 86% increase in prostate cancer risk compared to those with no use of statins.

This study suggests that statins increase the risk of prostate cancer and the higher the statin dose, the higher the risk of cancer.

Paper 118: Statin use associated with worse prognosis and erectile dysfunction for prostate cancer patients

Kontraros M et al Pathological characteristics, biochemical recurrence and functional outcome in radical prostatectomy patients on statin therapy. *Urologia Internationalis* 2013;90(3):263-9

This Greek study investigated the effects of statin use on radical prostatectomy patients. The study included 588 radical prostatectomy patients, average age 65.2 years.

The Greek investigators detected:

- Statin users of more than two years had a 2.76 times greater likelihood of a more aggressive cancer.
- Statin users of more than two years had a 5.39 times greater likelihood of having a postoperative Gleason score equal to seven or more. (The Gleason score provides an effective measurement that helps determine how severe the level of prostate cancer. Scores from two to four are very low on the cancer aggression scale. Scores from five to six are mildly aggressive. A score of seven indicates that the cancer is moderately aggressive. Scores from eight to ten indicate that the cancer is highly aggressive.)
- Statins were found to be an independent predictor of recurrence of the cancer.

- The probability of erectile dysfunction was significantly greater for statin users.

Paper 119: Long-term statin use increases the risk of basal cell carcinoma by 30%

Asgari MM et al Statin use and risk of basal cell carcinoma. *Journal of the American Academy of Dermatology* 2009 Jul;61(1):66-72

The objective of the study was to examine the association between statin use and basal cell carcinoma risk. (Basal cell carcinoma is known as non-melanoma skin cancer. Non-melanoma skin cancer refers to a group of cancers that slowly develop in the upper layers of the skin.) The study included 12,123 patients, average age 64 years, who had been diagnosed with basal cell carcinoma. They were followed for an average of 4.25 years and 6,381 patients developed a subsequent basal cell carcinoma during follow-up.

The head researcher of the study was dermatologist specialist Dr Maryam Asgari. Her findings pinpointed:

- Those that used statins had a 2% increased risk of subsequent basal cell carcinoma compared to those that did not use statins.
- Those that used statins for five years or more had a 30% increased risk of subsequent basal cell carcinoma compared to those that did not use statins.
- Those that used other cholesterol lowering drugs (such as gemfibrozil, niacin, cholestyramine, colestipol, niacinamide and fenofibrate) had a 10% increased risk of subsequent basal cell carcinoma compared to nonusers.

Paper 120: Statin users have a 14% increased risk of melanoma

Jagtap D et al Prospective analysis of association between use of statins and melanoma risk in the Women's Health Initiative. *Cancer* 2012 Oct 15;118(20):5124-3

Melanoma is the most lethal form of skin cancer. This Wayne State University study examined the association between statin use and the risk of melanoma. The study consisted of 119,726 postmenopausal white women who were followed for 11.6 years.

The study indicated:

- Statin users had a 14% increased risk of melanoma compared to nonusers.
- Statin users of more than five years had a 43% increased risk of melanoma compared to nonusers.

Paper 121:
Statin users have a 25% increased risk of developing Merkel cell carcinoma

Sahi H et al Increased incidence of Merkel cell carcinoma among younger statin users. *Cancer Epidemiology* 2012 Oct;36(5):421-4

Merkel cell carcinoma is a rare type of skin cancer. It develops in Merkel cells which are in the top layer of the skin.

The aim of the study, based at the Helsinki University Hospital, was to find out whether statin users have an increased incidence of Merkel cell carcinoma. The study included 454,935 men and women.

The study observed:

- Statin users had a 25% increased risk of developing Merkel cell carcinoma compared to non-statin users.
- Statin users aged below 60 had a 216% increased risk of developing Merkel cell carcinoma compared to non-statin users.

Paper 122:
The association between statins and thyroid cancer

Hung SH et al Statin Use and Thyroid Cancer: A Population-Based Case-Control Study. *Clinical Endocrinology (Oxf)* 2015 Jul;83(1):111-6

Otolaryngologists are physicians trained in the medical and surgical management and treatment of patients with diseases and disorders of the ear, nose, throat, and related structures of the head and neck.

This study, conducted by Dr Shih-Han Hung a specialist in Otolaryngology, aimed to evaluate the association of statin use with thyroid cancer. The study included 500 subjects with thyroid cancer as cases and 2,500 gender- and age-matched subjects without thyroid cancer as controls.

Dr Hung found:

- Women who used statins had a 43% increased risk of thyroid cancer compared to women not taking statins.
- Men who used statins had a 28% increased risk of thyroid cancer compared to men not taking statins.

Paper 123:
Statins and Cancer risk

Thompson JS et al Statins and Cancer: A Potential Link? *American Journal of Therapeutics* 2010 Jul-Aug;17(4):e100-4

Dr Joseph Thompson from the Chicago Medical School carried out a review of the scientific evidence concerning statins (and other cholesterol lowering drugs) and the risk of cancer.

Dr Thompson's review revealed:

- Results from the Simvastatin and Ezetimibe in Aortic Stenosis (SEAS) study unveiled a potential increased risk of cancer and cancer death for individuals taking the well-known drug combination of ezetimibe/simvastatin.
- There are numerous studies that have found potential links between statins and various forms of cancer.
- Many studies show small correlations between statin use and increased incidence of cancer.

Paper 124:
Statins And Cancer: Cause For Concern

Ravnskov U et al Statins And Cancer: Cause For Concern *British Medical Journal* 17 November 2001;323:1145

Dr Uffe Ravnskov has published over 80 scientific papers regarding the cholesterol, saturated fat, heart disease hypothesis. Here he questions the wisdom of recommending statin treatment for a large segment of the world's population simply because they have elevated cholesterol levels or are assumed to be at increased risk for coronary events because of the presence of other risk markers.

Dr Ravnskov comments:

- It is already known that statins may induce fatal rhabdomyolysis, cardiac insufficiency, peripheral polyneuropathy, hepatic toxicity, and mental disturbances.
- A much more momentous issue is that all statins have proven carcinogenic.
- In the Heart Protection Study (HPS) non-melanoma skin cancer was seen in 243 patients treated with simvastatin compared with 202 cases in the control group.
- In the Scandinavian Simvastatin Survival Study (4S) non-melanoma skin cancer was seen in 13 patients treated with simvastatin compared with six in the control group.
- Also disquieting was the significant increase in breast cancer rates in patients treated with pravastatin in the Cholesterol and Recurrent Events trial (CARE).

Paper 125: Statins may promote cancer in certain segments of the population

Goldstein MR et al Do statins prevent or promote cancer?
Current Oncology 2008 April; 15(2): 76–77

Dr Mark Goldstein and his colleagues highlight that prospective data suggest that statins actually increase cancer in certain segments of the population.

They state that close inspection of statin trials reveal the specific populations at risk for the development of incident cancer with statin treatment. These include:

- The elderly.
- People with a history of breast or prostate cancer.
- Statin-treated individuals undergoing immunotherapy for cancer may be at increased risk for worsening cancer.
- In over 75's at high risk for cardiovascular disease, cancer incidence is significantly increased in subjects randomized to pravastatin in the PROSPER trial.
- Likewise an analysis of the LIPID study, containing individuals with cardiovascular disease, revealed a significant increase in cancer incidence in the elderly subjects, age: 65–75 years, randomised to pravastatin.

- The elderly, when subjected to atorvastatin, a high-dose versus low-dose demonstrated a trend toward increased death, largely from an increase in cancer mortality in the TNT trial.
- An alarming increase in breast cancer incidence, some of which were recurrences, was seen in women randomized to pravastatin in the CARE trial.
- Long-term follow-up (ten years after trial completion) of the WOSCOPS trial revealed an increase in prostate cancer in the men who were randomised to pravastatin therapy. That finding indicates that cancers may become evident a decade or more after treatment with statins.
- Statin therapy has been associated with tumour progression leading to radical cystectomy in patients treated for bladder cancer with bacille Calmette–Guérin immunotherapy.

Dr Goldstein concludes: "*We feel that there is ample evidence that statins may promote cancer in certain segments of the population*".

The findings from this chapter offer evidence that statin use may be associated with an increased risk of cancer.

- There is a trend of increased cancer incidence with statin users.
- The longer the use of statins, the bigger the increase in risk of cancer.
- The elderly are particularly prone to cancer risk when taking statins.

Cholesterol and statin expert Dr Uffe Ravnskov commented on the findings of Drs Thomas Newman and Stephen Hulley regarding the link between statins and cancer in animals, and also the evidence with humans, statins and cancer: "*Caution should be used in the use of the statin drugs as there is much evidence to suggest that such treatment may lead to cancer in humans as well... The results from the statin trials are therefore disquieting*".

Chapter 5

The common association between statin use and muscle damage

The most significant and well-documented adverse effect with statins is muscle toxicity. Muscle symptoms may vary from mild problems, for example, pain, tenderness or weakness to more severe conditions of damage and cell death.

The problem is so widespread that the statin manufacturers have to issue a warning about the danger of muscle disease when selling the drugs.

The following papers analyse the incidence of statin induced muscle pain, where the pain occurs and the severity of the symptoms.

Paper 126:
Statins cause shoulder stiffness in nearly one-tenth of women

Harada K et al Shoulder stiffness: a common adverse effect of HMG-CoA reductase inhibitors in women? *Internal Medicine* 2001 Aug;40(8):817-8

This study, headed by Dr Kazuhiro Harada from Kasaoka Daiichi Hospital, investigated the effects of statins on shoulder stiffness. The study included 66 women aged 46 to 76 years.

- The study found that statins caused shoulder stiffness in 9.1% of the women taking statins.

Dr Harada concludes: "*The present study suggests that HMG-CoA reductase inhibitors (statins) can cause or worsen shoulder stiffness, commonly recognized in middle-aged women*".

Paper 127:
Statins increase the risk of musculoskeletal pain

Buettner C et al Statin use and musculoskeletal pain among adults with and without arthritis. *American Journal of Medicine* 2012 Feb;125(2):176-82

This study, set at the prestigious Harvard Medical School, evaluated the relationship between statin use and musculoskeletal pain. (The musculoskeletal system is made up of the body's bones (the skeleton), muscles, cartilage, tendons, ligaments, joints, and other connective tissue that supports and binds tissues and organs together.) The study included 8,228 adults aged 40 years or more.

- The study reported those taking statins had a 15% increased risk of musculoskeletal pain compared to nonusers.

Paper 128:
Statins and leg cramps

Garrison SR et al Nocturnal leg cramps and prescription use that precedes them: a sequence symmetry analysis. *Archives of Internal Medicine* 2012 Jan 23;172(2):120-6

Quinine is widely used as an effective therapy for leg cramps.

This study evaluated the association of various pharmaceutical drugs with muscle cramps. The study used databases containing the prescribing information about 4.2 million people to determine in adults 50 years or older whether new quinine prescriptions increase in the year following the start of various pharmaceutical drugs.

- Regarding statins, the study found that new quinine prescriptions increased by 16% in people who had started taking statins the previous year.

Paper 129:
Statin use linked to musculoskeletal diseases, joint pain and injuries

Mansi I et al Statins and Musculoskeletal Conditions, Arthropathies, and Injuries *Journal of the American Medical Association Internal Medicine* 2013 Jul 22;173(14):1-10

The lead author of the study was Dr Ishak Mansi whose research interests include statin effects and side effects. The objective of this study was to determine whether statin use is associated with musculoskeletal disorders. (Musculoskeletal disorders can affect the body's muscles, joints, tendons, ligaments and nerves.) This analysis compared 6,967 statin users with 6,967 nonusers.

The study pinpointed:

- Statin users had a 19% increased risk of all musculoskeletal diseases compared to nonusers.
- Statin users had a 13% increased risk of injury-related diseases (dislocation, sprain, strain) compared to nonusers.
- Statin users had a 9% increased risk of drug-associated musculoskeletal pain compared to nonusers.
- Statin users had a 7% increased risk of joint pain compared to nonusers.

Dr Mansi concludes: "*Musculoskeletal conditions, arthropathies, injuries, and pain are more common among statin users than among similar nonusers*".

Paper 130:
Statins implicated in muscular side-effects

Franc S et al A comprehensive description of muscle symptoms associated with lipid-lowering drugs. *Cardiovascular Drugs and Therapy* 2003 Sep-Nov;17(5-6):459-65

Paris based researchers set out to report on the muscular side-effects of cholesterol-lowering drugs. The study included 815 patients, average age 57 years, taking cholesterol-lowering drugs (~90% were taking statins).

The research indicated:

- 20.2% of the patients experienced muscle problems which they attributed to the cholesterol-lowering drugs.
- A clear chronological link between muscle symptoms and the cholesterol-lowering drugs was revealed, either because they appeared soon after drug initiation or because of an improvement after drug withdrawal.

- Cramps and stiffness were the most frequent symptoms, tendonitis-associated pain was also common; reported in almost half the cases.
- 39% of patients had used analgesics for pain relief.

Paper 131: After six months of taking statins, over 20% of people develop muscle pain

Smiderle L et al Evaluation of sexual dimorphism in the efficacy and safety of simvastatin/atorvastatin therapy in a southern Brazilian cohort. *Arquivos Brasileiros de Cardiologia* 2014 Jul;103(1):33-40

This study evaluated the effects of simvastatin/atorvastatin on men and women. The six month study included 495 patients, aged 25-82 years, (331 women and 164 men), who received simvastatin/atorvastatin.

When high levels of creatine phosphokinase (an enzyme found mainly in the heart, brain, and skeletal muscle) are detected in the blood, it is considered to be an abnormal result. High levels of the enzyme may occur due to the following conditions: Heart attack, pericarditis after a heart attack, polymyositis or dermatomyositis, heart muscle inflammation, myopathy (a disease of the muscles), rhabdomyolysis (a breakdown of muscle tissues), muscular dystrophies, convulsions, stroke, brain injury, delirium tremens, hypothyroidism (a decrease in the activity of the thyroid gland) or hyperthyroidism (an increase in activity of the thyroid gland), death of lung tissue.

After six months, the study found:

- 20.3% of the patients developed muscle pain.
  - 9% of the male patients developed muscle pain.
  - 25.9%of the female patients developed muscle pain.
- 11.1% of the patients had increased creatine phosphokinase levels and/or abnormal liver function.
  - 17.9% of the male patients had increased creatine phosphokinase levels and/or abnormal liver function.
  - 7.6% of the female patients had increased creatine phosphokinase levels and/or abnormal liver function.

Paper 132:
Statins cause muscle pain in 24% of patients

Palamaner Subash Shantha G et al Association of vitamin d and incident statin induced myalgia-a retrospective cohort study. *PLoS One* 2014 Feb 19;9(2):e88877

This study, led by Dr Ghanshyam Palamaner Subash Shantha an internist in Scranton Pennsylvania, assessed the association between vitamin D and statin induced myalgia (muscle pain). The study, which lasted for seven years, included 5,526 adult patients who attended a primary care clinic. 1,160 out of 5,526 patients were taking statins.

- Dr Palamaner Subash Shantha recorded that 24% of the statin taking patients developed statin induced myalgia.

Paper 133:
33% of statin users report having muscle problems

Riphagen IJ et al Myopathy during statin therapy in the daily practice of an outpatient cardiology clinic: prevalence, predictors and relation with vitamin D. *Current Medical Research and Opinion* 2012 Jul;28(7):1247-52

This Dutch study assessed the prevalence of myopathy (muscle disease) in statin users attending the outpatient clinic of the Department of Cardiology of a University Hospital. The study included 84 statin users who completed a questionnaire.

- The Dutch investigators revealed that 33% of the statin users reported that they suffered from myopathy.

Paper 134:
Statins increase the risk of muscle disease by 36% in diabetics

Koro CE et al The risk of myopathy associated with thiazolidinediones and statins in patients with type 2 diabetes: a nested case-control analysis. *Clinical Therapeutics* 2008 Mar;30(3):535-42

Dr Carol Koro, an epidemiologist, investigated the association of statins and various antidiabetic drugs with the risk of myopathy (muscle disease) in patients with type two diabetes. The study included 3,696 patients with myopathy who were matched with 21,871 controls.

- Dr Koro found that, compared with patients who did not use either statins nor antidiabetic drugs, those who used statins had a 36% increased risk of muscle disease.

Paper 135:
Muscular symptoms are common with statin therapy

Bruckert E et al Mild to moderate muscular symptoms with high-dosage statin therapy in hyperlipidemic patients—the PRIMO study. *Cardiovascular Drugs and Therapy* 2005 Dec;19(6):403-14

The lead author of the study was Professor Eric Bruckert. He is Professor of Endocrinology and Director of Endocrinology-Metabolism and Prevention of Cardiovascular Disease, Pitié-Salpêtrière Hospital, Paris, France. The study, (Prediction of Muscular Risk in Observational conditions, PRIMO), was an observational study of muscular symptoms in 7,924 patients receiving high-dosage statin therapy.

The French investigators observed:

- Overall, muscular symptoms were reported by 832 patients with onset normally about one month following initiation of statin therapy.
- Muscular pain prevented even moderate exertion during everyday activities in 38% patients.
- 4% of patients were confined to bed or unable to work.

Professor Bruckert concludes: "*PRIMO demonstrated that mild to moderate muscular symptoms with high-dosage statin therapy may be more common and exert a greater impact on everyday lives than previously thought*".

Paper 136:
In patients with muscle pain, statin use results in a 39% prevalence of structural muscle damage

Mohaupt MG et al Association between statin-associated myopathy and skeletal muscle damage. *Canadian Medical Association Journal* 2009 Jul 7;181(1-2):E11-8

This study was conducted by Dr Markus Mohaupt, head of the division of hypertension, department of nephrology/hypertension at the University of Bern.

Dr Mohaupt notes that many patients taking statins often complain of muscle pain and weakness and current consensus guidelines support continuation of the statin therapy as long as circulating levels of creatine phosphokinase (high levels are considered a marker of muscle damage) are less than 1950 U/L (10× the upper limit of normal).

The study sought to determine whether statin-associated myopathy (muscle pain) is associated with underlying structural muscle damage and whether the extent of muscle damage is reflected by the level of circulating creatine phosphokinase. The study included 44 patients with clinically diagnosed statin-associated myopathy, of which 29 were currently taking statins and 15 had stopped taking statins.

Dr Mohaupt's study found:

- There was a high prevalence of structural muscle damage in 25 of the 44 patients (39%) who had statin-associated myopathy.
- Only one patient with structural damage had a circulating level of creatine phosphokinase that was elevated more than 1950 U/L.
- Significant muscle damage was observed in 16 of 29 patients currently receiving statins.
- Significant muscle damage was observed in nine of 15 patients who had discontinued statins.
- Of the nine patients with significant muscle damage who had discontinued statins, six had stopped taking stains within 5–20 weeks, and three had stopped between one year and more than five years.

Dr Mohaupt concluded: "Persistent myopathy in patients taking statins reflects structural muscle damage. A lack of elevated levels of circulating creatine phosphokinase does not rule out structural muscle injury".

Paper 137: Statins are associated with an approximate doubling of the risk of muscle disease

Nichols GA et al Does statin therapy initiation increase the risk for myopathy? An observational study of 32,225 diabetic and nondiabetic patients. *Clinical Therapeutics* 2007 Aug;29(8):1761-70

The objective of this Portland based study was to determine the prevalence of myopathy (muscle disease) among subjects with or without diabetes, some of whom received statin treatment. The study included 32,225 subjects who were followed for nine years.

The study ascertained:

- Statins users with diabetes had a 43% increased risk of myopathy compared to nonusers with diabetes.
- Statin users without diabetes had a 143% increased risk of myopathy compared to nonusers without diabetes.

This study reveals that statins are associated with an approximate doubling of the risk of muscle disease.

Paper 138: Statin users suffer from significantly more musculoskeletal pain

Buettner C et al Prevalence of musculoskeletal pain and statin use. *Journal of General Internal Medicine* 2008 Aug;23(8):1182-6

The head researcher of this study was Dr Catherine Buettner. She has been practicing medicine for 15 years and specialises in Internal Medicine.

This study sought to evaluate whether statin use was associated with a higher prevalence of musculoskeletal pain. The study included 3,580 participants, aged 40 or over, without arthritis.

After analysing the data Dr Buettner and her team found:

- Compared to persons who did not use statins, those who used statins had a 50% increased risk for any musculoskeletal pain.
- Compared to persons who did not use statins, those who used statins had a 59% increased risk for lower back pain.
- Compared to persons who did not use statins, those who used statins had a 50% increased risk for lower extremity pain.

Dr Buettner concluded: "*Statin use is significantly associated with greater prevalence of musculoskeletal pain overall, lower extremity pain, and lower back pain*".

Paper 139:
Statins increase the risk of muscle pain by 90%

Parker BA et al The Effect of Statins on Skeletal Muscle Function. *Circulation* 2013 Jan 1;127(1):96-103

This Hartford Hospital study assessed the effects of statins on muscle function. The study included 420 healthy subjects, who had never previously taken statins, who received either 80 mg of atorvastatin or placebo for six months.

The study observed:

- The creatine kinase levels of those who received statins increased by 20.8 U/L. (The appearance of creatine kinase in blood has been generally considered to be an indirect marker of muscle damage.)
- Those who received statins had a 90% increased risk of muscle pain compared to those who received placebo.

Paper 140:
Statins are significantly associated with increased myositis risk

McClure DL et al Statin and statin-fibrate use was significantly associated with increased myositis risk in a managed care population. *Journal of Clinical Epidemiology* 2007 Aug;60(8):812-8

This four-year study quantified the risk of myositis (myositis cases were defined as creatine kinase levels more than 10x upper limit of normal and a myopathy (muscle disease) diagnosis) associated with statin and fibrate drug use within a managed care organization population. The study included 15,033 subjects aged 40-89 years.

The study identified:

- Statin users had a 177% increased risk of myositis compared to nonusers.
- Statin-fibrate combination users had a 806% increased risk of myositis compared to nonusers.

Paper 141:
Statins increase the risk of muscle adverse reactions

El-Salem K et al Prevalence and risk factors of muscle complications secondary to statins. *Muscle and Nerve* 2011 Dec;44(6):877-81

The aim of the study, headed by Professor Khalid El-Salem of Jordan University of Science and Technology, was to investigate the prevalence of muscle complications among patients using statins. The study included 345 patients receiving statins who were compared with an age- and gender-matched control group of 85 nonusers.

- Professor El-Salem's study found that statin users had a 256% increased risk of muscle adverse reactions compared to nonusers.

Paper 142:
Statins increase the risk of chronic muscle diseases by 286%

Sailler L et al Increased exposure to statins in patients developing chronic muscle diseases: a two-year retrospective study. *Annals of the Rheumatic Diseases* 2008 May;67(5):614-9

Myositis means inflammation of the muscles. Polymyositis affects many areas, mainly the larger muscles like those around your shoulders, hips and thighs. When polymyositis develops alongside a skin rash, the condition is called dermatomyositis. Both conditions are autoimmune diseases; which means your immune system attacks your body's own tissues.

Investigators from the Paul Sabatier University in Toulouse evaluated the association between chronic muscle diseases and prior exposure to cholesterol lowering drugs. The study, which lasted for two years, included 37 patients with chronic muscle diseases such as dermatomyositis and polymyositis who were compared to 185 control subjects.

- The Toulouse researchers discovered that those who were exposed to statins had a 286% increased risk of dermatomyositis and polymyositis.

Paper 143:
The use of a statin may be associated with the occurrence of polymyalgia rheumatica

de Jong HJ et al Statin-associated polymyalgia rheumatica. An analysis using WHO global individual case safety database: a case/non-case approach. *PLoS One* 2012;7(7):e41289

Polymyalgia rheumatica is a condition that causes pain, stiffness and inflammation in the muscles around the shoulders, neck and hips.

Dr Hilda de Jong was the lead author in this study. Dr de Jong's PhD was in pharmacoepidemiology from Maastricht University Medical Centre. The objective of the study was to assess whether there is an association between statin use and the occurrence of polymyalgia rheumatica in the spontaneous reporting database of the World Health Organisation (WHO). The study was conducted on a case/non-case basis on individual case safety reports in the WHO global individual case safety reports database (VigiBase). Case reports containing the adverse event term polymyalgia rheumatica were defined as cases. Non-cases were all case reports containing other adverse event terms. In VigiBase, Dr de Jong identified 327 reports of polymyalgia rheumatica (cases) that were matched with 1,635 reports of other adverse drug reactions.

- The study found that statins were more often reported, by 1,321%, in patients with polymyalgia rheumatica in comparison with patients who had experienced other adverse drug reactions.

Dr de Jong concluded: "*The results of this study lends support to previous anecdotal case reports in the literature suggesting that the use of a statin may be associated with the occurrence of polymyalgia rheumatica*".

Paper 144: Podiatrist sees an increasing number of mainly female patients are being diagnosed with polymyalgia rheumatic. In every case the patient is taking statins

Turnbull PA Management of polymyalgia rheumatic. *British Medical Journal* 2010;340:c620

Pat Turnbull a podiatrist from Cheshire in the UK made the following observations regarding statins and polymyalgia rheumatica: "*As a Podiatrist, I am seeing an increasing number of mainly female patients being diagnosed with polymyalgia rheumatica, who are being treated with prednisolone. In every case thus far the patient is taking statins often in high doses*".

Paper 145:
Statins trigger latent neuromuscular disorders

Tsivgoulis G et al Presymptomatic neuromuscular disorders disclosed following statin treatment. *Archives of Internal Medicine* 2006 Jul 24;166(14):1519-24

This paper, published in the prestigious *Archives of Internal Medicine,* describes four cases of how statins may trigger underlying neuromuscular diseases.

Case 1

- A 48-year-old man was started on pravastatin.
- Three months later, he complained of general fatigue, muscular aches and stiffness.
- His creatine kinase levels were elevated.
- Discontinuation of pravastatin treatment resulted in mild symptom improvement and a moderate fall in creatine kinase levels.
- Examination and tests revealed that pravastatin had triggered myotonic dystrophy. (Myotonic dystrophy is characterized by progressive muscle wasting and weakness. People with this disorder often have prolonged muscle contractions (myotonia) and are not able to relax certain muscles after use. For example, a person may have difficulty releasing their grip on a doorknob or handle. Also, affected people may have slurred speech or temporary locking of their jaw, cataracts and abnormalities in heartbeat and, in men, hormonal changes that may lead to early balding and infertility.)

Case 2

- A 62-year-old man had been given simvastatin for three years.
- He had been experiencing symptoms of fatigue for two years.
- He had elevated creatine kinase levels.
- Despite discontinuing simvastatin his creatine kinase levels remained elevated.
- Examination and tests revealed that simvastatin had triggered McArdle's disease. (Patients with McArdle's disease have an enzyme deficiency (myophosphorylase) which renders them

unable to release glucose from glycogen in muscle. This makes patients susceptible to muscle weakness, and fatigue and muscle cramps after exercise. Myoglobinuria (dark urine which indicates rhabdomyolysis or muscle destruction) occurs in about one third of patients with McArdle's disease following intense exercise.)

Case 3

- A 51-year-old man who had been taking atorvastatin for 18 months was hospitalised for rhabdomyolysis.
- Tests revealed he had elevated creatine kinase levels.
- He stopped atorvastatin and his symptoms improved over the next two months, but his creatine kinase levels remained elevated.
- Three months after discontinuation of statin treatment, he still reported exercise intolerance and muscle fatigue.
- Examination and tests revealed that atorvastatin had triggered mitochondrial myopathy. (Mitochondrial myopathy is a disease caused by damage to the mitochondria—small, energy-producing structures that serve as the cells' "power plants". Symptoms include muscle weakness or exercise intolerance, heart failure or rhythm disturbances, dementia, movement disorders, stroke-like episodes, deafness, blindness, droopy eyelids, limited mobility of the eyes, vomiting, and seizures.)

Case 4

- A 58-year-old man had been taking pravastatin 20 mg per day for six months.
- This was increased to 40 mg per day and shortly afterwards he experienced muscle twitching, frequent muscle cramps, and difficulty in climbing stairs.
- His creatine kinase levels were significantly elevated.
- Discontinuation of pravastatin was associated with mild improvement.
- Four months later, examination and tests revealed that pravastatin had triggered Kennedy's disease. (Kennedy's disease is a motor neuron disease that affects males. It is one of a group of disorders called *spinal muscular atrophy*. Early

> symptoms include tremor of the outstretched hands, muscle cramps with exertion, and fasciculation's (fleeting muscle twitches visible under the skin.) Eventually, individuals develop limb weakness which usually begins in the pelvic or shoulder regions. Weakness of the facial and tongue muscles may occur later in the course of the disease and often leads to dysphagia (difficulty in swallowing), dysarthria (slurring of speech), and recurrent aspiration pneumonia. Some individuals develop gynecomastia (excessive enlargement of male breasts) and low sperm count or infertility. Others develop diabetes.

These cases illustrate that statins may trigger symptoms in patients with a latent neuromuscular disease. These symptoms may have never been triggered if the patients had not taken the statins.

Paper 146: Statins induce partial paralysis in patients with neurological diseases

Dobkin BH Underappreciated statin-induced myopathic weakness causes disability. *Neurorehabilitation and Neural Repair* 2005 Sep;19(3):259-63

Dr Bruce Dobkin, a neurologist from the University of California Los Angeles, conducted a study on the effects of statins on the strength in patients with stroke or other neurologic diseases. The study included eight patients that had had a stroke affecting one side, and ten patients with other neurologic diseases who developed difficulty in walking by three to 12 months after starting statins. All patients had started taking statins three to 12 months earlier.

- Examination revealed the patients had paresis (partial paralysis).
- They stood up with difficulty, walked with difficulty and had imbalance on turns.
- No improvement in strength or mobility was found six weeks after initiating resistance exercises.
- Statins were stopped.
- By three months off statin, all patients recovered their normal strength. Walking improved, and they arose from a chair without pushing off with their arms.

Dr Dobkin concludes that statin-induced muscle weakness: *"may be underappreciated"*.

Paper 147:
Statins unmask McArdle's disease

Livingstone C et al McArdle's disease diagnosed following statin-induced myositis. *Annals of Clinical Biochemistry* 2004 Jul;41(Pt 4):338-40

This paper, authored by Dr Callum Livingstone of the Royal Surrey County Hospital, describes the case of a man where statin use induced myositis and led to a diagnosis of McArdle's disease. McArdle's disease is the inability to break down glycogen. Glycogen is an important source of energy that is stored in all tissues, but especially in the muscles and liver. Symptoms include burgundy-coloured urine, fatigue, exercise intolerance, poor stamina, muscle cramps, muscle pain, muscle stiffness and muscle weakness.

- A 69-year-old man taking statins had an episode of myositis (inflammation of the muscles) and was diagnosed with McArdle's disease.
- This case shows how statin use may "unmask" previously clinically silent or clinically tolerated conditions, such as McArdle disease.

Dr Livingstone concluded: *"In patients who develop a raised plasma creatine kinase level or muscular symptoms during lipid-lowering (statin) therapy, the clinician should be alert to the possibility of an underlying myopathy"*.

Paper 148:
Polymyositis may be induced by statins and fenofibrates

Fauchais AL et al Polymyositis induced or associated with lipid-lowering drugs: five cases. *Revue de Medecine Interne* 2004 Apr;25(4):294-8

In this paper, Professor Anne-Laure Fauchais from the Limoges University Hospital describes five patients who developed polymyositis due to cholesterol lowering drugs. (Polymyositis is an inflammatory disease (of many muscles) that leads to muscle weakness, swelling (inflammation), tenderness, and damage.)

- All five patients with polymyositis had been taking cholesterol lowering drugs (four with statins, one with fenofibrates).
- All had proximal muscular weakness (shoulders, hips etc) and increased muscle enzyme levels.
- One patient had antisynthetase syndrome (an autoimmune disease affecting the muscles, lungs and joints).
- Another patient had hard skinned swollen hands.
- Four patients were tested positive for antinuclear antibodies (suggesting they had an autoimmune disease).
- Muscle biopsies in four patients revealed polymyositis.
- All patients discontinued their statins and fenofibrates.
- Three patients showed partial clinical improvement.

Professor Fauchais concluded: *"Muscular symptoms in patients with cholesterol lowering drugs treatment (statins and fenofibrates) could be the first symptom of polymyositis".*

Paper 149:
Polymyositis linked with statins

Takagi A et al Pravastatin-associated polymyositis, a case report *Rinsho Shinkeigaku* 2004 Jan;44(1):25-7

This paper describes the case of a man who developed polymyositis after starting pravastatin treatment.

- A 69-year-old man complained of general muscle pain, joint pain and muscle weakness in two weeks after he started to take 10 mg per day pravastatin.
- Investigations revealed he had elevated levels of creatine kinase and muscle inflammation.
- He tested positive for antinuclear antibodies. (Antinuclear antibodies are substances produced by the immune system that attack the body's own tissues.)
- He stopped taking pravastatin and was given anti-inflammatory drugs.
- His symptoms as well as creatine kinase levels improved.
- Polymyositis was diagnosed.
- He restarted statin treatment with atorvastatin and had similar symptoms.

Paper 150:
Report highlights the connection between statin treatment and considerable muscular weakness

Thual N et al Fluvastatin-induced dermatomyositis.
Annales de Dermatologie et de Venereologie
2005 Dec;132(12 Pt 1):996-9

This report from Caen University Hospital depicts a case of dermatomyositis occurring after fluvastatin intake. (Dermatomyositis is a muscle disease characterized by inflammation and a skin rash.)

- A 76-year-old male patient sought medical attention for a skin rash and considerable muscular weakness present for one month.
- Two months earlier, fluvastatin had been prescribed.
- Creatine phosphokinase levels were elevated.
- Dermatomyositis was diagnosed.
- All clinical and laboratory abnormalities diminished spontaneously within one month of the final intake of fluvastatin.

Paper 151:
Statins and focal myositis

Asbach P et al Statin-associated focal myositis.
International Journal of Cardiology
2009 Mar 20;133(1):e33-4

This paper, published in *The International Journal of Cardiology* describes the case of a man who had muscle damage to his hip while on statin therapy.

- A man on statin therapy was admitted to hospital with hip symptoms.
- He was examined by magnetic resonance imaging. (Magnetic resonance imaging is a medical imaging technique used to visualize internal structures of the body in detail and can create more detailed images of the human body than possible with X-rays.)
- This revealed focal myositis in his hip muscle. (Focal myositis is an inflammatory pseudotumor of skeletal muscle.)
- The damage to his hip was attributed to his statin intake.

Paper 152:
Muscle disease associated with statin therapy

Needham M et al Progressive myopathy with up-regulation of MHC-I associated with statin therapy. *Neuromuscular Disorders* 2007 Feb;17(2):194-200

Dr Merrilee Needham and her team from the University of Western Australia investigated the phenomenon whereby statins induce muscle damage, which persists or even worsens after stopping the drug. The study included eight patients who continued to display muscle damage despite stopping the statins.

The Australian researchers found:

- Examination revealed all patients had necrosis (death) of some of their muscle cells, but only three showed signs of inflammation.
- All patients had elevated levels of major histocompatibility complex-I even in non-necrotic muscle cells. (Major histocompatibility complex-I is a cell surface molecule that interacts with white blood cells to destroy diseased cells.)
- Progressive improvement occurred after commencement of immunosuppressive drugs. (Drugs that inhibit the immune system.)

The elevated major histocompatibility complex-I and improvement with immunosuppressive drugs suggests that statins caused abnormal activity in the patients' immune system, which resulted in the immune system to start attacking the muscle cells.

Dr Needham concludes: "*These observations suggest that statins may initiate an immune-mediated myopathy (muscle disease) that persists after withdrawal of the drug*".

Paper 153:
Statin use may provoke an immune reaction that leads to destruction of muscle fibres

Grable-Esposito P et al Immune-mediated necrotizing myopathy associated with statins. *Muscle and Nerve* 2010 Feb;41(2):185-90

This study, based at the world renowned Harvard Medical School, investigated the association between statin use and immune-mediated necrotizing myopathy. (Immune-mediated diseases are conditions which result from abnormal activity of the body's immune system where the immune system may overreact or start attacking the body.)

Necrotizing myopathy is a disorder in which the muscle fibres suffer destruction (necrosis). The study included 25 patients, who received statins for an average of three years, who met the following criteria:

- o Muscle weakness occurring during or after treatment with statins.
- o Elevated creatine kinase levels.
- o Persistence of muscle weakness and elevated creatine kinase levels despite discontinuation of the statin.
- o Improvement with immunosuppressive agents. (Immunosuppressive agents are drugs that inhibit or prevent activity of the immune system.)
- o A muscle biopsy showing necrotizing myopathy without significant inflammation.

The study found:

- 16 patients developed muscle weakness while on statins and nine patients developed muscle weakness following discontinuation of the medication.
- When comparing patients with statin exposure to those without, 82% of patients with necrotizing myopathy had statin exposure.
- Of the 25 patients, 24 required more than one immunosuppressive agent.
- 15 patients relapsed after being tapered off immunosuppressive therapy.

The Harvard study shows that statin use may provoke an immune reaction that leads to destruction of muscle fibres. This destruction may develop while taking statins or occur after discontinuing statins and required aggressive treatment with immunosuppressive therapy to be controlled.

Paper 154:
Statin use is associated with necrotizing myopathy

Khattri S Statin-Associated Necrotizing Myopathy in an Older Woman. *Journal of Musculoskeletal Medicine* Vol. 29 No. 4: 112-113: 2012

This case report, from the Albert Einstein College of Medicine in New York, describes the case of a woman who developed necrotizing myopathy due to statin therapy.

- An 81-year-old woman was admitted to the hospital with progressive shortness of breath and generalized weakness that had started three weeks earlier.
- The patient had been taking simvastatin, 40 mg per day, for the previous 11 years.
- Blood tests revealed elevated levels of:
- Creatine phosphokinase 3510 U/L (normal range, 20 to 200 U/L).
- Aspartate aminotransferase 205 U/L (normal range, 9 to 36 U/L).
- Alanine aminotransferase 335 U/L (normal range, 5 to 40 U/L).
- Urine myoglobin 8,620 ng/mL (normal range, 0 to 49 ng/mL).
- Lactate dehydrogenase 947 U/L (normal range, 110 to 210 U/L).
- Examination found she was breathing rapidly, had an elevated heart rate, impaired lung function and poor muscle strength.
- She was given steroid treatment.
- Tests revealed she had muscle damage and a muscle biopsy showed features consistent with necrotizing myopathy without significant inflammation.
- She was diagnosed with statin-induced necrotizing myopathy.
- Simvastatin was discontinued.
- Her creatine phosphokinase, aspartate aminotransferase, alanine aminotransferase, urine myoglobin and actate dehydrogenase levels normalised and she was discharged.

This case reveals that statin use may be associated with necrotizing myopathy.

Paper 155:
Muscle complaints associated with statins

Soininen K et al Muscle symptoms associated with statins: a series of twenty patients. *Basic and Clinical Pharmacology and Toxicology* 2006 Jan;98(1):51-4

Muscle disease (myopathy) is usually defined as pain and/or weakness in skeletal muscles and creatine kinase levels higher than ten times the upper limit of the normal range (5 – 130 U/L). The presence of normal or only slightly elevated creatine kinase levels is often used as an argument that it is not statins that have caused myopathy in patients with muscle complaints during statin therapy.

The aim of this study, headed by expert in internal medicine Dr Kari Soininen, was to examine the creatine kinase levels of patients with muscle complaints while on statin therapy. The study included 20 patients who reported muscle complaints that limited daily functioning during statin use. 18 patients had their creatine kinase levels measured.

This Finnish study revealed:

- Of the 18 patients that had their creatine kinase levels measured:
    - Seven had a major increase in levels.
    - Six had a minor increase in levels.
    - Five had normal levels.
- All patients muscle complaints resolved after discontinuation of statins.

Dr Soininen concluded: *"This case series confirms previous studies showing that statins may cause muscle complaints that limit daily activities, without causing a marked creatine kinase elevation"*.

Paper 156:
Statin-associated muscle disease with normal creatine kinase levels

Trøseid M et al Statin-associated myopathy with normal creatine kinase levels. Case report from a Norwegian family. *Acta Pathologica, Microbiologica, et Immunologica Scandinavica* 2005 Sep;113(9):635-7

This paper, authored by Dr Marius Trøseid of the Akershus University Hospital in Norway, describes four members of the same family who developed muscle disease after starting statin therapy.

- Four memebers of a family, developed statin-associated muscle symptoms although they had normal creatine kinase levels.
- In two out of the four patients (mother and son), investigations suggested muscle disease, and muscle biopsies showed evidence of mitochondrial damage.

- In a third patient (daughter), investigations revealed evidence of slight muscle disease.
- All four patients discontinued the statins.
- The symptoms in all four patients diminished after discontinuation of the statin drugs.

Paper 157:
Statins and muscle damage

Phillips PS et al Statin-associated myopathy with normal creatine kinase levels. *Annals of Internal Medicine* 2002 Oct 1;137(7):581-5

Muscle damage is associated with high creatine kinase levels.

This study investigated if statins cause muscle damage despite patients having normal creatine kinase levels. The study included four patients with muscle symptoms that developed during statin therapy and reversed during placebo use. The study measured:

- o Patients' ability to identify blinded statin therapy from placebo.
- o Muscle strength and functional capacity.

The observations on the four patients revealed:

- All four patients repeatedly distinguished blinded statin therapy from placebo.
- Strength testing confirmed muscle weakness during statin therapy that reversed during placebo use.
- Muscle biopsies showed evidence of mitochondrial dysfunction which reversed in the three patients who had repeated biopsy when they were not receiving statins.
- Creatine kinase levels were normal in all four patients despite the presence of significant muscle damage.

Statins were found to cause muscle damage in patients despite normal creatine kinase levels.

Paper 158:
Simvastatin induced muscle pain

Cooper JM et al Neuroleptic malignant syndrome or a statin drug reaction? A case report. *Clinical Neuropharmacology* 2009 Nov-Dec;32(6):348-9

This Australian paper reports the case of a woman who developed muscle pain while on statin treatment.

- A 60-year-old woman was admitted to hospital with delirium, fever, marked limb rigidity and elevated creatinine kinase level.
- She was diagnosed with neuroleptic malignant syndrome, and was successfully treated with medication. (Neuroleptic malignant syndrome is a life-threatening neurological disorder most often caused by an adverse reaction to neuroleptic or antipsychotic drugs. It generally presents with muscle rigidity, fever, fainting and cognitive changes such as delirium, and is proven on raised levels of creatine phosphokinase.)
- Eight years later, she is again admitted to hospital with symptoms suggesting recurrence of neuroleptic malignant syndrome including elevated creatine phosphokinase levels and muscle pain, but without limb rigidity.
- The patient was taking simvastatin and antibiotics.
- She stopped taking simvastatin.
- There was a rapid decrease in creatine phosphokinase levels and resolution of symptoms.

Discontinuation of simvastatin led to cessation of muscle pain and other symptoms, which superficially resembled neuroleptic malignant syndrome.

This case reveals that statin treatment may result in elevated creatine phosphokinase levels, muscle pain and other symptoms that may be confused with neuroleptic malignant syndrome.

Paper 159:
Muscle disease is a dangerous side-effect of statin drugs

Edholm B Statin-induced dysphagia. *Ugeskrift for Laeger* 2010 Feb 15;172(7):544-5

Dysphagia is the medical term for swallowing difficulties.

This paper from the Slagelse Hospital reports of a man who developed dysphagia and muscle fatigue after statin therapy.

- A 68-year-old man was referred to hospital with progressive dysphagia.

- The patient further developed muscle fatigue (it was difficult for him to lift his arms above his head) and additional signs of myopathy (muscle disease) such as high levels of creatine kinase.
- The dysphagia was diagnosed as a late-onset side-effect of statin therapy.
- He stopped taking statins and 14 days later, the power to his arms returned, his swallowing function was significantly better and his creatine kinase levels normalised.

The author of the paper, Bjarke Edholm (a specialist in Ear, nose and throat) from the Slagelse Hospital in Denmark, concluded: "*As an increasing number of patients are being treated with lipid-lowering drugs (statins), it is important to recall that myopathy is a dangerous side-effect which may have either quick or delayed onset, and that dysphagia can be the initial symptom*".

Paper 160:
Sporadic rippling muscle disease unmasked by simvastatin

Baker SK et al Sporadic rippling muscle disease unmasked by simvastatin. *Muscle and Nerve* 2006 Oct;34(4):478-81

This case report describes a man who developed rippling muscle disease after starting simvastatin. Rippling muscle disease is characterized by painful muscle stiffness involving skeletal muscle contractions which produces a visible rippling effect.

- A 53-year-old-man developed rippling muscle disease two months after starting simvastatin.
- He experienced stiffness, myalgias (muscle pains), and classic rippling, which was confirmed on clinical examination.
- Discontinuation of the statin improved his symptoms.
- Simvastatin therapy was resumed and resulted in a prompt and severe return of his symptoms.

Paper 161:
Statins may cause permanent bladder muscle damage

Yokoyama T et al Statin-Associated Underactive Bladder. *Lower urinary tract symptoms* May 2014 Volume 6, Issue 2, pages 124–125

Dr Teruhiko Yokoyama reports the case of a woman in which statin use may have caused bladder muscle damage resulting in underactive bladder with permanent urinary retention.

- A 69 year-old woman started taking statins.
- Two months later, she sought medical attention for urinary retention and thigh and calf muscle pain.
- She discontinued the statins and reported modest improvement in her symptoms.
- Her medical treatment consisted of clean intermittent catheterization (insertion of a small tube into the urethra) four times a day to drain her urine.
- However, 36 months later, she still required catheterization on a daily basis.

Dr Yokoyama concluded: *"The findings of this case support the potential risk of permanent bladder smooth muscle damage due to statin that can induce retention and underactive bladder"*.

Paper 162:
Muscular Side Effects of Statins

Sinzinger H et al Muscular Side Effects of Statins.
Journal of Cardiovascular Pharmacology August 2002 –
Volume 40 – Issue 2 – pp 163-171

Dr Helmut Sinzinger from the University of Vienna reviewed the scientific literature concerning the muscular side effects of statins.

His review found:

- The side-effects of statins may be by far more prevalent than so far suspected.
- Strict adherence to the measures of life-style change and performance of regular exercise can even further worsen significantly these side effects.
- More and more subtypes of muscle damage are been identified.

The data from this review paper reveals that the side effects of statins are under-reported (especially muscle problems).

The studies in this chapter confirm that statins cause widespread damage to the muscles.

- In many studies, over a quarter of the participants (sometimes a much larger percentage) reported statin induced muscle problems.
- The statin associated muscle disease was widespread over many areas of the body including the: Shoulder, neck, back, leg, hip and in multiple areas concurrently.
- Statin users suffered from muscular weakness, joint pain and cramps.
- Walking and balance problems, and sometimes partial paralysis were experienced by those prescribed statins.
- The muscle damage is so severe in some patients taking statins that cell death occurred.
- Statins may elevate levels of liver enzymes (indicating muscle damage) and cause mitochondrial damage.
- Autoimmune reactions have been induced by statins where the body attacks and destroys its own tissue.
- Muscle adverse side effects (and other adverse side effects) are under-reported.

Professor Eric Bruckert commented *(see paper 135)*: "*Mild to moderate muscular symptoms with statin therapy may be more common and exert a greater impact on everyday lives than previously thought*".

Chapter 6

Low thyroid, Rhabdomyolysis and multiorgan failure

This chapter touches on the dangers of prescribing statins to people with an under-active thyroid, but focuses mainly on rhabdomyolysis, the most life threatening form of statin induced muscle disease.

Paper 163:
Analysis of 119 statin randomized controlled trials find that statins users have a 59% increased risk of rhabdomyolysis
McClure DL et al Systematic review and meta-analysis of clinically relevant adverse events from HMG CoA reductase inhibitor trials worldwide from 1982 to present. *Pharmacoepidemiology and Drug Safety* 2007 Feb;16(2):132-43

Rhabdomyolysis is the breakdown of muscle tissue that leads to the release of muscle fibre contents (such as the protein myoglobin) into the blood. These substances are harmful to the kidney and may cause kidney failure.

The objective of this analysis, led by Clinical Epidemiologist Dr David McClure, was to determine the association of adverse events from a systematic review and meta-analysis of statin randomized controlled trials. The analysis included over 86,000 participants from 119 studies.

Regarding rhabdomyolysis Dr McClure found:

- Statin users had a 59% increased risk of rhabdomyolysis (the breakdown of muscle fibres that leads to the release of muscle fibre contents into the bloodstream and may cause kidney damage) compared to nonusers.

Paper 164:
Doctor says patients with low thyroid must not use statins

Tokinaga K et al HMG-CoA reductase inhibitors (statins) might cause high elevations of creatine phosphokinase (CK) in patients with unnoticed hypothyroidism. *Endocrine Journal* 2006 Jun;53(3):401-5

Hypothyroidism (underactive thyroid gland) is the term used to describe a condition in which there is a reduced level of thyroid hormone (thyroxine) in the body. This can cause various symptoms, the most common being: tiredness, weight gain, constipation, aches, dry skin, lifeless hair and feeling cold.

This study, conducted by Dr Kotaro Tokinaga and his team of researchers from Matsudo City Hospital, investigated the effects of statins in patients with unnoticed hypothyroidism. The study included 77 patients with hypothyroidism of which nine patients accidentally received statins without diagnosis of hypothyroidism.

The study observed:

- In the patients accidentally receiving statins levels of creatine kinase were 223% higher than those in patients not receiving statins. (When creatine kinase levels are high, it usually means there has been damage or stress to muscle tissue, the heart, or the brain.)
- Patients with high creatine kinase levels (over 1000 U/L) were five times more frequent in patients accidentally receiving statins than in those not receiving statins.

Dr Tokinaga concludes: *"The present study confirms that statins enhances levels of creatine kinase in patients with hypothyroidism. We must not begin and continue to use these drugs without checking the possibility of hypothyroidism... (statins) might be a risk factor for severe myopathy and rhabdomyolysis in patients with hypothyroidism".*

Paper 165:
Simvastatin-induced compartment syndrome

Ramdass MJ et al Simvastatin-induced bilateral leg compartment syndrome and myonecrosis associated with hypothyroidism. *Postgraduate Medical Journal* 2007 Mar;83(977):152-3

Compartment syndrome is a painful and potentially serious condition caused by bleeding or swelling within an enclosed bundle of muscles (a muscle 'compartment'). Acute compartment syndrome must be treated in hospital using a surgical procedure called an emergency fasciotomy. The doctor will make an incision to cut open the skin and fascia surrounding the muscles, to immediately relieve the pressure inside the muscle compartment and prevent permanent tissue damage. The wound will be closed 48-72 hours later.

This paper, authored by vascular surgeon Dr Michael Ramdass, reports the case of a hypothyroid man who developed compartment syndrome in both legs after starting statins.

- A 54-year-old hypothyroid man started to take simvastatin.
- After one month, he developed generalised muscle pains and was unable to walk and had intense pain in both legs.
- Examination revealed both legs were tense, swollen and tender.
- He stopped taking simvastatin.
- Urgent fasciotomies were performed and the patient made a recovery.

Dr Ramdass concluded: *"It is likely that this complication will be seen more often with the increased worldwide use of this drug"*.

Paper 166: Rhabdomyolysis due to the additive effect of statins and hypothyroidism

Yeter E et al Rhabdomyolysis due to the additive effect of statin therapy and hypothyroidism: a case report. *Journal of Medical Case Reports* 2007 Nov 10;1:130

This Turkish paper describes a case of rhabdomyolysis due to atorvastatin in a patient without any precipitating factors other than hypothyroidism.

- Two weeks after starting to take atorvastatin, a 56-year-old man was admitted to hospital with complaints of severe muscle pain and proximal muscle weakness of the extremities, with difficulty in exercise and climbing stairs.
- Physical examination revealed he had puffiness around his eyes, lip swelling and mild goitre. All his limbs were swollen and he had pitting edema.

- His levels of alanine transaminase, aspartate aminotransferase and creatine kinase were elevated.
- Thyroid function tests confirmed the diagnosis of hypothyroidism.
- The diagnosis was rhabdomyolysis secondary to the additive effect of hypothyroidism and atorvastatin.
- Atorvastatin was stopped.
- His symptoms progressively improved in a few days.
- On discharge, two week after admission, his alanine transaminase, aspartate aminotransferase and creatine kinase levels had decreased.
- His thyroid stimulating hormone level was in the normal range after six weeks.

Paper 167:
Statins may cause rhabdomyolysis and kidney failure

Qari FA Severe rhabdomyolysis and acute renal failure secondary to use of simvastatin in undiagnosed hypothyroidism. *Saudi Journal of Kidney Diseases and Transplantation* 2009 Jan;20(1):127-9

Dr Faiza A. Qari, an Associate Professor in the Medical Department at the King Abdul Al Aziz University Hospital, chronicles the account of a woman with undiagnosed hypothyroidism who developed rhabdomyolysis after receiving statin therapy.

- A 52-year-old woman was admitted to a hospital's emergency department with complaints of generalized, dull, and constant muscle pain. She expressed an "inability to put her weight on her feet". These symptoms persisted for three days and were associated with weakness and fatigue.
- 20 days earlier, she had started taking Simvastatin, 80 mg daily.
- Laboratory evaluation revealed creatine kinase levels of 81,660 U/L (normal levels are between 24-195 U/L. High creatine kinase levels indicate muscle damage) and thyroid stimulating hormone levels of 22.7 U/L (normal levels are between .5-3.0. High thyroid stimulating hormone levels indicate hypothyroidism).
- The patient was found to be hypothyroid and was diagnosed to have rhabdomyolysis and kidney failure.

- Simvastatin was discontinued and 15 days after hospitalisation, the laboratory results showed that creatine kinase levels had fallen to 1,865 U/L.
- At the patient's follow-up visit one month after hospitalisation, she continued to report some mild residual weakness.
- At six weeks her creatine kinase levels and thyroid stimulating hormone levels had normalised to 151 U/L and 2.06 U/L respectively.

This case reveals that statins may cause rhabdomyolysis and kidney failure especially in individuals with hypothyroidism.

Paper 168:
Simvastatin can induce rhabdomyolysis and is linked to under active thyroid

Kiernan TJ et al Simvastatin induced rhabdomyolysis and an important clinical link with hypothyroidism. *International Journal of Cardiology* 2007 Jul 31;119(3):374-6

This report by cardiologist Dr Thomas Kiernan details the case of a woman who developed rhabdomyolysis after starting statin treatment.

- An 85-year-old woman with kidney impairment and under active thyroid commenced on simvastatin 80 mg per day.
- Shortly after this she developed severe muscular weakness and laboratory evidence of rhabdomyolysis.
- Despite having hypothyroidism controlled for years with L-thyroxine (100 mcg per day), her biochemistry now reflected a hypothyroid state with inadequate thyroid replacement.
- On discontinuing her simvastatin to treat her rhabdomyolysis, the patient's thyroid state returned to normal within four weeks without any change in L-thyroxine dosage.

This case shows that simvastatin may induce rhabdomyolysis and is linked to under active thyroid.

Paper 169:
Rhabdomyolysis induced by statins

Manoukian AA et al Rhabdomyolysis secondary to lovastatin therapy. *Clinical Chemistry* 1990 Dec;36(12):2145-7

This case report by Dr Anthony Manoukian from the University of Hawaii illustrates how statins may induce rhabdomyolysis.

- A 59-year-old woman was admitted to hospital with a two-day history of shortness of breath and difficulty walking. She had been discharged from hospital two weeks earlier for congestive heart failure and, since discharge, had experienced progressive weight gain and swelling of the feet and ankles such that walking had become difficult.
- For 13 days before admission to hospital she had been taking lovastatin, 20 mg orally twice a day.
- On the second hospital day she complained of profound muscle weakness in her lower extremities which progressed over several hours to include the upper extremities. In addition she could no longer walk because of severe pain.
- Creatine kinase levels increased from 157 U/L two weeks before admission to 176,500 U/L on the twelfth hospital day. (High creatine kinase levels are a marker for rhabdomyolysis.)
- The patient's symptoms and creatine kinase levels resolved after discontinuation of the statin drug.

As well as inhibiting the body from producing cholesterol, statins also repress the production of several other biologically essential compounds such as coenzyme Q10 and heme A, which are important components in the system of mitochondrial energy production.

Mitochondria are known as the powerhouses of the cell. They are tiny cellular organelles that take in nutrients, break them down, and create energy for the cells.

Dr Manoukian concluded: "*We speculate that the rhabdomyolysis was due to mitochondrial damage secondary to inadequate synthesis of coenzyme Q and heme A*".

Paper 170:
Statins with pomegranate juice may increase the risk of rhabdomyolysis

Sorokin AV et al Rhabdomyolysis associated with pomegranate juice consumption. *American Journal of Cardiology* 2006 Sep 1;98(5):705-6

Internist, Dr Alexey Sorokin outlines the case of a man who developed rhabdomyolysis after drinking pomegranate juice while taking statins.

- A 48-year-old man had been taking ezetimibe and rosuvastatin for 17 months.
- Three weeks before admission to hospital, he began drinking pomegranate juice (200 ml twice weekly).
- On admission he had thigh pain and elevated serum creatine kinase level (138,030 U/L, normal is less than 200 U/L) and was diagnosed with rhabdomyolysis.

Dr Sorokin concludes: *"This report suggests that pomegranate juice may increase the risk of rhabdomyolysis during rosuvastatin treatment"*.

Paper 171:
Rhabdomyolysis induced by a single dose of a statin

Jamil S et al Rhabdomyolysis induced by a single dose of a statin. *Heart* 2004 Jan;90(1):e3

Statins have been shown to cause toxic effects on muscles and rhabdomyolysis. In most cases, rhabdomyolysis occurs following the use of these drugs for at least one week.

Researchers from the Chesterfield and North Derbyshire Royal Hospital chronicle a case of rhabdomyolysis after just a single dose of simvastatin.

- A 54-year-old man was admitted to hospital with a one-week history of shortness of breath and was found to have high blood pressure.
- He was treated with various drugs including simvastatin (40 mg/day).
- After one dose of simvastatin he was found to have a raised creatinine kinase concentration of 11,290 μ/l (normal 10-120 μ/l) with a raised urine myoglobin concentration of 46,560 μg/ml (normal 0–50 μg/ml). (Raised levels of creatinine kinase and urine myoglobin are associated with rhabdomyolysis.)
- All his parameters improved when simvastatin treatment was stopped.

This case highlights that rhabdomyolysis may be caused by a reaction to simvastatin.

The UK researchers concluded: *"Clinicians should be aware of this possible complication presenting in the early days of the use of statins"*.

Paper 172: Doctor says that statins cause rhabdomyolysis, which is a dreadful condition for patients

Waness A et al Simvastatin-induced rhabdomyolysis and acute renal injury. *Blood Purification* 2008;26(4):394-8

Dr Abdulkarim Waness (whose research interests include lung and cardiovascular diseases) and his colleagues describe the case of a woman who developed rhabdomyolysis after taking simvastatin.

- A 63-year-old was admitted to hospital in April 2007 with the chief complaint of severe generalized muscle pain.
- She had been taking simvastatin 10 mg daily for the past one year.
- The dose was increased to 40 mg daily, ten days prior to her initial first visit to hospital.
- After a few days, she started experiencing fatigue, malaise, poor appetite and vomiting.
- Subsequently, she developed severe muscle pain in her extremities and abdomen, followed by urine discoloration (red urine noted by relatives) with a low output of urine. At this point she was admitted to hospital.
- On physical examination, the patient was drowsy, had severe muscular tenderness and decreased strength.
- Laboratory evaluation revealed she had high levels of creatine kinase, potassium and phosphate, with low levels of sodium and calcium.
- Based on the examination and laboratory findings, she was diagnosed with rhabdomyolysis complicated by acute kidney injury caused by simvastatin treatment.
- This diagnosis was further confirmed by the elevation noticed in her liver enzymes, a well-known complication of all statins.
- The patient was admitted to the medical ward, simvastatin was stopped and urgent treatment with haemodialysis was started.
- Within ten days of stopping simvastatin, her creatine kinase levels normalised and her potassium, sodium, calcium and phosphate, also progressively improved.
- Her severe muscle pain resolved and she started having better urine output.

- Her kidney function fully recuperated within one month of stopping simvastatin.

Dr Abdulkarim Waness concludes: "*Rhabdomyolysis remains a dreadful condition for both patients and physicians. Indeed, its symptoms of severe myalgia (muscle pain), urine discoloration, decreased urine output, acute renal failure, and other complications are not easily forgotten by any patient who experiences this potentially fatal condition... simvastatin, among other HMG-CoA reductase inhibitors (statins), is known to cause rhabdomyolysis. Physicians should always keep in mind the possibility of this complication occurring*".

Paper 173: Use of statins are a risk factor for the onset of rhabdomyolysis

Ram R et al Rhabdomyolysis induced acute renal failure secondary to statins. *Indian Journal of Nephrology* 2013: 23: 3: 211-213

This paper reports the case of an elderly lady who developed rhabdomyolytic acute kidney failure one week after starting statins.

- A 65-year-old lady with chronic kidney disease was admitted to hospital with complaints of severe generalized muscle pain, difficulty in assuming upright posture from sitting position, and difficulty in walking of one-week duration. She also complained of swelling of feet and face, nausea, loss of appetite and noticed decreased urine output, and reddish discoloration to urine for the last three days.
- A week before admission, she had started atorvastatin 10 mg per day.
- Neurological examination showed 2/5 power in all four limbs, absent deep tendon reflexes, and muscle tenderness.
- Tests showed she had raised urea levels of 192 mg/dL indicating kidney damage (normal levels are 10-20 mg/dL).
- She had low T3 (triiodothyronine) and T4 (thyroxine) levels with high thyroid stimulating hormone levels, and was diagnosed with hypothyroidism.
- The patient was initiated on haemodialysis.

- Muscle pain, reddish discoloration to urine, deterioration of renal function, elevated serum glutamic oxaloacetic transaminase, creatinine kinase, and increased urine myoglobin led to the diagnosis of rhabdomyolysis.
- Atorvastatin was stopped.
- After seven sessions of haemodialysis, the urine output improved and creatine kinase and serum glutamic oxaloacetic transaminase levels returned to normal. She regained power in all limbs. Deep tendon reflexes appeared again.

This case shows that use of statins may be a risk factor for the onset of rhabdomyolysis.

Paper 174: Lovastatin associated with rhabdomyolysis, kidney failure and liver disease

Fernández Zatarain G et al Rhabdomyolysis and acute renal failure associated with lovastatin. *Nephron* 1994;66(4):483-4

Dr Gonzalo Fernández Zatarain from the General Hospital of Castellón outlines the case of a woman who developed rhabdomyolysis, kidney failure and liver disease after starting statins.

- A 65-year-old woman started to take lovastatin at 20 mg per day.
- Two weeks later, she noticed widespread muscle pain, strength loss and dark urine.
- A week later, she sought medical treatment as she was immobile and could not pass urine (anuria).
- Examination and laboratory tests led to a diagnosis of rhabdomyolysis, kidney failure and liver disease.
- She stopped taking lovastatin.
- She started to pass urine after two weeks.
- Her muscular symptoms began to improve after three weeks.
- She was able to get out of bed after four weeks.
- After two months, her kidney function returned.
- She achieved complete recovery after three months.

Dr Fernández Zatarain Concluded: "*This severe rhabdomyolysis case with secondary acute renal failure associated to lovastatin... shows the potential risk during lovastatin use, even at low doses*".

Paper 175: Statin therapy leads to rhabdomyolysis and severe obstructive sleep apnea

Ebben MR et al Severe obstructive sleep apnea after cerivastatin therapy: a case report. *Journal of Clinical Sleep Medicine* 2008 Jun 15;4(3):255-6

This report by Dr Matthew Ebben, who has clinical expertise in sleep apnea, chronicles the case of a woman who developed rhabdomyolysis and severe obstructive sleep apnea while taking statins. (Sleep apnea is a disorder in which you have one or more pauses in breathing or shallow breaths while you sleep. As a result, the quality of your sleep is poor, which makes you tired during the day.)

- An 85-year-old woman sought treatment at a sleep medicine clinic for evaluation for sleep apnea syndrome.
- She complained that after taking statins, approximately five years previously, she began sleeping for 12 hours per night.
- However, even after 12 hours of sleep per night, she suffered from excessive daytime sleepiness and took naps for about two hours each afternoon.
- After initiation of the statin therapy, she also developed symptoms of rhabdomyolysis, which included muscle pain and muscle weakness for which she was subsequently hospitalised.
- After stopping statins, she slowly regained her muscle strength back, but her excessive daytime sleepiness persisted.

Dr Ebben concludes: "*We hypothesize that weakness in the upper airway dilator muscles or the diaphragm due to cerivastatin-induced myopathy (muscle damage) might have been responsible for her severe apnea*".

Paper 176: Risk for fatal statin-induced rhabdomyolysis

Eriksson M et al Risk for fatal statin-induced rhabdomyolysis as a consequence of misinterpretation of 'evidence-based medicine'. *Journal of Internal Medicine* 2005 Mar;257(3):313-4

Researchers from Karolinska University Hospital illustrate the case of an elderly woman who developed rhabdomyolysis and died after taking statins.

- An 80-year-old woman was given 40 mg daily of simvastatin after having a heart attack.
- She was readmitted to hospital six months later because of weakness and severe muscle pain.
- Tests revealed high myoglobin levels indicating she had rhabdomyolysis (Rhabdomyolysisis is the breakdown of muscle fibres. Muscle breakdown causes the release of myoglobin into the bloodstream) and she died of multiple organ insufficiency after a month.

The researchers concluded: *"Our opinion is that 40 mg simvastatin was the causative agent for this severe rhabdomyolysis and death"*.

Paper 177:
Fatal rhabdomyolysis associated with simvastatin

Weise WJ et al Fatal rhabdomyolysis associated with simvastatin in a renal transplant patient. *American Journal of Medicine* 2000 Mar;108(4):351-2

This paper, published in *The American Journal of Medicine,* discusses the case of a woman who died from rhabdomolysis while taking statins.

- A 55-year-old woman was hospitalised in September 1998 for profound weakness and fatigue of two weeks duration.
- She had been taking simvastatin 10 mg per day before receiving a kidney transplant in November 1995.
- Simvastatin was restarted in March 1998 and the dose was increased to 20 mg per day in June 1998.
- An examination found she had severe muscle weakness.
- Laboratory studies showed she had myoglobin in the urine and abnormally high levels of creatine kinase, potassium and phosphate.
- She was diagnosed with simvastatin induced rhabdomolysis.
- The patients muscle weakness continued despite discontinuation of simvastatin.
- She died ten days later.

Paper 178:
Statins trigger rhabdomyolysis

Gama MP et al High doses statins administration causing rhabdomyolysis: case report. *Arquivos Brasileiros de Endocrinologia e Metabologia* 2005 Aug;49(4):604-9

Brazilian researchers outline the case of an elderly woman who died from statin-induced rhabdomyolysis.

- A 71-year-old woman was admitted to the emergency room at hospital after suffering shortness of breath for ten days and worsening muscle pain in the region of the thighs and hips.
- She had initially been taking simvastatin for two years at 20 mg per day. This had been raised to 40 mg per day for six months and then raised again to 80 mg per day for the last 40 days.
- The patient had been referred to a neurologist who diagnosed myositis (inflammation of the muscles).
- She discontinued use of simvastatin, which led to a slight improvement of muscle pain. However, her shortness of breath had worsened which led to her admission to hospital.
- A physical examination of the patient revealed she was in a poor general condition with an abnormally slow heart rate and edema in her lower limbs.
- Tests revealed elevated levels of creatinine, aspartate aminotransferase, and alanine aminotransferase.
- Further tests revealed an enlarged heart and fluid in the lungs.
- She was diagnosed with rhabdomyolysis with kidney failure.
- Despite treatment the patient died.
- A review of the case led to a diagnosis of statin-induced rhabdomyolysis.

Paper 179:
Statins with grapefruit juice can be fatal

Karch AM The grapefruit challenge: the juice inhibits a crucial enzyme, with possibly fatal consequences. *American Journal of Nursing* 2004 Dec;104(12):33-5

This paper describes the case of a man who died after drinking grapefruit juice whilst taking statins.

- A 59-year-old man started to take atorvastatin.
- Eight months later, he was admitted to an emergency department complaining of the sudden onset of muscle pain, fatigue and fever.
- The only major change his lifestyle had been drinking two or three glasses of fresh grapefruit juice every day.

- The man became critically ill as a result of the interaction between grapefruit juice and his cholesterol-lowering medication.
- He was diagnosed with rhabdomyolysis and stopped taking atorvastatin.
- The patient ended up going into kidney failure and ultimately died.

"*The potential of drug interactions with grapefruit juice has been out there a long time, but most people just aren't aware of it,*" says the author of the paper, Amy Karch, a Clinical Associate Professor of Nursing. "*There is so much information bombarding people all the time that a lot of people may have heard this but forgotten it. But the problems can be life-threatening.*"

Paper 180: Statin treatment linked to rhabdomyolysis

Baek SD et al Fatal rhabdomyolysis in a patient with liver cirrhosis after switching from simvastatin to fluvastatin. *Journal of Korean Medical Science* 2011 Dec;26(12):1634-7

This Korean paper chronicles the case of a man with liver cirrhosis who died due to statin-induced rhabdomyolysis complicated by liver failure.

- A 56-year-old man with liver cirrhosis was admitted to hospital in December, 2008 for evaluation of weakness in his lower legs of one-week duration. He first experienced discomfort and myalgia in his lower legs, which worsened over time and made him unable to walk.
- He had been taking simvastatin (20 mg per day) regularly for ten years.
- He was diagnosed with liver cirrhosis one year ago.
- Ten days before admission to hospital he was switched from simvastatin to fluvastatin (20 mg per day) by his doctor, as the patient was concerned about his liver disease.
- The patient had mild tenderness of the lower extremities.
- Laboratory findings included aspartate transaminase 1,303 IU/L (normal is less than 40), alanine transaminase 354 IU/L (normal is less than 40), alkaline phosphatase 145 IU/L (normal is 40 to 120), creatine kinase 36,804 IU/L (normal is

50 to 250 IU/L) and his creatine kinase muscle brain fraction was 157.0 ng/mL (normal is less than 5 ng/mL).

- The patient was diagnosed with fluvastatin-induced rhabdomyolysis and fluvastatin was discontinued.
- He was given intravenous treatment, but despite this his rhabdomyolysis worsened.
- His creatine kinase levels increased to 166,160 IU/L, and kidney failure occurred.
- He underwent continuous kidney replacement therapy on day seven, but his kidney function did not recover and liver function worsened.
- He died due to rhabdomyolysis complicated by liver failure on day 15.

To conclude: This patient was diagnosed with liver cirrhosis nine years after starting simvastatin. He was worried about his liver disease and was switched to fluvastatin by his doctor. Twenty-five days later, he died of rhabdomyolysis complicated by liver failure.

Paper 181:
Statin and NSAID drugs lead to the death of a patient from kidney damage and severe skin lesions

Noordally SO et al A fatal case of cutaneous adverse drug-induced toxic epidermal necrolysis associated with severe rhabdomyolysis. *Annals of Saudi Medicine* 2012 May-Jun;32(3):309-11

Toxic epidermal necrolysis is a life-threatening skin condition that is usually induced by a reaction to medications. Atorvastatin is a recognized cause of rhabdomyolysis (the breakdown of muscle fibres that leads to kidney damage). Naproxen is a widely used nonsteroidal anti-inflammatory (NSAID) drug that is a known cause of skin lesions.

This paper reports a fatal case of drug-induced toxic epidermal necrolysis associated with severe muscle necrosis (death of muscle cells) due to the use of naproxen and a statin.

- A 61-year-old female patient was admitted to hospital with complaints of breathing difficulties, vomiting, and diarrhoea that started two days prior to admission.
- Her medications included atorvastatin 10 mg once daily and naxproxen 500 mg three times a day.

- Acute kidney injury and rhabdomyolysis were present on admission to the hospital.
- She had very high levels of creatine phosphokinase (indicating muscle damage by statins).
- Naproxen treatment had started ten days before admission and had led to the rapid onset of skin lesions.
- The patient rapidly developed multiple organ failure with respiratory failure, and complete skin necrosis (death of skin tissue). Despite treatment she died the following day.

The paper concludes that the patient died of drug induced toxic epidermal necrolysis associated with severe muscle necrosis due to the use of naproxen and statin drugs leading to acute kidney damage and complete skin necrosis.

Paper 182:
Simvastatin implicated in rhabdomyolysis and death

Hare CB et al Simvastatin-nelfinavir interaction implicated in rhabdomyolysis and death. *Clinical Infectious Diseases* 2002 Nov 15;35(10):e111-2

Dr C. Bradley Hare, an Assistant Clinical Professor of Medicine at The University of California San Francisco UCSFT portrays the case of a man with HIV who developed rhabdomyolysis and died after starting statins.

- A 70-year-old man was admitted to hospital after suffering with muscle weakness, muscle pains, and diarrhoea.
- He was HIV infected and his antiretroviral therapy regimen consisted of zidovudine, lamivudine and nelfinavir. This regimen had not been changed in more than two years.
- The patient had been on simvastatin (10 mg per day). Six months before admission, the patient's statins were changed to pravastatin (40 mg per day). Then one month prior to admission, this was changed to simvastatin (80 mg per day).
- Three weeks after the initiation of treatment with the higher simvastatin dosage, the patient noted the development of new worsening muscle weakness, which caused him to fall several times, and an increase in the severity of diarrhoea, which before had only been mild.
- Laboratory tests revealed he had rhabdomyolysis.

- The patient developed worsening kidney failure and oliguria that required haemodialysis. (Oliguria is defined as passing a reduced urine volume. It is a clinical characteristic of acute kidney injury.)
- When he subsequently developed abdominal pain, laboratory findings demonstrated metabolic acidosis (metabolic acidosis occurs when the body produces too much acid, or when the kidneys are not removing enough acid from the body).
- The patient died suddenly, and an autopsy found he had suffered a heart attack.

Paper 183:
Statin use is associated with an 80% higher risk of multiple organ failure in severely injured blunt trauma patients

Neal MD et al Preinjury statin use is associated with a higher risk of multiple organ failure after injury: a propensity score adjusted analysis. *Journal of Trauma* 2009 Sep;67(3):476-82; discussion 482-4

This study, led by Dr Matthew Neal from The University of Pittsburgh Medical Centre, sought to determine the relationship between preinjury statin use and outcome in severely injured blunt trauma patients. (Blunt trauma is a usually serious injury caused by a blunt object or collision with a blunt surface, as in a vehicle accident or fall from a building.) Data was obtained from 295 blunt injured adults with hemorrhagic shock. Patients aged 55 years and older were analysed.

- The study found preinjury statin use was associated with an 80% higher risk of multiple organ failure in severely injured blunt trauma patients.

Paper 184:
Multiorgan failure induced by atorvastatin

Sreenarasimhaiah J et al Multiorgan failure induced by atorvastatin. *American Journal of Medicine* 2002 Sep;113(4):348-9

This Washington University School of Medicine paper illustrates the case of a woman who had multiorgan failure and died after starting statins.

- Eight months before she was hospitalised, a 65-year-old woman started to take atorvastatin.
- She had stopped taking atorvastatin because it caused jaundice.
- However, one month before admission, she restarted the statin and she developed profound weakness in her lower extremities, a decreased urine output and shortness of breath.
- Physical examination in hospital revealed she had jaundice, swelling in the feet and legs, (peripheral oedema), fluid in the lungs (pulmonary oedema) and muscle weakness.
- Investigations found she had elevated levels of creatinine, bilirubin, alanine aminotransferase, aspartate aminotransferase and creatine kinase.
- Laboratory results revealed she had kidney failure, a heart attack, pancreatitis and anaemia.
- Despite stopping atorvastatin and receiving medical support, her mental function deteriorated and she died of multiorgan failure.

Paper 185: Hepatitis, rhabdomyolysis and multiorgan failure resulting from statin use

Rajaram M Hepatitis, rhabdomyolysis and multiorgan failure resulting from statin use. British Medical Journal Case Reports 2009;2009. pii: bcr07.2008.0412

Dr Muthuram Rajaram, from the St Helens and Knowsley Hospitals NHS Trust, describes the case of a woman who developed hepatitis, rhabdomyolysis and multiorgan failure resulting from the use of statins.

- A 77-year-old female patient was admitted to hospital with malaise, anorexia and generally feeling unwell for a week.
- She was taking atorvastatin 80 mg daily.
- The dose of atorvastatin was increased from 40 mg to 80 mg daily approximately six months before admission.
- Examination revealed she was jaundiced.
- Laboratory tests revealed the following abnormalities (normal levels in brackets):
    - o Creatine kinase: 523 iu/l (25–200)
    - o Lactate dehydrogenase: 1241 iu/l (240–525)

- o Total bilirubin: 284 μmol/l (2–22)
- o Alanine transaminase: 2314 iu/l (11–55)
- o γ glutamyl transferase: 132 iu/l (5–50)
- o Aspartate transaminase: 1269 iu/l (12–42)
- o Alkaline phosphatase: 438 iu/l (40–125)
- o Urea: 15.9 mmol/l (3.6–7.3)
- o Creatinine: 290μmol/l (45–110)

- A diagnosis of hepatitis related to statin use with accompanying kidney failure was made.
- The statin was stopped and her liver biochemistry improved.
- However, on the fourth day after admission, her kidney function deteriorated.
- Examination revealed excess fluid around the lungs and abdominal areas.
- The patient was transferred to the intensive care unit and required haemofiltration. (Hemofiltration is a kidney replacement therapy similar to haemodialysis.)
- Despite improvement in her kidney function, the creatine kinase levels continued to rise and peaked at 107,178 iu/l.
- Two weeks after admission to the hospital, the patient died of multiorgan failure.

Dr Rajaram concludes: *"The cause of hepatitis, rhabdomyolysis, and acute renal failure in this patient was the increase in dose of atorvastatin and subsequent elevation of serum atorvastatin concentration. We suggest that the elevation of atorvastatin concentrations resulted in skeletal muscle damage and rhabdomyolysis, as indicated by the elevation of creatine kinase and subsequent deposition of myoglobin in the kidneys, causing acute renal failure as indicated by the elevation of urea and creatinine"*.

The horrific consequences of statin induced rhabdomyolysis are described in this chapter. The dangers of prescribing statins to anyone with an under-active thyroid are also portrayed and the adverse implications of statin elevated enzyme values are illustrated.

- Rhabdomyolysis is a very serious and often fatal repercussion of statin therapy.
- Prescribing statins to patients with an under-active thyroid may increase the risk of rhabdomyolysis.

- Consuming pomegranate juice or grapefruit juice whilst taking statins may also elevate rhabdomyolysis risk.
- Statin induced rhabdomyolysis could result in kidney failure, liver disease, liver cirrhosis, hepatitis, pancreatitis and multiorgan failure.
- Severe muscle weakness and muscle pain are associated with rhabdomyolysis.
- Other conditions can be triggered with statins and rhabdomyolysis such as anorexia, sleep apnea, anaemia, malaise, breathing difficulties, diarrhoea, jaundice, swelling in the feet and legs, fluid in the lungs, metabolic acidosis and heart attack.

I shall leave Dr Abdulkarim Waness to describe rhabdomyolysis: *"Rhabdomyolysis remains a dreadful condition for both patients and physicians. Indeed, its symptoms of severe myalgia (muscle pain), urine discoloration, decreased urine output, acute renal failure, and other complications are not easily forgotten by any patient who experiences this potentially fatal condition"*.

Chapter 7

Statins interfere with liver function

The package insert for statin drugs advises that a liver enzyme test *(see Glossary)* should be perfomed before taking statins. The inserts also recommend: "*Patients are advised to consult their health care professional if they have symptoms that include unusual fatigue, loss of appetite, right upper abdominal discomfort, dark urine or yellowing of the skin or whites of the eyes*".

Data from more than two million 30-84 year-olds from England and Wales identified a 53% increased risk of liver disease in statin users *(see paper 411)*.

This chapter examines more of the scientific evidence to assess the effects of statin toxicity on the liver.

Paper 186:
Statins can cause significant liver toxicity

Ballarè M et al Hepatotoxicity of hydroxy-methyl-glutaryl-coenzyme A reductase inhibitors. *Minerva Gastroenterologica e Dietologica* 1992 Jan-Mar;38(1):41-4

This Italian based study investigated the relationship between statins and liver toxicity. The study included 100 patients taking simvastatin and 90 patients treated with pravastatin who were followed-up for six months.

- The study found that in 5% of simvastatin-treated patients and 4.5% of pravastatin-treated patients significant liver toxicity was observed, which required drug discontinuation.

Paper 187:
Statin users have a 26% increased risk of liver function test abnormalities

de Denus S et al Statins and liver toxicity: a meta-analysis. *Pharmacotherapy* 2004 May;24(5):584-91

Liver function tests measure various chemicals in the blood made by the liver. An abnormal result indicates the presence of liver disease.

The research interests of lead author of this study, Dr Simon de Denus, are mainly in the field of cardiovascular pharmacotherapy. The objective of the study was to assess the risk of liver function test abnormalities with the use of statins. Dr de Denus conducted a search of the scientific literature for published randomised, placebo-controlled statin clinical trials which revealed 13 trials including 49,275 patients.

- This meta-analysis of 13 trials found that statin users had a 26% increased risk of liver function test abnormalities compared to nonusers.

Paper 188: Statins increase the risk of liver damage

Sattam Z et al Comparative Effects of Lovastatin and Simvastatin on Liver Function tests in Hyperlipidaemic Patients. *Medical Journal of Basrah University* Vol: 25, No: 1 2007

Drug-induced liver damage has become an important public health problem, contributing to more than 50% of acute liver failure cases, and there have been observations of a large number of liver failure cases on statin therapy.

In liver function tests, liver damage is confirmed with increased levels of bilirubin and the liver enzymes; Alanine transaminase, aspartate aminotransferase and alkaline phosphatase.

This study measured the effects of statins on liver function tests. The study included:

- 53 patients, aged 35-60 years, took simvastatin therapy. The simvastatin dose ranged from 10 to 20mg a day. Duration of treatment ranged from one month to four years. (Simvastatin group.)
- 42 patients, aged 38-60, took lovastatin therapy. The lovastatin dose ranged from 10 to 20mg a day. Duration of treatment ranged from one month to three years. (Lovastatin group.)
- A control group of 50 subjects, aged 35-58 who did not take statins. (No-statin group.)

The study found:

- The alanine transaminase levels of the lovastatin group were 113% higher than the no-statin group.
- The aspartate aminotransferase levels of the lovastatin group were 90% higher than the no-statin group.
- The alkaline phosphatase levels of the lovastatin group were 11% higher than the no-statin group.
- The bilirubin levels of the lovastatin group were 40% higher than the no-statin group.
- The alanine transaminase levels of the high dose (20 mg a day) lovastatin group were 181% higher than the no-statin group.
- The aspartate aminotransferase levels of the high dose (20 mg a day) lovastatin group were 151% higher than the no-statin group.
- The alkaline phosphatase levels of the high dose (20 mg a day) lovastatin group were 20% higher than the no-statin group.
- The bilirubin levels of the high dose (20 mg a day) lovastatin group were 72% higher than the no-statin group.
- The alanine transaminase levels of the long-term usage (over 12 months) lovastatin group were 333% higher than the no-statin group.
- The aspartate aminotransferase levels of the long-term usage (over 12 months) lovastatin group were 321% higher than the no-statin group.
- The alkaline phosphatase levels of the long-term usage (over 12 months) lovastatin group were 24% higher than the no-statin group.
- The bilirubin levels of the long-term usage (over 12 months) lovastatin group were 145% higher than the no-statin group.
- The alanine transaminase levels of the simvastatin group were 103% higher than the no-statin group.
- The aspartate aminotransferase levels of the simvastatin group were 60% higher than the no-statin group.
- The alkaline phosphatase levels of the simvastatin group were 6% higher than the no-statin group.
- The bilirubin levels of the simvastatin group were 45% higher than the no-statin group.

- The alanine transaminase levels of the high dose (20 mg a day) simvastatin group were 150% higher than the no-statin group.
- The aspartate aminotransferase levels of the high dose (20 mg a day) simvastatin group were 102% higher than the no-statin group.
- The alkaline phosphatase levels of the high dose (20 mg a day) simvastatin group were 3% higher than the no-statin group.
- The bilirubin levels of the high dose (20 mg a day) simvastatin group were 55% higher than the no-statin group.
- The alanine transaminase levels of the long-term usage (over 12 months) simvastatin group were 255% higher than the no-statin group.
- The aspartate aminotransferase levels of the long-term usage (over 12 months) simvastatin group were 240% higher than the no-statin group.
- The alkaline phosphatase levels of the long-term usage (over 12 months) simvastatin group were 3% higher than the no-statin group.
- The bilirubin levels of the long-term usage (over 12 months) simvastatin group were 83% higher than the no-statin group.

The results from this study revealed significant increases of alanine transaminase, aspartate aminotransferase and bilirubin levels in the lovastatin group compared with the control group and significant increases of alanine transaminase and bilirubin in the simvastatin group when compared with the control group.

The study also revealed that the higher the dose of the statin or the longer the dose of the statin generally correlated with increased levels of the liver enzymes.

Paper 189:
Anicteric hepatitis associated with treatment with lovastatin

Bruguera M et al Hepatitis associated with treatment with lovastatin. Presentation of 2 cases. *Gastroenterologia y Hepatologia* 1998 Mar;21(3):127-8

This paper describes two women who developed anicteric hepatitis after starting statin treatment. (Anicteric hepatitis is hepatitis without jaundice.)

- Two women of 57 and 59 years of age were admitted to hospital with anicteric hepatitis.
- They had initiated lovastatin treatment (20 mg per day) nine months ago and three years ago respectively.
- Investigations led to the diagnosis of statin induced anicteric hepatitis in both cases.
- They both discontinued lovastatin.
- Within a few weeks, their conditions resolved.

Paper 190:
Statins and liver damage

Li L et al Drug-Induced Acute Liver Injury Within 12 Hours After Fluvastatin Therapy. *American Journal of Therapeutics* 2014 Jan 21 1536-3686

This paper outlines the case of a man who developed liver damage after starting statins.

- A 52-year-old man suffered liver damage, which appeared 12 hours after beginning treatment with fluvastatin.
- The patient complained of increasing nausea, anorexia, and upper abdominal pain.
- Laboratory tests revealed he had elevated creatine kinase and transaminases (liver enzymes).
- He stopped taking fluvastatin and within three weeks his liver enzymes normalized.

The lead researcher of the paper Dr Li Li from Hebei Medical University concluded: *"When prescribing statins, the possibility of hepatic damage should be taken into account"*.

Paper 191:
Statins involved with development of acute hepatitis

Oteri A et al Reversible acute hepatitis induced by rosuvastatin. *Southern Medical Journal* 2008 Jul;101(7):768

Dr Alessandro Oteri from the University of Milan depicts the case of a man who developed acute hepatitis after treatment with rosuvastatin.

- In January 2007, a 62-year-old man started taking rosuvastatin 10 mg per day.

- Two months later, the patient experienced nausea, asthenia (loss or lack of bodily strength) and jaundice; he was hospitalized with a diagnosis of acute hepatitis.
- Laboratory tests revealed increased aspartate aminotransferase (1430 U/L; normal range 15-45 U/L) and alanine aminotransferase (2,317 U/L; normal range 10-70 U/L).
- He stopped taking rosuvastatin.
- Aspartate aminotransferase and alanine aminotransferase levels decreased to normal values within three weeks, thus suggesting a potential statin drug involvement.

Dr Oteri concludes: *"As drug-induced liver toxicity has a high morbidity and mortality, regular transaminase screening should be performed in patients treated with statins"*.

Paper 192:
Acute hepatitis induced by lovastatin

Grimbert S et al Acute hepatitis induced by HMG-CoA reductase inhibitor, lovastatin. *Digestive Diseases and Sciences* 1994 Sep;39(9):2032-3

The case of an adult who suffered from clinical hepatitis three months after the onset of lovastatin administration is chronicled by Dr Sylvie Grimbert a specialist in Gastroenterology and Hepatology.

The patient suffered:

- Loss of strength and energy.
- Jaundice.
- Increased aminotransferase levels. (Elevated levels of aminotransferase (an enzyme) suggest the existence of medical problems such as viral hepatitis, diabetes, congestive heart failure, liver damage and bile duct problems.)
- Increased alkaline phosphatase levels. (Elevated levels of alkaline phosphatase (an enzyme) indicate the presence of liver disease or bone disorders.)

Examination of the patients liver cells revealed:

- Cell death.
- Blocked bile ducts.
- Increased white blood cell levels. (Elevated white blood cells in the liver, suggest the existence of liver damage.)

Withdrawal of lovastatin was followed by complete normalization of liver tests within two months.

Paper 193:
Acute cholestatic hepatitis linked to atorvastatin

de Castro ML et al Acute cholestatic hepatitis after atorvastatin reintroduction. *Gastroenterologia y Hepatologia* 2006 Jan;29(1):21-4

Cholestasis (cholestatic hepatitis, cholestatic jaundice) is where the normal flow of bile from the liver to the small intestine is interrupted by either a blockage in the duct system or a side effect of medications.

This Spanish paper illustrates the case of a man who developed cholestatic hepatitis while on statins.

- In October 2003, a 72-year-old man was admitted to hospital after suffering for three days with jaundice and dark urine.
- In February 2003 he had started taking 20 mg of atorvastatin daily.
- He stopped atorvastatin three months ago, and restarted at a dose of 40 mg per day a week before his hospitalisation.
- Physical examination revealed jaundiced skin and mucus membrane.
- Laboratory test revealed elevated liver function tests of aspartate aminotransferase, alanine transaminase, gamma-glutamyl transpeptidase and alkaline phosphatase.
- Investigations led to a diagnosis of cholestatic hepatitis.
- He discontinued atorvastatin and his symptoms and laboratory abnormalities normalised.

Paper 194:
Cholestatic jaundice induced by atorvastatin

Minha S et al Cholestatic jaundice induced by atorvastatin: a possible association with antimitochondrial antibodies. *Israel Medical Association Journal* 2009 Jul;11(7):440-1

Dr Saar Minha, an interventional cardiologist, portrays the case of a man who developed cholestatic jaundice while taking atorvastatin.

- A 68-year-old man was admitted to hospital complaining of fever, dark urine and hives (itchy rash).

- He was taking atorvastatin 20 mg per day.
- Physical examination revealed he had jaundice and large areas of hives.
- Abnormal laboratory results included elevated liver function tests with a cholestatic pattern:
    - o total bilirubin 7.4 mg/dl (normal 0.2–1.0 mg/dl)
    - o alkaline phosphatase 555 U/L (normal 39–117 U/L)
    - o alanine aminotransferase 250 U/L (normal 4–41 U/L)
    - o aspartate aminotransferase 50 U/L (normal 5–38 U/L)
    - o lactate dehydrogenase 540 U/L (normal 240–480 U/L)
- A diagnosis of drug-induced liver damage was made.
- The patient stopped taking atorvastatin and he had a rapid biochemical and clinical improvement.
- During the following four weeks the patient was discharged and readmitted twice with similar clinical and laboratory findings.
- A liver biopsy revealed on his next admission revealed severe inflammation.
- Further investigation revealed that between admissions and prior to each recurrent bout of cholestatic hepatitis the patient had renewed his treatment with atorvastatin.
- Complete cessation of atorvastatin was followed by a return to normal values of liver function tests and a complete clinical recovery.

Paper 195:
Lovastatin induces cholestatic jaundice

Spreckelsen U et al Cholestatic jaundice during lovastatin medication. *Deutsche Medizinische Wochenschrift* 1991 May 10;116(19):739-40

This German paper describes the case of a man who developed cholestatic jaundice after starting lovastatin therapy.

- A 48-year-old man started lovastatin therapy at 20 mg per day.
- After two months on the statin drug, cholestatic jaundice developed. His total bilirubin levels were 6.15 mg/dL (normal bilirubin levels are less than 1.5 mg/dL).
- He discontinued lovastatin.
- Within two weeks of discontinuing lovastatin, the jaundice and abnormal biochemical findings resolved.

Paper 196:
Cholestasis can be an adverse effect of lovastatin

Yoshida EM et al Lovastatin and cholestasis. *Canadian Medical Association Journal* 1993 Feb 1;148(3):374

Dr Eric Yoshida, Chairman of the Canadian Liver Foundation Medical Advisory Committee, outlines the case of a man who developed cholestasis after taking lovastatin.

- A 43-year-old man with kidney disease was given lovastatin therapy.
- After two months of therapy, he experienced nausea, vomiting, abdominal pain, and had pale stools.
- Examination revealed he had elevated levels of alkaline phosphatase and gamma-glutamyl transpeptidase which led to a diagnosis of cholestasis.
- He stopped taking lovastatin.
- Two weeks later, his alkaline phosphatase and gamma-glutamyl transpeptidase levels had started to return towards normal levels.

Paper 197:
Acute cholestatic hepatitis induced by statins

Torres M et al Acute cholestatic hepatitis induced by cerivastatin. *Medicina Clinica* 2002 May 18;118(18):717

This case of a man who developed cholestatic hepatitis after starting statin therapy is chronicled by Dr Miguel Torres head of Internal Medicine at Hospital de l'Esperit.

- A 67-year-old man was admitted to hospital with nausea.
- Physical examination showed he had jaundiced skin and mucous membranes.
- Three weeks earlier, he had started statin treatment.
- Laboratory tests revealed he had elevated liver enzymes of aspartate aminotransferase, alanine aminotransferase, gamma-glutamyltransferase and alkaline phosphatase.
- A liver biopsy revealed inflammation.
- A diagnosis of statin induced acute cholestatic hepatitis was made.
- He stopped taking statins.

- One month later, tests revealed normalisation of aspartate aminotransferase, alanine aminotransferase, gamma-glutamyltransferase and alkaline phosphatase levels.

Paper 198:
Atorvastatin can induce cholestasis and bile duct damage

Merli M et al Atorvastatin-induced prolonged cholestasis with bile duct damage. *Clinical Drug Investigation* 2010;30(3):205-9

Investigators from The University of Rome depict the case of a man who developed cholestasis after starting statin treatment.

- A 72–year-old man started taking atorvastatin 20 mg per day.
- He was admitted to hospital 40 days later with jaundice, lack of bodily strength, nausea, vomiting, lack of bile in his faeces and dark urine.
- Laboratory analysis showed a dramatic increase in levels of bilirubin and alkaline phosphatase.
- The analysis also revealed he had elevated levels of aspartate aminotransferase, alanine aminotransferase and gamma-glutamyltransferase.
- Examination revealed an enlarged liver.
- A liver biopsy found inflammation and bile duct damage.
- Atorvastatin induced cholestasis was diagnosed.
- The patient stopped taking atorvastatin.
- His aspartate aminotransferase, alanine aminotransferase gamma-glutamyltransferase and bilirubin levels normalised within five months.
- His alkaline phosphatase took eight months to normalise.

Paper 199:
Autoimmune hepatitis can be triggered by statins

Alla V et al Autoimmune hepatitis triggered by statins. *Journal of Clinical Gastroenterology* 2006 Sep;40(8):757-61

Autoimmune hepatitis is inflammation of the liver that occurs when immune cells mistake the liver's normal cells for harmful invaders and attack them.

The author of the paper, Dr Vamsee Alla, has expertise in hepatitis. Dr Alla illustrates the cases of three patients in whom it is probable that statins initiated the development of autoimmune hepatitis.

- Two men (aged 47 and 51) and one woman (aged 57) developed autoimmune hepatitis after the initiation of statin therapy.
- The woman developed hepatitis due to statins on two separate occasions: the first in 1999, due to simvastatin, and the second in 2001 to 2002, due to atorvastatin, which was severe and persisted even after discontinuing medication.
- In the two men, exposure to statins preceded development of autoimmune hepatitis, which persisted despite discontinuing medications.
- Three similar previously reported cases were noted.

Dr Alla concluded: "*The three cases reported here, and three similar previously reported cases, indicate that severe, persistent autoimmune hepatitis can be triggered by statins*".

Paper 200:
Overlap syndrome of autoimmune hepatitis and primary biliary cirrhosis triggered by fluvastatin

Nakayama S et al Overlap syndrome of autoimmune hepatitis and primary biliary cirrhosis triggered by fluvastatin. *Indian Journal of Gastroenterology* 2011 Mar;30(2):97-9

Primary biliary cirrhosis is a liver disease that damages the small bile ducts in the liver.

Dr Satoshi Nakayama from Mishuku Hospital portrays the case of a man who developed overlap syndrome of autoimmune hepatitis and primary biliary cirrhosis after initiation of statin therapy.

- A 59-year-old man was prescribed fluvastatin 20 mg per day.
- One month later, blood tests showed liver damage that continued one month after discontinuation of fluvastatin.
- Laboratory tests revealed elevated levels of the liver enzymes: aspartate aminotransferase, alanine aminotransferase, gamma glutamyl transferase and alkaline phosphatase.
- These results suggested fluvastatin-induced liver injury.

- In addition, investigations showed evidence of autoimmune liver disease.
- A liver biopsy revealed liver damage, inflammation, cell death and bile duct damage.
- The patient was diagnosed with fluvastatin induced overlap syndrome of autoimmune hepatitis and primary biliary cirrhosis.
- Subsequently, the patient developed jaundice and received treatment.
- Four months later, his liver enzyme levels had returned to normal, but tests found he still had autoimmune liver disease.

Dr Nakayama concluded: "*Autoimmune liver disease should be considered as a possible diagnosis in patients with evidence of prolonged liver damage after discontinuation of statins*".

Paper 201:
Statins increase the risk of gallstone disease

Chiu HF et al Statin use and the risk of gallstone disease: a population-based case-control study. *Expert Opinion on Drug Safety* 2012 May;11(3):369-74

The aim of this study, carried out by Professor Hui-Fen Chiu and colleagues at Kaohsiung Medical University, was to investigate the association between the use of statins and the risk of gallstone disease. The study included 1,014 gallstone disease cases and 1,014 controls aged 50 years or older.

The study found:

- Those who used statins had a 14% increased risk of developing gallstone disease compared to those who did not take statins.
- Those with the highest cumulative statin use had a 30% increased risk of developing gallstone disease compared to those who did not take statins.

The evidence from this chapter confirms that statin drugs confer an increased risk of hepatic (liver) disease.

- Statin induced liver disease may manifest with or without jaundice.
- Auto-immune hepatitis may be triggered by statins which still persists even after discontinuing the statin drug.

- Bile duct damage, inflammation and cellular death in the liver have been found in statin users.
- Symptoms from statin induced liver disease include: Abdominal pain, anorexia, asthenia, hives, jaundice, nausea, and loss of energy and strength.
- Liver function tests revel statin users are more likely to have elevated readings (indicating liver damage).
- Statin users also have an increased risk of gallstone disease.

Dr Malcolm Kendrick, a UK doctor who has specialised in heart disease and is a peer-reviewer for the *British Medical Journal*, comments on the relationship between statins and liver damage: "*Cholesterol drugs, including statins, all interfere with liver function to a greater or lesser degree. Some people have an immediate and severe reaction, in others it is milder. There is some evidence that, over time, liver damage will worsen*".

Chapter 8

Clinicians should be aware of the association of statins with acute pancreatitis

The medical literature contains reports of pancreatitis in patients taking statins. The next 13 papers review this literature to evaluate the increased risk of pancreatitis and the symptoms and adverse health effects that may manifest in patients prescribed statins.

Paper 202:
Statins increase the risk of acute pancreatitis
Lancashire RJ et al Discrepancies between population-based data and adverse reaction reports in assessing drugs as causes of acute pancreatitis. *Aliment Pharmacology and Therapeutics* 2003 Apr 1;17(7):887-93

Pancreatitis is inflammation of the pancreas. There are two types of pancreatitis: acute – when the pancreas is inflamed and causes short-term illness – and chronic – when the pancreas is irreversibly damaged and causes ongoing, long-term illness or bouts of acute symptoms.

Acute pancreatitis can be a life-threatening illness with severe complications. Symptoms come on suddenly or develop over a few days. Symptoms include:

- Severe pain in your upper abdomen.
- Loss of appetite.
- Feeling sick and vomiting.
- Temperature higher than 37.5°C.
- Swollen abdomen.
- Rapid pulse.

If acute pancreatitis is very severe, it may also lead to dehydration and a drop in blood pressure.

If the inflammation is severe or recurrent, the pancreas can be permanently damaged.

Complications of acute pancreatitis can include:

- o Some of the pancreatic tissue dying, which can lead to an abscess.
- o Fluid-filled cysts developing around your pancreas.
- o Bleeding in the pancreas.

Complications of chronic pancreatitis can include the above, as well as:

- o Type 1 diabetes.
- o Increased risk of developing pancreatic cancer.
- o Malnutrition.

This study, headed by data scientist Robert Lancashire, investigated the risk of various types of drugs with pancreatitis. The study included 3,673 patients with acute pancreatitis and around 11,000 controls.

- Regarding statins, the study found those who were prescribed statins had a 10% increased risk of acute pancreatitis compared to those who never used statins.

Paper 203:
Statin use increases the risk of pancreatitis by 41% Singh S et al Statins and pancreatitis: a systematic review of observational studies and spontaneous case reports. *Drug Safety* 2006;29(12):1123-32

This paper from Wake Forest University is an analysis of the controlled observational studies in the scientific literature that assessed the risk of pancreatitis in patients receiving statins.

The analysis found:

- Patients with a past history of exposure to statins had a 41% increased risk of acute pancreatitis compared with nonusers of statins.
- Pancreatitis can occur at both high and low doses of statins.

- Statin-induced pancreatitis can occur at any time but seems to be very uncommon early on and more likely to occur after many months of therapy.

Paper 204:
Statins increase the risk of acute pancreatitis by 44%

Thisted H et al Statins and the risk of acute pancreatitis: a population-based case-control study. *Aliment Pharmacology and Therapeutics* 2006 Jan 1;23(1):185-90

The aim of this Danish study was to examine if statins are associated with risk of acute pancreatitis. The study included 2,576 patients with acute pancreatitis and 25,817 controls from the general population.

- The study revealed that statin users had a 44% increased risk of pancreatitis.

Paper 205:
Atorvastatin-induced acute pancreatitis

Deshpande PR et al Atorvastatin-induced acute pancreatitis. *Journal of Pharmacology and Pharmacotherapeutics* 2011 Jan;2(1):40-2

Dr Prasanna Deshpande from Manipal University reports the case of a statin-induced acute pancreatitis.

- A 53-year-woman was admitted to hospital with complaints of severe abdominal pain and vomiting on the day before admission.
- She had started to take atorvastatin therapy (10 mg/day) about six weeks previously.
- Tests revealed she had pancreatic abnormalities.
- She stopped taking atorvastatin
- After withdrawal of statins the patient recovered.
- Extensive investigations revealed there was no other reason for the acute pancreatitis apart from the statin therapy.
- She was advised not to take atorvastatin.

Dr Deshpande concluded: "*This case further strengthens the fact that statins may cause acute pancreatitis*".

Paper 206: Lovastatin linked to pancreatitis

Pluhar W A Case of possible lovastatin-induced pancreatitis in concomitant Gilbert syndrome. *Wiener Klinische Wochenschrift* 1989 Sep 1;101(16):551-4

This paper outlines the case of a patient who developed pancreatitis after taking a statin drug.

- A 46-year-old male patient with Gilbert's syndrome (a hereditary cause of raised bilirubin and may lead to bouts of jaundice) was prescribed lovastatin 20 mg twice daily.
- After one week, this led to a slight to moderate elevation of amylase (elevated amylase indicates a diseased pancreas) and bilirubin with the occurrence of symptoms attributable to mild pancreatitis.
- These symptoms were sufficiently severe to require discontinuation of the drug.
- Statins were restarted and the pancreatitis recurred.
- The patient discontinued the statins and the symptoms resolved.

Paper 207: Pancreatitis induced by all statins

Singh S et al Recurrent acute pancreatitis possibly induced by atorvastatin and rosuvastatin. Is statin induced pancreatitis a class effect? *Journal of the Pancreas* 2004 Nov 10;5(6):502-4

The head researcher of this paper, Dr Sonal Singh, is a recipient of the prestigious Society of General Internal Medicine Clinician-Investigator award for the mid-Atlantic region and the Bruce Squires Award for the Best Research paper of the year from the Canadian Medical Association Journal.

Dr Singh chronicles the case of a woman who developed pancreatitis after treatment with statins.

- A 77-year-old female was presented to a medical facility with abdominal discomfort, nausea and vomiting for the past few days.
- She had recently been started on rosuvastatin (Crestor) and her dose increased from 10 to 20 mg daily.

- Statin induced pancreatitis was diagnosed and the patient improved with discontinuation of rosuvastatin.
- Her medical history revealed that she had a similar episode of pancreatitis precipitated by atorvastatin (Lipitor) a year ago. A pimply rash and skin inflammation accompanied that episode.
- She was advised to avoid all statins in the future.

Dr Singh concludes: "*The occurrence of pancreatitis with two different statins in the patient argues that statins induced pancreatitis may be a class-effect of statins (side-effect of all statins)*".

Paper 208: Simvastatin associated with pancreatitis

Johnson JL et al A Case of Simvastatin-Associated Pancreatitis and Review of Statin-Associated Pancreatitis. *Pharmacotherapy* Volume: 26 Issue: 3 March 2006 Page(s): 414-422

This paper depicts the case of a middle-aged man who developed pancreatitis after taking statins.

- A 58-year-old man who was hospitalized with idiopathic pancreatitis four months after starting simvastatin therapy.
- He stopped the statins and was discharged from hospital after five days.
- He restarted simvastatin therapy and was again admitted to hospital 16 months later with a second diagnosis of acute pancreatitis.
- He stopped the statins and was discharged from hospital after three days.
- Simvastatin was restarted on discharge, but the patient stopped taking it after experiencing muscle soreness and weakness in his arms.
- He recalled having similar arm pain that preceded the previous episode of acute pancreatitis.
- All other causes of the pancreatitis had been ruled out; thus, the correlation between simvastatin-induced muscle pain and onset of acute pancreatitis on two separate occasions made simvastatin the suspected instigating agent.

Paper 209: Patient develops acute pancreatitis due to pravastatin therapy

Anagnostopoulos GK et al Acute pancreatitis due to pravastatin therapy. *Journal of Pancreatology* 2003 May;4(3):129-32

The author of the paper, Dr George Anagnostopoulos, is a fellow of the European Board of Gastroenterology and Hepatology.

Dr Anagnostopoulos portrays the case of a man who developed pancreatitis after statin therapy.

- A 56-year-old man presented at the Emergency Room at hospital complaining that he had had abdominal pain radiating to the back for the previous two days. The pain was accompanied by nausea and vomiting. The patient had been treated for the previous six months with pravastatin 20 mg once daily. No other medication was regularly used.
- Laboratory data on admission showed increased levels of amylase (1,615 U/L; normal values: 25-115 U/L). (When the pancreas is diseased or inflamed, amylase is released into the blood.)
- Pravastatin was discontinued and amylase levels became normal after three days.
- The patient was discharged from the hospital five days later.
- Five months after this episode, the patient reintroduced pravastatin 40 mg once daily, on his own initiative.
- Three days later, the patient again felt abdominal pain radiating to the back.
- Laboratory examination revealed an increased serum amylase level (2,334 U/L).
- Pravastatin was discontinued and the patient was discharged six days later.

Dr Anagnostopoulos concluded that the paper: "*further reinforces the fact that statins may cause acute pancreatitis*".

Paper 210: Atorvastatin may induce pancreatitis

Prajapati S et al Atorvastatin-induced pancreatitis. *Indian Journal of Pharmacology* 2010 Oct;42(5):324-5

This paper describes the case of a man who developed pancreatitis and starting statin therapy.

- A 58-year-old man sought medical treatment for severe vomiting and abdominal pain.
- He had been taking atorvastatin 10 mg for last six months.
- Physical examination revealed severe abdominal tenderness and bloating.
- Laboratory investigations revealed elevated lipase levels 137 IU/dL (normal range: 16–63 IU/dL) and amylase levels 501 IU/dL (normal range: 0–85 IU/dL).
- A computerised tomography (CT) scan showed inflammation of the pancreas.
- The patient was diagnosed as a case of atorvastatin acute pancreatitis and hospitalised.
- Atorvastatin was stopped.
- The patient improved (lipase levels normalised to 48 IU/dL) and he was discharged from the hospital after ten days.

Paper 211:
Pravastatin associated with pancreatitis

Tsigrelis C et al Pravastatin: a potential cause for acute pancreatitis. *World Journal of Gastroenterology* 2006 Nov 21;12(43):7055-7

Dr Constantine Tsigrelis from Saint Peter's University Hospital in New Brunswick illustrates the case of a woman who developed acute pancreatitis after initiation of statin therapy.

- A 50-year-old female was admitted to hospital after suffering from abdominal pain, nausea, and vomiting for one day.
- Four days prior to admission, she was started on 10 mg pravastatin, though the patient stopped this medication the day prior to admission as she attributed her symptoms to the new medication.
- Of note, she was on atorvastatin years years prior to admission for a period of three days, though this was discontinued because it caused generalised body pain.
- She developed respiratory problems and a scan found inflammation in the pancreas.
- Laboratory tests revealed severe pancreatitis.

- She was admitted to the intensive care unit and after treatment improved significantly and was discharged after 14 days.
- She did not restart any statins and remained free of any adverse effects.

Dr Tsigrelis concluded: *"Clinicians should be aware of the association of statins with acute pancreatitis"*.

Paper 212:
The association between simvastatin and pancreatitis

Murinello A et al Acute pancreatitis due to simvastatin. *Jornal Português de Gastrenterologia* 2006, 13: 92-96

This Portuguese paper reports the case of a woman who developed pancreatitis after statin therapy.

- A 74-year-old woman was admitted to hospital with a diagnosis of acute pancreatitis.
- She had been prescribed simvastatin one year prior to admission.
- Just one day before admission, the patient began to complain of increasingly intense abdominal and back pain along with anorexia, nausea and vomiting.
- Investigations found excess fluid in the pancreatic area.
- Simvastatin was stopped, and within a few days the patient improved.
- Three weeks later, the patient was discharged from hospital and a scan revealed a reduction in the fluid in the pancreatic area.
- The patient was advised not to restart statins again.

Paper 213:
The link between statins and pancreatitis

Tysk C et al Acute pancreatitis induced by fluvastatin therapy. *Journal of Clinical Gastroenterology* 2002 Nov-Dec;35(5):406-8

Professor of Medicine, Dr Curt Tysk, outlines the case of a man who developed pancreatitis after statin treatment and conducts a review of other reports of statins and pancreatitis.

- A 36-year-old male patient, after three months' treatment with fluvastatin 40 mg per day, presented with acute pancreatitis.
- The statin was stopped and the patient recovered.
- Some months later, the patient reintroduced fluvastatin on his own initiative, which caused a recurrence of pancreatitis within a few days.
- A review of previous reports shows that statin-induced pancreatitis may occur within the first day of therapy or after several months.

Paper 214:
Pancreatitis associated with simvastatin

McDonald KB et al Pancreatitis associated with simvastatin plus fenofibrate. *Annals of Pharmacotherapy* 2002 Feb;36(2):275-9

This paper describes the case of a man who developed acute necrotizing pancreatitis associated with simvastatin and fenofibrate use.

- A 70-year-old man was admitted to hospital with rapid onset of abdominal pain, nausea, and vomiting.
- Six months prior to admission, he had been taking simvastatin three days of the week and fenofibrate the other days days of the week.
- He was diagnosed with acute pancreatitis.
- His condition deteriorated and he was transferred to a hospital's intensive care unit.
- His pancreatic tissue died off and had to be surgically removed.
- His condition was now simvastatin and fenofibrate induced acute necrotizing pancreatitis.
- After a hospital stay of 121 days, including multiple intensive care unit admissions, the patient died.

These 13 papers suggest there may be an association between statins and pancreatitis.

- Studies show statin users have more than a 40% increased risk of pancreatitis compared to nonusers.

- Statin-induced pancreatitis can develop from hours to years after initiation of therapy.
- Reports have revealed statin use has resulted in pancreatic tissue die-off and death.
- Symptoms of pancreatitis caused by statins include: Abdominal pain, nausea, vomiting, muscle soreness, weakness in the arms, back pain, anorexia, skin inflammation and rash.

Dr Constantine Tsigrelis from Saint Peter's University Hospital commented: "*Clinicians should be aware of the association of statins with acute pancreatitis*".

Chapter 9

Statins linked to peripheral neuropathy

Peripheral neuropathy is a neurological condition often manifesting in the lower limbs, and is often encountered in the patients of podiatrists. Brenton West, a podiatrist from Australia, noticed that peripheral neuropathy was an increasingly common occurrence in his practice. He researched the medical literature and found the reported incidence rate of peripheral neuropathy ranges between 4-14 times more likely for those on statins compared to control groups.

In this chapter of the book, the medical research is scrutinised to verify Brenton West's findings and to describe the side effects and symptoms caused by statin induced neuropathy.

Paper 215:
Statins cause definite damage to the peripheral nerves

Otruba P et al Treatment with statins and peripheral neuropathy: results of 36-months a prospective clinical and neurophysiological follow-up. *Neuro Endocrinology Letters* 2011;32(5):688-90

Neuropathy is a collection of disorders that occurs when nerves of the peripheral nervous system (the part of the nervous system outside of the brain and spinal cord) are damaged. The condition is generally referred to as peripheral neuropathy, and it is most commonly due to damage to nerve axons.

The peripheral nervous system includes different types of nerves with their own specific functions, including:

- o Sensory nerves – responsible for transmitting sensations, such as pain and touch.
- o Motor nerves – responsible for controlling muscles.
- o Autonomic nerves – responsible for regulating automatic functions of the body, such as blood pressure and bladder function.

The symptoms of peripheral neuropathy can include:

- o Numbness and tingling in the feet or hands.
- o Burning, stabbing or shooting pain in affected areas.
- o Loss of balance and co-ordination.
- o Muscle weakness, especially in the feet.
- o Bone degeneration.
- o Changes in the skin, hair and nails.

Peripheral neuropathy may affect only one nerve (mononeuropathy), several nerves (mononeuritis multiplex), or many nerves in the body (polyneuropathy).

This Czech Republic study investigated the effects of statin treatment on lower-limb peripheral nerves. The study included 42 patients on statin therapy who were followed for three years.

- The study found that long-term treatment with statins caused definite damage to peripheral nerves when the treatment lasts longer than two years.

Paper 216:
Statins and fibrates are associated with an increased risk of peripheral neuropathy

Corrao G et al Lipid lowering drugs prescription and the risk of peripheral neuropathy: an exploratory case-control study using automated databases. *Journal of Epidemiology and Community Health* 2004 Dec;58(12):1047-51

The lead author of the study, Professor Giovanni Corrao, is a past President of the Italian Society of Medical Statistics and Clinical Epidemiology.

His study explored the association between prescription of cholesterol lowering drugs and the risk of peripheral neuropathy. 2,040 patients with peripheral neuropathy and 36,041 controls were included in the study.

The study revealed:

- Those that took statins had a 19% increased risk of peripheral neuropathy.
- Those that took fibrates had a 49% increased risk of peripheral neuropathy.
- Those that had higher doses of statins and fibrates had a higher risk of peripheral neuropathy.

Professor Corrao concluded: "*The use of both statins and fibrates was associated with the risk of peripheral neuropathy*".

Paper 217:
Statin users have a 30% increased risk of polyneuropathy

Anderson JL et al Do statins increase the risk of idiopathic polyneuropathy? *American Journal of Cardiology* 2005 May 1;95(9):1097-9

This study, published in the prestigious *American Journal of Cardiology*, examined the relationship between statins and polyneuropathy. The study included 272 patients with polyneuropathy and 1,360 matched controls.

- The study identified that statin users had a 30% increased risk of polyneuropathy compared to nonusers.

Paper 218:
Statins increase the risk of peripheral neuropathy by 30%

Tierney EF et al The association of statin use with peripheral neuropathy in the US population 40 years of age or older. *Journal of Diabetes* 2013 Jun;5(2):207-15

Researchers from the Centres for Disease Control and Prevention in Atlanta assessed the connection between statin use and peripheral neuropathy. They used data collected in the 1999-2004 National Health and Nutrition Examination Survey (NHANES) on people aged 40 or over.

- The Atlanta researchers observed that those on statins had a 30% increased risk of peripheral neuropathy.

Paper 219:
Statin use increases the risk of peripheral neuropathy

Gaist D et al Are users of lipid-lowering drugs at increased risk of peripheral neuropathy? *European Journal of Clinical Pharmacology* 2001 Mar;56(12):931-3

The objective of this Odense University study was to estimate the risk of peripheral neuropathy associated with the use of cholesterol-lowering drugs. The study lasted for six years and included 96,193 participants, aged 40-74 years, who comprised of:

- o 17,219 persons who received at least one prescription for cholesterol-lowering drugs (cholesterol lowering drug group).
- o 28,974 persons with "high cholesterol" who had not been prescribed cholesterol-lowering drugs (high cholesterol group).
- o 50,000 individuals from the general population (general population group).

The cholesterol lowering drugs included: Cholestyramine, colestipol, bezafibrate, ciprofibrate, clofibrate, fenofibrate, gemfibrozil, pravastatin, fluvastatin, atorvastatin, cervastatin, simvastatin, acipimox and nicotinic acid.

The Odense University investigators reported:

- Those taking statins had a 150% increased risk of peripheral neuropathy compared to the general population.
- Those taking any cholesterol lowering drugs had a 60% increased risk of peripheral neuropathy compared to the general population.
- Those with "high cholesterol" had a 10% decreased risk of peripheral neuropathy compared to the general population.

Paper 220:
Health care professionals should be aware of the possible role of statin drugs in neuropathy

de Langen JJ et al HMG-CoA-reductase inhibitors and neuropathy: reports to the Netherlands Pharmacovigilance Centre. *Netherlands Journal of Medicine* 2006 Oct;64(9):334-8

Dr Joyce de Langen, a manager at The Netherlands Pharmacovigilance Centre *Lareb*, (*Lareb* collect details of adverse drug reactions in the Netherlands) analysed the *Lareb* database of reported adverse drug reactions for reports concerning neuropathy associated with the use of statin drugs.

- The *Lareb* database revealed that neuropathy is significantly more reported by 270% during treatment with statins as compared with any other drug.
- Time to onset of neuropathy was up to six years from initiation of statin therapy.

- Reports of various pharmacovigilance centres worldwide are forwarded to the database of the World Health Organisation Collaborating Centre for International Drug Monitoring in Uppsala, Sweden. Uppsala found that neuropathy, peripheral neuropathy or polyneuropathy is more reported by 186% during treatment with statins as compared with any other drug.

Dr De Langen concludes: "*The average time to onset supports conclusions of previous studies and case reports that especially long-term exposure increases the risk for peripheral neuropathy. Considering the increasing number of patients taking HMG-CoA-reductase inhibitors (statins), health care professionals should be aware of the possible role of these drugs in neuropathy*".

Paper 221:
Long-term exposure to statins may substantially increase the risk of polyneuropathy

Gaist D et al Statins and risk of polyneuropathy: a case-control study. *Neurology* 2002 May 14;58(9):1333-7

This Danish study analysed the risk of polyneuropathy in statin users. The authors of the study used a patient registry to identify first-time-ever cases of polyneuropathy. They found 166 cases of polyneuropathy and each case was compared with 25 control subjects. The cases were classified as definite (35), probable (54), or possible (77).

The study ascertained:

- In all cases of polyneuropathy, statin users had a 270% increased risk of developing the disease compared to nonusers.
- In definite cases of polyneuropathy, statin users had a 1320% increased risk of developing the disease compared to nonusers.
- In all cases of polyneuropathy, current statin users had a 360% increased risk of developing the disease compared to nonusers.
- In definite cases of polyneuropathy, current statin users had a 1510% increased risk of developing the disease compared to nonusers.
- In definite cases of polyneuropathy, patients treated with statins for two or more years had a 2640% increased risk of developing the disease compared to nonusers.

The lead author of the study, Dr David Gaist an epidemiologist from Odense University Hospital, concluded: *"Long-term exposure to statins may substantially increase the risk of polyneuropathy"*.

Paper 222:
Lovastatin and peripheral neuropathy

Ahmad S Lovastatin and peripheral neuropathy.
American Heart Journal 1995 Dec;130(6):1321

This paper, published in the *American Heart Journal,* describes two patients who developed neuropathy while taking statin drugs.

Patient 1

- A 54-year-old woman had been taking lovastatin for around a year.
- She became unsteady and noticed weakness in her arms and legs.
- She also had painful tingling and numbness in her arms and legs.
- Examinations revealed decreased sensation to touch in her arms and legs.
- She had no reflexes in her ankles, knees and wrists.
- Electrophysiologic studies found she had neuropathy.
- Lovastatin was stopped.
- Over the next six weeks she was able to walk unaided and the pain in her arms and legs receded.
- She started taking lovastatin again and her symptoms recurred.
- She again stopped lovastatin and was advised to avoid all statin drugs.

Patient 2

- A 62-year-old man had been taking lovastatin for nine months.
- He complained of painful tingling and numbness in his feet.
- Examination showed a decreased sensation to touch on his legs.
- He had no ankle and knee reflexes.
- Statin induced neuropathy was diagnosed.

- Lovastatin was discontinued.
- His painful tingling and numbness receded over the next six weeks.

Paper 223:
Statin therapy linked to small fibre neuropathy

Lo YL et al Statin therapy and small fibre neuropathy: a serial electrophysiological study. *Journal of the Neurological Sciences* 2003 Apr 15;208(1-2):105-8

Associate Professor Yew Long Lo, a Senior Consultant Neurologist, describes three patients who developed small fibre neuropathy after statin therapy. (Small fibre neuropathy is a condition characterized by severe pain attacks that typically begin in the feet or hands.) (Large fibre neuropathy is characterized by numbness, tingling, weakness and loss of deep tendon reflexes.)

- The small fibre neuropathy began in the patients after one month of statin therapy.
- All patients showed abnormal sympathetic skin responses. (Sympathetic skin responses are the recorded response of the sympathetic nervous system evoked by an electrical stimulus.)
- The statin drugs were withdrawn and sympathetic skin responses returned to normal in tandem with clinical improvement.
- Statin therapy was readministered in one patient who redeveloped small and large fibre neuropathy.

Paper 224:
Doctor says that simvastatin should be considered among the causes of peripheral neuropathy

Phan T et al Peripheral neuropathy associated with simvastatin. *Journal of Neurology, Neurosurgery and Psychiatry* 1995 May;58(5):625-8

This Australian paper describes four patients who developed sensorimotor neuropathy (sensorimotor neuropathy is a type of peripheral neuropathy that damages the motor nerves and the sensory nerves) while being treated with simvastatin and had complete or partial recovery after the withdrawal of statin treatment.

Case 1

- A man aged 52 started treatment with simvastatin (10 mg/day).
- Soon after he noticed generalised muscle weakness and fatigue. The weakness became progressively worse and he had difficulty in ascending stairs and running. After six months, his right foot and subsequently his left foot became numb.
- Treatment with simvastatin was withdrawn and on review six weeks later, muscle cramps and weakness had improved although he still had the symptoms and signs of peripheral neuropathy.
- On his last review, 18 months after the withdrawal of simvastatin, there had been further clinical improvement.

Case 2

- A woman of 66 had started two years previously with simvastatin (10 mg/daily) which was subsequently gradually increased to 40 mg/daily after one year.
- After the two years of statins, the woman had weakness of the lower limbs and difficulty in rising from a chair. After three more months, she was severely incapacitated and confined to a wheelchair. By four months she was unable to feed herself or to comb her hair and was admitted to a nursing home. She had pain in the fingers, the front of her legs, lower chest and abdominal wall.
- Simvastatin was stopped and improvement followed. Nine months later, she could feed herself, comb her hair and walk with the aid of a stick. Power in all muscle groups in the lower limbs also increased greatly.

Case 3

- A woman of 65 had started two years previously with simvastatin (10 mg/daily) which was subsequently increased to 20 mg/daily after one year.
- After two years of statins, the woman developed upper and lower limb weakness. Initially she had difficulty in rising out of chairs and climbing stairs and weakness progressed over a period of six weeks until she was unable to lift her arms

above her head, rise from a chair unaided, or walk without support. She complained of a burning sensation in her left foot.

- Simvastatin treatment was withdrawn and four months later she had completely recovered clinically.

Case 4

- A woman aged 39 was given a daily dose of 10 mg of simvastatin.
- Within 24 hours of starting the drug she developed pain in her right calf, and later pain in her right groin and pains down both arms. These symptoms were followed by the development of a sensation of pins and needles in her fingertips and later the toes.
- Simvastatin was discontinued after a total dose of 180 mg. On review three months later, she reported almost complete recovery from her symptoms except for a few patches of tenderness over her body.

The researchers suggest that statins may damage the peripheral nerves because they block the production of ubiquinone (Coenzyme Q10). Without the presence of ubiquinone within the body's cells, cellular energy cannot be generated or sustained.

The head of the study, Dr Tai Phan, concluded that: *"Simvastatin should be considered among the causes of peripheral neuropathy"*.

Paper 225:
Long-term statin treatment may be associated with chronic peripheral neuropathy

Jeppesen U et al Statins and peripheral neuropathy. *European Journal of Clinical Pharmacology* 1999 Jan;54(11):835-8

Specialist in neurology at Odense University Hospital Unni Jeppesen reports of seven cases of peripheral neuropathy associated with long-term statin therapy.

- Diagnosis of neuropathy by statin therapy was confirmed after all other causes of neuropathy were thoroughly excluded.
- Neuropathy symptoms manifested up to seven years after initiation of statin therapy.

- In all seven cases the neuropathy affected the nerve fibres and with affection of both thick and thin nerve fibres.
- The symptoms of neuropathy persisted during an observation period lasting from 10 weeks to one year in four cases after statin treatment had been withdrawn.

Jeppesen concluded: *"Long-term statin treatment may be associated with chronic peripheral neuropathy"*.

Paper 226:
Guillain-Barre syndrome may be a serious side-effect of statin treatment

Rajabally YA et al Disorder resembling Guillain-Barré syndrome on initiation of statin therapy. *Muscle and Nerve* 2004 Nov;30(5):663-6

Guillain–Barré syndrome is an acute polyneuropathy, a disorder affecting the peripheral nervous system. It occurs when the body's immune system attacks part of the nervous system. It can cause life-threatening complications and is the most common cause of acute non-trauma-related paralysis.

This paper reports the case of a man who developed a Guillain-Barre type syndrome after starting statins.

- On initiation of simvastatin therapy a disorder resembling Guillain-Barre syndrome occurred in a 58-year-old man.
- He had experienced a similar but milder episode after starting pravastatin six months earlier.

This case suggests that Guillain-Barre syndrome may be a serious side-effect of statin treatment.

Paper 227:
Statins can cause the peripheral nerves to malfunction

Abellán-Miralles I et al Multiple mononeuropathy associated to treatment with pravastatin. *Revista de Neurologia* 2006 Dec 1-15;43(11):659-61

Multiple mononeuropathy (mononeuritis multiplex) is the simultaneous malfunction of two or more peripheral nerves in separate areas of the body. It causes abnormal sensations and weakness. Multiple mononeuropathy typically affects only a few nerves, often in different areas of the body. In contrast, polyneuropathy affects many nerves, usually in about the same areas on both sides of the body.

Dr Inmaculada Abellán-Miralles from the Marina Baixa Hospital outlines the case of a woman who was diagnosed with multiple mononeuropathy after beginning pravastatin therapy.

- A 51-year-old female patient who, after beginning therapy with pravastatin, suffered with abnormal sensations in the limbs and developed an unstable gait.
- Multiple mononeuropathy was diagnosed.
- Her condition improved on withdrawing from the statin treatment and it became worse again when statins were restarted.
- When pravastatin therapy was stopped for good, the patient's condition progressively improved until she was practically free of symptoms.

Paper 228:
Simvastatin can induce mononeuropathy multiplex

Scola RH et al Simvastatin-induced mononeuropathy multiplex: case report. *Arquivos de Neuro psiquiatria* 2004 Jun;62(2B):540-2

This Brazilian paper chronicles the case of a man who developed mononeuropathy multiplex after starting to take statins.

- A 63-year-old man was admitted to hospital with a history of pain in the right thigh that started three weeks prior to his admission.
- In a few days, he also developed paresthesias (sensation of tickling, tingling, burning, pricking, or numbness of a person's skin) in his fingers and toes and difficulty in walking.
- He had been taking simvastatin 40 mg a day for the past six months and had increased the dosage to 80 mg a day in the past month.
- He had weakness of his hands and feet, with the left hand and left foot more distinctively compromised.
- He also had diminished tactile sensation in the left hand as well as in his lower legs, mostly on the left.
- The patient walked with left foot drop. (Foot drop is the inability to lift the foot and toes properly when walking. It is

caused by weakness or paralysis of the muscles that lift the foot.)

- Investigations found abnormalities were present, consistent with simvastatin induced mononeuropathy multiplex. Namely nerve damage was found in his: Left hand, left elbow, both feet and both lower legs.
- Simvastatin was discontinued and the symptoms started to improve in two weeks.
- After one month, the patient reported an improvement of strength in both hands and left foot and better tactile sensation in his hands and feet.
- Four weeks later, he had no complaints regarding the use of his hands for daily life activities.

Paper 229:
Simvastatin-induced meralgia paresthetica

Sasson M et al Simvastatin-induced meralgia paresthetica.
Journal of the American Board of Family Medicine
2011 Jul-Aug;24(4):469-73

Meralgia paresthetica (a type of mononeuropathy) is numbness or pain in the outer thigh not caused by injury to the thigh, but by injury to a nerve that extends from the thigh to the spinal column.

This paper portrays the case of a man who developed meralgia paresthetica while on statin therapy.

- A 58-year-old man complained of a burning pain along his right thigh for the past two months. The pain worsened when he stood erect.
- He had been taking simvastatin for about two years.
- Physical examination found a hypoesthetic area (an abnormally low sensitivity to stimuli) on his right thigh.
- A month later, he returned with an exacerbation of the burning pain of both thighs, with a pain intensity level of 10 of 10.
- Again a hypoesthetic area was diagnosed, though this time on both of his thighs.
- Tests revealed impaired function of the left lateral femoral cutaneous nerve.
- The patient continued to suffer from the burning pain, especially when standing with an erect posture and after long

periods of walking. He was prescribed amitriptyline 20 mg to be taken at night before sleep. The patient reported use of amitriptyline and improvement of the pain during his next visit two months later. However, he discontinued the amitriptyline because he could not suffer the sedation side effect.

- A year after the first encounter the patient returned and reported that he has stopped the use of simvastatin 20 mg, which had been prescribed about three years before. He was afraid of the side effects after reading a newspaper article.
- The burning pain subsided a week after simvastatin cessation and reached a pain level of 0 of 10 after a month.
- He restarted simvastatin and after a few days the same burning pain began and increased, reaching a pain level of 10 of 10 after two weeks.
- He stopped taking simvastatin and the pain decreased again gradually, disappearing completely after a few weeks.
- Half a year after cessation of the statin use the pain had not returned.

Paper 230:
Simvastatin-induced polyneuropathy

Camargos EF et al My legs are getting old: simvastatin-induced polyneuropathy. *British Medical Journal Case Reports* 2011 Mar 3;2011. pii: bcr0920103340

Polyneuropathy is a serious, unpredictable, occasionally progressive, and life threatening neurological disorder that occurs when many nerves throughout the body malfunction simultaneously. It may affect the feet and hands, causing weakness, loss of sensation, pins-and-needle sensations or burning pain.

Dr Einstein Francisco Camargos from Brasilia University depicts the case of a woman who developed statin-induced polyneuropathy.

- An 82-year-old woman was evaluated at Hospital in response to a complaint of weakness and discomfort in the legs.
- She had taken simvastatin for seven years and said jokingly, "*I feel that my legs are getting old*".
- Examinations revealed she had impaired reflexes in the lower limbs.

- Tests found elevated levels of creatinine phosphokinase. (Elevated creatinine phosphokinase levels usually mean there has been injury or stress to muscle tissue, the heart, or the brain.)
- An electromyographic (EMG) study was compatible with polyneuropathy (sensorimotor axonal neuropathy – moderate to severe).
- She discontinued simvastatin and one month later, her symptoms were reduced and the level of creatinine phosphokinase normalised.

Dr Camargos concluded: "*Given the results of the EMG, the absence of other causes of polyneuropathy, and the substantial clinical improvement after withdrawal of medication, we conclude that our patient suffered from simvastatin-induced polyneuropathy*".

Paper 231:
Atorvastatin can induce neuropathy

Vaughan TB et al Statin neuropathy masquerading as diabetic autoimmune polyneuropathy. *Diabetes Care* 2005 Aug;28(8):2082

Dr Tom Brooks Vaughan (an expert in diabetes) illustrates the case of a young woman who developed neuropathy after starting statin treatment.

- An 18-year-old female, with diabetes, over several months developed restless legs followed by parasthesias (sensation of tickling, tingling, burning, pricking, or numbness of a person's skin), diarrhoea, incontinence and gastroparesis (delayed emptying of the stomach) leading to weight loss.
- She was taking atorvastatin.
- Examination revealed loss of sensation to the upper arms and thighs, loss of reflexes, loss of vibration sense (loss of the ability to feel mechanical vibrations on or near the body), a fast heart rate and orthostatic hypotension (a form of low blood pressure in which a person's blood pressure suddenly falls when standing up or stretching).
- Statin induced neuropathy was diagnosed.
- Atorvastatin was discontinued.
- Within one week, her symptoms improved dramatically.

- Within six months, the low blood pressure, diarrhoea, and delayed emptying of the stomach had resolved.

This case shows that statins can cause neuropathy that, in the diabetic patient, will almost invariably be attributed to diabetes. Awareness of this association and removal of the statin could result in restoration of neurological function and a much-improved quality of life in the diabetic patient.

Paper 232:
Studies and case reports show a risk of peripheral neuropathy associated with statin use

Chong PH etal Statin-associated peripheral neuropathy: review of the literature. *Pharmacotherapy* 2004 Sep;24(9):1194-203

Dr Pang Chong notes that case reports of peripheral neuropathy in patients treated with statins may have gone unnoticed by health care professionals. To evaluate the possible link between statins and peripheral neuropathy Dr Chong and his colleagues from the University of Illinois reviewed the scientific literature.

- Dr Chong found that evidence in studies as well as case reports shows a risk of peripheral neuropathy associated with statin use may exist.

Dr Chong concludes: *"These findings should alert prescribers to a potential risk of peripheral neuropathy in patients receiving any of the statins"*.

Paper 233:
Statin use is linked to an increased risk of peripheral neuropathy

Backes JM et al Association of HMG-CoA reductase inhibitors with neuropathy. *Annals of Pharmacotherapy* 2003 Feb;37(2):274-8

Dr James M Backes, a Clinical Assistant Professor from University of Kansas Medical Centre, reviewed the scientific literature between 1984 and 2002 concerning the association between statins and peripheral neuropathy.

Dr Backes review revealed:

- Studies and case reports suggest an increased risk of peripheral neuropathy with statin drugs.

- Most patients were receiving long-term therapy, although the onset was highly variable.
- The majority of cases were at least partially reversible with drug cessation.

Dr Backes concludes: "*Observational data suggest a link between chronic statin use and increased risk of peripheral neuropathy*".

The scientific research in this chapter correlates closely with the findings of the Australian podiatrist Brenton West.

- Statin users have a substantially increased risk of neuropathy and long-term statin users may have a 27-fold increase in risk.
- The side effects and symptoms of statin induced neuropathy include: Fatigue, unsteadiness, burning sensation, muscle cramps, generalised muscle weakness especially in the arms and legs, painful tingling and numbness in the feet, foot drop, loss of reflexes in the ankles knees and wrists, decreased sensation to touch in the legs, pins and needles in the fingers and toes, and pain in the calf groin and arms.

Statin drugs expert Dr Duane Graveline comments: "*Being placed on statin drugs is another more recent cause of peripheral neuropathy. Muscle weakness is frequently a symptom of neuropathy and the muscle weakness may develop in a matter of days or may slowly progress over weeks or months. Other symptoms of neuropathy include numbness, tingling and pricking sensations, burning pain (especially at night) and/or sensitivity to touch. Many people report loss of balance and incoordination. If left undiagnosed, neuropathy can lead to deterioration of the muscles and paralysis. In the extreme, severe neuropathy as a side effect to statin use can lead to death*".

Chapter 10

Lupus and skin abnormalities are being reported by statin drug users

Lupus and many cases of various types of skin abnormalities are being reported by statin drug users. The nature of these abnormalities differ widely; from various types of rashes and pimples with or without itching, to erupting fluid from skin lesions.

Chapter 10 reviews the scientific literature regarding the relationship of statins with lupus and skin abnormalities.

Paper 234:
Study suggests a link between statin exposure and lupus induction

Moulis G et al Statin-induced lupus: a case/non-case study in a nationwide pharmacovigilance database. *Lupus* 2012 Jul;21(8):885-9

Lupus (lupus erythematosus) is an autoimmune disease where the body's immune system becomes hyperactive and attacks normal, healthy tissue.

- o Lupus causes swelling and tissue damage, and can attack any part of the body.
- o It most commonly affects the heart, joints, skin, lungs, blood vessels, kidneys and the brain/nervous system.

Common symptoms include:

- o Chest pain when taking a deep breath
- o Fatigue
- o Fever with no other cause
- o General discomfort, uneasiness, or ill feeling (malaise)
- o Hair loss

- o Mouth sores
- o Sensitivity to sunlight
- o Skin rash
- o Swollen lymph nodes

The goal of this study was to detect a safety signal regarding statin-induced lupus. Dr Guillamue Moulis and his team of researchers from the University Hospital of Toulouse conducted a case/non-case study in the French PharmacoVigilance Database from January 2000 until December 2010. Cases were drug-induced lupus reports. Non-cases were all reports of other adverse drug reactions. Exposure to statins at the time of adverse drug reactions was screened in each report. Data from 235,147 adverse drug reports were analysed by the investigators.

- The researchers found those who developed lupus were 67% more likely to be taking statins compared to those who had other adverse drug reactions.

Dr Moulis concluded: "*This pharmacoepidemiological study suggests a link between statin exposure and lupus induction*".

Paper 235:
Association found between reporting of statins and lupus-like syndrome

de Jong HJ et al Association between statin use and lupus-like syndrome using spontaneous reports. *Seminars in Arthritis Rheumatism* 2011 Dec;41(3):373-81

The study assessed whether there was an association between statin use and the occurrence of lupus-like syndrome. A case/noncase study based on individual case safety reports listed in the World Health Organization global individual case safety reports database (VigiBase) was conducted by Dr Hilda de Jong. Cases were defined as reports of lupus-like syndrome and noncases were reports of other adverse drug reactions. Dr de Jong identified 3,362 reports of lupus-like syndrome as cases that were matched with 27,092 reports of other adverse drug reactions as noncases.

- The statistics from the database revealed that statin use was more often reported, by 101%, in patients with lupus-like syndrome in comparison with patients who had experienced other adverse drug reactions.

Dr de Jong concluded: "*We found an association between reporting of statins and lupus-like syndrome*".

Paper 236:
Lupuslike syndrome associated with simvastatin

Bannwarth B et al Lupuslike syndrome associated with simvastatin. *Archives of Internal Medicine* 1992 May;152(5):1093

Dr Bernard Bannwarth, a Professor of Therapeutics & Rheumatologist, reports the case of a woman who developed a lupus-like syndrome while taking statin drugs.

- A 70-year-old woman had been taking simvastatin for 18 months.
- For three months she had been suffering from worsening fatigue, multiple joint pain of her upper limbs, and morning stiffness.
- A physical examination revealed she had swelling and tenderness of the wrists and small joints of the hands.
- She had an erythrocyte sedimentation rate of 49 mm/h (normal is less than 30 mm/h) and a C-reactive protein level of 32 mg/L (normal is less than 6 mg/L). A high erythrocyte sedimentation rate and elevated C-reactive protein levels are indicative of inflammation of the body.
- She tested positive for antinuclear antibodies. (The presence of antinuclear antibodies suggests the patient may have an auto immune disease such as lupus.)
- She stopped taking simvastatin.
- Within three days, her joint pain disappeared and her symptoms completely resolved within two weeks.

Dr Bannwarth concluded: "*Our case may confirm that long-term treatment with various HMG-CoA reductase inhibitors, including lovastatin and simvastatin, is a potential cause of drug induced lupus syndrome*".

Paper 237:
Link between Atorvastatin and lupus-like syndrome with autoimmune hepatitis

Graziadei IW et al Drug-induced lupus-like syndrome associated with severe autoimmune hepatitis. *Lupus* 2003;12(5):409-12

This Austrian paper describes the case of a patient who developed severe autoimmune hepatitis and lupus-like syndrome while taking statins.

- A patient was diagnosed with atorvastatin-induced severe autoimmune hepatitis and lupus-like syndrome.
- Atorvastatin was withdrawn.
- Despite the withdrawal of the statin drug the disease persisted and even deteriorated with evidence of acute liver failure.
- The patient failed to respond to conventional immunosuppression treatment.
- Only the introduction of intense immunosuppressive therapy, as used in solid organ transplantation, led to a complete and sustained recovery of the patient.

Paper 238:
Simvastatin induces lupus erythematosus

Khosla R et al Simvastatin-induced lupus erythematosus. *Southern Medical Journal* 1998 Sep;91(9):873-4

Dr Raman Khosla, who specialises in internal medicine, chronicles the case of a man who developed lupus erythematosus after starting statin therapy.

- A 79-year-old man had fatigue, muscle pain, and chest pain three months after initiation of therapy with simvastatin.
- He had signs of inflammation in the tissues around his heart and lungs.
- He was diagnosed with simvastatin-induced lupus erythematosus.

Dr Khosla concludes: *"This should alert clinicians to this possible adverse effect of simvastatin and other statins"*.

Paper 239:
Lupus-like syndrome associated with simvastatin

Hanson J et al Lupus-like syndrome associated with simvastatin. *Lancet* 1998 Sep 26;352(9133):1070

Antinuclear antibodies are a type of protein manufactured by the immune system that attacks and causes damage to the cell's nucleus.

High levels of antinuclear antibodies are found in more than 98% of patients with lupus.

Raynaud's phenomenon is excessively reduced blood flow, causing discoloration of the fingers, toes, and occasionally other areas. Raynaud's phenomenon occurs in about one-third of patients with lupus.

Dr Jonathan Hanson from Harrogate District Hospital illustrates the case of a man who developed a lupus-like syndrome and Raynaud's phenomenon while taking statins.

- A 39-year-old self-employed food worker sought medical attention with a six-week history of numbness, predominantly in his right hand when extracting food from the deep freeze.
- He also reported pallor and numbness on exercise to the extent that he would have difficulty in releasing the grip on his tennis racquet.
- Further inquiry revealed occasional joint pain.
- He had been taking simvastatin 20 mg daily for four years.
- Examination revealed evidence he had Raynaud's phenomenon.
- Tests revealed he was positive for antinuclear antibodies.
- He stopped taking simvastatin.
- After two months all symptoms were improving, although after five months, mild Raynaud's persisted with slight restriction of flexion in his fingers and after one year, he was still positive for antinuclear antibodies.

Dr Hanson concludes: *"This observation does suggest that similar problems, of varying severity, may be affecting patients taking this class of drug (statins)"*.

Paper 240:
Long-term exposure to statins may be associated with drug-induced lupus erythematosus and other autoimmune disorders

Noel B Lupus erythematosus and other autoimmune diseases related to statin therapy: a systematic review. *Journal of the European Academy of Dermatology and Venereology* 2007 Jan;21(1):17-24

Dr Bernard Noel reviewed the scientific literature concerning statin-induced autoimmune diseases including lupus erythematosus.

The review revealed:

- Statins were associated with various autoimmune diseases such as systemic lupus erythematosus, subacute cutaneous lupus erythematosus, dermatomyositis, polymyositis and lichen planus pemphigoides.
- Autoimmune hepatitis was observed in some patients with systemic lupus erythematosus.
- The average time of exposure before disease onset was 12 months, with a range from one month to six years.
- Aggressive immunosuppressive therapy was required in the majority of cases to aid clinical recovery.
- Some patients died despite the immunosuppressive therapy.

Dr Noel concludes: *"Long-term exposure to statins may be associated with drug-induced lupus erythematosus and other autoimmune disorders. Fatal cases have been reported despite early drug discontinuation and aggressive systemic immunosuppressive therapy"*.

Paper 241:
13-year study of nearly one million individuals shows that statins significantly increase the risk of shingles in older people

Antoniou T et al Statins and the risk of herpes zoster: a population-based cohort study. *Clinical Infectious Disease* 2014 Feb;58(3):350-6

Dr Tony Antoniou (a Clinical Pharmacy Specialist), and his team of researchers from St. Michael's Hospital in Toronto, examined the relationship between statin use and incidence of herpes zoster (shingles). The study included 494,651 individuals treated with a statin and an equal number of untreated individuals. The participants were aged 66 years of age or older and the study lasted for 13 years.

The Canadian study ascertained:

- Those who used statins had a 13% increased risk of shingles compared to nonusers.
- Those with diabetes who used statins had an 18% increased risk of shingles compared to nonusers.
- Those who used statins had a 4% increased risk of knee arthroplasty compared to nonusers.

Dr Antoniou concluded: "*In this population-based study of nearly one million older individuals, we found that statin-treated patients were at an increased risk of developing herpes zoster*".

Paper 242:
Pravastatin-associated inflammatory muscle weakness

Schalke BB et al Pravastatin-associated inflammatory myopathy. *New England Journal of Medicine* 1992 Aug 27;327(9):649-50

This paper illustrates the case of a woman who developed a syndrome resembling dermatomyositis while on statin therapy. (Dermatomyositis is an inflammatory disease marked by muscle weakness and a distinctive skin rash. Symptoms include; difficulty swallowing, muscle weakness stiffness or soreness, purple or violet coloured upper eyelids, purple-red skin rash, shortness of breath.)

- A 66-year-old woman had been taking pravastatin for five months.
- She developed a syndrome resembling dermatomyositis over a period of five weeks.
- She was admitted with severe muscle weakness in the upper limbs and had prominent skin lesions on her face, neck, shoulder, chest, and arms.
- Her creatine kinase levels were elevated. (Indicating muscle damage.)
- Muscle biopsy revealed inflammation and damage.
- Pravastatin was discontinued, which was followed by clinical improvement in her weakness, regression of the skin lesions, and normalization of the creatine kinase levels.

Paper 243:
Dermatomyositis-like syndrome linked to statin intake

Vasconcelos OM et al Dermatomyositis-like syndrome and HMG-CoA reductase inhibitor (statin) intake. *Muscle and Nerve* 2004 Dec;30(6):803-7

Dr Olavo Vasconcelos, a neurologist in Bethesda, outlines the case of a patient who developed dermatomyositis while taking simvastatin.

- A patient developed an adult-onset dermatomyositis-like syndrome characterized by skin rash and progressive proximal

(shoulder and hip) muscle weakness concurrent with the intake of simvastatin.
- The patient discontinued simvastatin and initiated steroid therapy which resolved the symptoms.

Dr Vasconcelos concluded: "*Caregivers are urged to be alert regarding the early recognition and proper care of the spectrum of neuromuscular complications linked to statin intake*".

Paper 244:
Simvastatin associated with dermatomyositis

Rasch A et al Simvastatin-induced dermatomyositis. *Der Hautarzt* 2009 Jun;60(6):489-93

This paper portrays the case of a woman who developed dermatomyositis while taking statin drugs.

- A 71-year-old woman was admitted to hospital in March after suffering for six months with a rash, back pain, weak muscles of the upper shoulder girdle, swelling in her fingers and eyelids and a general malaise.
- She had been taking simvastatin for six years.
- Tests revealed positive Mi-2-Antibodies which are associated with dermatomyositis.
- She had elevated creatine kinase levels.
- A muscle biopsy found necrotizing myopathy (muscle cell death) and inflammation.
- She was diagnosed with simvastatin induced dermatomyositis.
- Simvastatin was withdrawn.
- After four weeks, the patient reported a significant improvement in her symptoms.

Paper 245:
Simvastatin can induce dermatomyositis

Zaraa IR et al Simvastatin-induced dermatomyositis in a 50-year-old man. *British Medical Journal Case Reports* 2011 Mar 29;2011. pii: bcr0220113832

The author of this paper Dr Inés Rania Zaraa is a prominent Associate Professor in the Department of Dermatology at Rabta Hospital. Dr Zaraa depicts a case of dermatomyositis occurring after simvastatin intake.

- A 50-year-old male sought medical attention for a rash and considerable muscular weakness which he had suffered for three months.
- Laboratory tests showed raised levels of creatine kinase and lactate dehydrogenase.
- Examination of a muscle biopsy led to a diagnosis of dermatomyositis.
- Simvastatin was discontinued.
- His clinical and laboratory abnormalities improved within one month.

Dr Zaraa concluded: "*Our case of dermatomyositis in a patient receiving simvastatin adds to the previous reported cases in the literature and highlights the potential role of statins as triggers of immune systemic diseases*".

Paper 246:
Simvastatin can induce amyopathic dermatomyositis

Inhoff O et al Simvastatin-induced amyopathic dermatomyositis. *British Journal of Dermatology* 2009 Jul;161(1):206-8

Amyopathic dermatomyositis is a variant of dermatomyositis that is characterized by the typical skin rash but without the muscle abnormalities.

This paper highlights the case of a woman who developed amyopathic dermatomyositis while on statin therapy.

- A 70-year-old woman, treated for several years with simvastatin, sought medical attention for itching, rashes and plaques on sun-exposed parts of her body.
- The patient did not have muscle weakness.
- A skin biopsy revealed dermatitis and lesions coupled with thin and wrinkled skin.
- A diagnosis of simvastatin induced amyopathic dermatomyositis was made.
- Simvastatin was discontinued.
- Five months later, the skin lesions had almost completely cleared.

Paper 247:
Atorvastatin-induced dermatomyositis

Noël B et al Atorvastatin-induced dermatomyositis. *American Journal of Medicine* 2001 Jun 1;110(8):670-1

Dr Bernard Noel, a specialist in dermatology, describes the case of a man who developed dermatomyositis while on statin drugs.

- A 44-year-old man was hospitalised with difficulty in swallowing and talking and severe lack of strength.
- He had been taking atorvastatin for one year.
- Examination revealed a purple and violet rashes, purple spots, skin lesions and loss of muscle mobility.
- He had elevated creatine kinase levels and tested positive for antinuclear antibodies. (High creatine kinase levels indicate muscle damage and antinuclear antibodies are associated with inflammation and rheumatic diseases.)
- Necrosis (death) of skin and muscle cells was observed on a biopsy.
- Atorvastatin was discontinued and the improvement in the patient was rapid and spontaneous.
- Normalisation of creatine kinase levels but not of antinuclear antibodies was observed.
- Nine months later, he was still positive for antinuclear antibodies.

Dr Noel concluded: "*Two important clinical implications can be drawn from this case report. First, high plasma levels of antinuclear antibody may be due to statins long after patients stop taking them. Second, screening for both plasma creatine kinase concentration and antinuclear antibody may be useful in unexplained fatigue or skin eruption*".

Paper 248:
Pravastatin-induced dermatomyositis

Zuech P et al Pravastatin-induced dermatomyositis. *La Revue de Medecine Interne* 2005 Nov;26(11):897-902

Dr Pierre Zuech from the Poissy-Saint-Germain-en-Laye Hospital reports of nine patients who developed dermatomyositis while on statins.

- A 69-year-old woman developed dermatomyositis two years after she started a treatment with pravastatin.
- She stopped taking pravastatin and slowly improved.
- In three of the other eight patients, the discontinuation of statins was followed by spontaneous clinical and biological improvement.
- The other patients received high doses of corticosteroids and improved, except one patient who died of respiratory failure (pulmonary fibrosis).

Dr Zuech concludes: "*In these patients, dermatomyositis can be considered as a severe adverse reaction to HMG-CoA reductase inhibitors (statins)... and highlights the potential role of statins as triggers of immune systemic diseases*".

Paper 249:
Statins and erupting skin lesions

Stoebner PE et al Simvastatin-induced lichen planus pemphigoides. *Annales de Dermatologie et de Venereologie* 2003 Feb;130(2 Pt 1):187-90

Lichen planus pemphigoides is a rare autoimmune blistering disease that is characterized by the development of erupting fluid from skin lesions.

Dr Pierre-Emmanuel Stoebner from Saint-Eloi Hospital highlights the case of a man who suffered lichen planus pemphigoides after starting statins.

- A 63-year-old man started to take simvastatin.
- One month later, he developed a pruriginous (pale, dome-shaped papules that itch severely) and bullous lichenoid eruption.
- Examinations and tests led to a diagnosis of lichen planus pemphigoides.
- All the lesions progressively disappeared after statins were discontinued.

With the increasing use of statins Dr Stoebbner concludes: "*An association between simvastatin and lichen planus pemphigoides should be kept in mind*".

Paper 250:
Pravastatin may induce lichenoid dermatitis

Pua VS et al Pravastatin-induced lichenoid drug eruption. *Australasian Journal of Dermatology* 2006 Feb;47(1):57-9

Lichenoid dermatitis is an allergic reaction that causes a purple, itchy rash on the skin. It is caused by damage to the outer layer of the skin, which results in inflammation.

This paper reports the case of a woman who developed lichenoid dermatitis after statin therapy.

- A 64-year-old woman on pravastatin therapy sought treatment for a rash over large areas of her face and upper back.
- Examination of a biopsy of the rash revealed lichenoid dermatitis.
- Cessation of pravastatin resulted in gradual fading of the rash.

Paper 251:
Statins may be associated with skin lesions

Adams AE et al Statins and "chameleon-like" cutaneous eruptions: simvastatin-induced acral cutaneous vesiculobullous and pustular eruption in a 70-year-old man. *Journal of Cutaneous Medicine and Surgery* 2010 Sep-Oct;14(5):207-11

The authors of the paper note that statins are associated with many types of cutaneous eruptions (skin lesions and rashes) such as Stevens-Johnson syndrome, toxic epidermolytic necrolysis, porphyria cutanea tarda, linear IgA bullous dermatosis, and reaction patterns (lupus and dermatomyositis-like and pustular).

The paper presents the case of a man covered with skin lesions after taking simvastatin (zocor) drugs.

- A 70-year-old man was prescribed simvastatin and began to suffer with chronic vesiculobullous (blisters) and pustular annular lesions (pus filled lesions), on his arms, legs, hands, and feet.
- After two years, the man stopped taking simvastatin and his condition improved.
- He later restarted simvastatin and the lesions recurred.
- He eventually discontinued simvastatin and the lesions cleared.

Paper 252:
Skin lesions due to treatment with simvastatin

Feldmann R et al Skin lesions due to treatment with simvastatin (Zocor). *Dermatology* 1993;186(4):272

This paper depicts the case of a man who developed skin lesions after starting to take statins.

- A 50-year-old healthy man sought medical attention for itchy skin lesions.
- Five months earlier, he had started to take simvastatin.
- He then gradually developed extensive skin lesions, first beginning on the legs and hands.
- Physical examination revealed he had dry skin and scaly lesions on his legs, thighs, buttocks, trunk, face and fingertips.
- Simvastatin was discontinued.
- Within three months, the lesions on the trunk and legs had totally cleared.
- Two months later, the rest of the lesions had disappeared.
- He was still free of all lesions at a 15 month check-up.

Paper 253:
Cholesterol-lowering drugs can induce eczema, ichthyosis, or psoriasis as side effects

Proksch E et al Antilipemic drug-induced skin manifestations. *Hautarzt* 1995 Feb;46(2):76-80

Dr Ehrhardt Proksch (an expert in eczema and psoriasis) from Hautklinik Kiel University conducted a review of the scientific literature concerning the association between cholesterol-lowering drugs and skin abnormalities.

His review unearthed:

- The statin drugs, lovastatin (Mevacor), simvastatin (Zocor) and pravastatin (Selipram) can cause eczema.
- Triparanol and diazacholesterol can induce ichthyosis (a long-term condition that results in persistently thick, dry, "fish-scale" skin) or palmoplantar hyperkeratosis (disorder characterized by thickening of the skin of the palms and the soles).
- Gemfibrozil can cause an exacerbation of psoriasis (skin condition that causes red, flaky, crusty patches of skin covered with silvery scales).

Paper 254:
Simvastatin associated with cheilitis

Mehregan DR et al Cheilitis due to treatment with simvastatin. *Cutis* 1998 Oct;62(4):197-8

The author of the paper, Dr Darius Mehregan, is a board certified dermatologist in Monroe, Michigan. His paper reports two patients who developed cheilitis after beginning simvastatin therapy. (Cheilitis is inflammation of the lips. This inflammation may include the skin around the mouth and/or the inner lining of the lips (labial mucosa).

- The patients' rash resolved after discontinuation of simvastatin and subsequent treatment with moisturizers and steroids.

Dr Mehregan concludes: "*Epidermal cholesterol synthesis (cholesterol made by the skin) has been shown to be essential for maintaining the cutaneous (skin) barrier function. We suspect that skin barrier dysfunction may occur in the mucosa from inhibitors of HMG-CoA reductase (statins) in a manner analogous to the epidermis*".

Paper 255:
Chronic actinic dermatitis associated with simvastatin

Holme SA et al Chronic actinic dermatitis secondary to simvastatin. *Photodermatology, Photoimmunology and Photomedicine* 2002 Dec;18(6):313-4

This paper reports the case of a man who developed chronic actinic dermatitis after starting statin therapy. (Chronic actinic dermatitis is an eczema type eruption confined to sun-exposed skin areas.)

- A 54-year-old man (with itchy skin in the affected areas) sought treatment for persistent photosensitive eruption (skin disorders on sun-exposed skin) affecting his face, neck and back of his hands.
- The onset had occurred three weeks after commencing simvastatin therapy.
- After one more week, he stopped taking simvastatin and the condition slowly resolved.
- Eight months later, he was on vacation, and on the first day following exposure to sunlight the eruption recurred on sun-exposed areas of his skin.

- Investigations revealed a diagnosis of chronic actinic dermatitis due to photosensitivity to simvastatin.
- The patient was advised to avoid statins.

Paper 256:
Statins cause chronic actinic dermatitis

Granados MT et al Chronic actinic dermatitis due to simvastatin. *Contact Dermatitis* 1998 May;38(5):294-5

This Spanish paper describes the case of a man who developed chronic actinic dermatitis after simvastatin therapy.

- A 66-year-old man sought treatment at a clinic for persistent photosensitivity (sun allergy) of more than one year.
- Examination revealed thick and leathery eczema type plaques on the exposed areas of skin on his face, neck and back of his hands.
- Tests revealed inflammation was present.
- The patient had been taking simvastatin intermittently, the last period having been for one month, seven months before attending the clinic.
- Investigations led to the diagnosis of chronic actinic dermatitis due to systemic photosensitivity to simvastatin.

This case shows that even seven months after discontinuation of the drug, dermatitic reactions to sunlight can still occur in patients who have used statin drugs.

Paper 257:
Statins provoke outbreak of blisters

Morimoto K et al Photosensitivity to simvastatin with an unusual response to photopatch and photo tests. *Contact Dermatitis* 1995 Oct;33(4):274

Dr Kohkichi Morimoto from the Department of Dermatology at the National Defence Medical College in Japan chronicles the case of a woman who became photosensitive (abnormal reaction of the skin to light) after starting to take statin drugs.

- A 50-year-old woman started to take simvastatin.
- Three weeks later, she developed reddish blisters on the sun exposed areas of her skin.

- Tests revealed that she was photosensitive to UVA radiation.
- She stopped taking simvastatin.
- Four weeks later, tests found that photosensitivity to UVA of the patient had become normal.

Paper 258: Atorvastatin can induce drug reaction with eosinophilia and systemic symptoms (DRESS)

Gressier L et al Atorvastatin-induced drug reaction with eosinophilia and systemic symptoms (DRESS). *Annales de Dermatologie et de Venereologie* 2009 Jan;136(1):50-3

Drug reaction with eosinophilia and systemic symptoms (DRESS) describes a group of severe adverse reactions to medications. Diagnostic symptoms of DRESS include rash, fever, involvement of at least one internal organ and blood count abnormalities.

This paper illustrates the case of a woman who developed drug reaction with eosinophilia and systemic symptoms after starting statin therapy.

- A 58-year-old woman was admitted to hospital with a fever, skin rash and fluid retention in the face.
- She had started taking atorvastatin six weeks earlier.
- Examination revealed she had skin lesions, fever, abdominal pain, diarrhoea and aches and pains in many joints.
- Blood tests found her eosinophilia levels were elevated; she had inflammation and anicteric cholestasis. (Anicteric cholestasis is where bile cannot flow to the liver to the small intestine and the patient does not have jaundice.)
- The patient was diagnosed with atorvastatin induced DRESS.
- She stopped taking atorvastatin.
- Her condition improved after cessation of atorvastatin.

Paper 259: Acute generalised exanthematous pustulosis may be induced by simvastatin

Dobriţoiu AM et al Acute Generalised Exanthematous Pustulosis Induced By Simvastatin. *Therapeutics, Pharmacology and Clinical Toxicology* Vol XIV, Number 4, December 2010 Pages 306-308

Acute generalized exanthematous pustulosis is a skin eruption characterised by the rapid appearance of areas of red skin studded with small blisters filled with white/yellow fluid.

Dermatology specialist Dr Adina Dobriţoiu describes the case of a man who developed acute generalized exanthematous pustulosis while on statin therapy.

- A 67-year-old man was admitted to hospital with an extensive rash and pus filled lesions of sudden onset associated with fever and malaise. The lesions started on the face and neck and later spread to the rest of the skin. The patient complained of itching.
- He was on simvastatin therapy.
- Investigations found he had inflammation.
- Tests revealed simvastatin as the cause of acute generalized exanthematous pustulosis.
- He stopped taking simvastatin.
- His symptoms resolved within two weeks.

Dr Dobriţoiu concludes: "*Statins can be added to the list of potential causes of acute generalized exanthematous pustulosis*".

Paper 260: Statins and eosinophilic fasciitis

Dugonik A et al Eosinophilic Fasciitis. *Acta Dermatovenerologica Alpina, Pannonica et Adriatica* Vol 12, 2003, No 2 72-75

Eosinophilic fasciitis is a disease in which muscle tissue under the skin, called fascia, becomes swollen and thick. The fascia is inflamed with the eosinophil type of white blood cells which leads to symptoms of progressive thickening and often redness, warmth, and hardness of the skin surface.

Dermatologist Dr Aleksandra Dugonik outlines the case of a woman who developed eosinophilic fasciitis after starting simvastatin.

- A 58-year-old woman was evaluated for hard – skin type lesions which started on her upper extremities and progressed rapidly, involving her trunk and lower extremities.
- A few days later, she developed joint pain, edema of legs and a slightly elevated temperature.

- The first skin lesions appeared one month after she had started simvastatin.
- Clinical and histopathological findings corresponded to the diagnosis eosinophilic fasciitis.
- Simvastatin was discontinued.
- After two weeks, the patient's temperature normalised, joint pains and edema of legs subsided, and skin lesions softened. The percentage of eosinophils dropped to normal.

Paper 261:
Low blood pressure, facial swelling and abnormally high amounts of white blood cells induced by atorvastatin

Hampson JP et al Hypotension and eosinophilia with atorvastatin. *Pharmacy World and Science* 2005 Aug;27(4):279-80

The case of a man who collapsed and was in shock while on statin therapy is portrayed by Dr John Hampson from Maelor Hospital in Wales.

- A 67-year-old man suffered a hypersensitivity reaction to statin therapy. He collapsed and was in shock which was characterised by marked low blood pressure, facial swelling and eosinophilia. (Eosinophilia refers to conditions in which abnormally high amounts of eosinophils (white blood cells) are found in either the blood or in body tissues.
- The patient stopped taking atorvastatin.
- He restarted atorvastatin and facial swelling again recurred.

Dr Hampson concludes: "*Statin hypersensitivity reactions can occur several months after commencing therapy... prescribers and pharmacists should be aware of this important reaction which can be quite debilitating*".

Paper 262:
Family physicians should be aware of the possibility of dermographism with atorvastatin

Adcock BB et al Dermographism: an adverse effect of atorvastatin. *Journal of the American Board of Family Practice* 2001 Mar-Apr;14(2):148-51

Dermographism is a form of chronic hives (skin rash) called physical urticaria. The rash is caused by stroking the skin with an object. Dermographism is also known as "skin writing".

This paper, authored by Dr Bobbi Adcock at the University of Alabama, chronicles the case of a woman who developed dermographism after starting atorvastatin therapy.

- A 40-year-old woman visited her physician with a four-month history of skin rash.
- She had started to take atorvastatin five months previously.
- One month after atorvastatin was started, the patient reported mild itching with red spots appearing within seconds to minutes after application of light pressure to the skin. The rash resolved spontaneously within one hour.
- She then noticed a similar response after carrying books or shopping bags over her arms for a short distance. She drew a "happy face" on her forearm, and, as expected, a rash developed immediately and then faded within an hour. The same "happy face" reappeared the next day when she became overheated.
- There had been only mild irritation on localized areas of her body without interfering with usual activities until the day before her visit to her physician's office. At this time, she reported a widespread rash associated with nausea, vomiting, abdominal cramping, and diarrhoea.
- Dermographism was confirmed when a line was drawn on her forearm with an ink pen.
- Atorvastatin was identified as the offending cause and was discontinued.
- The following day, the patient developed a widespread itchy skin rash with gastrointestinal distress and new-onset left wrist pain with angioedema and tenderness of her soles. (Angioedema is the swelling of the deeper layers of the skin, caused by a build-up of fluid.)
- Erythema multiforme (skin lesions) was noted on her lower trunk and thighs.
- Within two to three days, angioedema and erythema multiforme had resolved.
- Episodes of dermographism became less frequent with complete resolution within three months.

- She did not start taking any statins again and had no further episodes.

Dr Adcock concluded: *"Family physicians should be aware of the possibility of dermographism with atorvastatin"*.

Paper 263:
Atorvastatin leads to urticaria

Anliker MD et al Chronic urticaria to atorvastatin.
Allergy 2002 Apr;57(4):366

Urticaria (also known as hives, welts or nettle rash) is a raised, itchy rash that appears on the skin.

This paper describes the case of a man who developed urticaria after starting statins.

- A 59-year-old man started to take atorvastatin. After eight weeks, he suffered from chronic urticaria.
- An allergy test showed a strong positive response for atorvastatin.
- The patient stopped taking atorvastatin and the urticaria subsided over the next ten days.

Paper 264:
Statins cause severe skin reaction after radiation treatment

Abadir R et al Radiation reaction recall following simvastatin therapy: a new observation.
Clinical Oncology (Royal College of Radiologists) 1995;7(5):325-6

This paper chronicles the case of a woman at Bothwell Regional Health Centre who had a severe skin reaction after starting statins.

- A 60-year-old woman with gall bladder cancer was treated with radiotherapy.
- No skin reaction was seen during radiotherapy or in one year of follow-up.
- A year after radiotherapy she was started on simvastatin.
- Within two to three days, a severe skin reaction developed.
- She stopped taking simvastatin and her condition improved.

Paper 265:
Statins linked to thrombocytopenic purpura

Lin ZW et al Rosuvastatin-Induced Thrombocytopenic Purpura-A Case Report. *Dermatologica Sinica* 27: 235-240, 2009

Thrombocytopenic purpura is a bleeding disorder in which the immune system destroys platelets, which are necessary for normal blood clotting. Persons with the disease have too few platelets in the blood. This results in bleeding into the skin which causes a characteristic skin rash that looks like pinpoint red spots (petechial and purpural rash). The symptoms can vary from mild bruising to severe bleeding.

Dr Zheng-Wei Lin from the Chang Gung Memorial Hospital illustrates the case of a man who developed thrombocytopenic purpura after starting statin therapy.

- A 57-year-old man started to take rosuvastatin.
- Nineteen days after he began taking rosuvastatin, he developed generalized petechiae.
- Rosuvastatin-induced thrombocytopenic purpura was diagnosed.
- The statin was stopped and his symptoms cleared within four weeks.

Dr Lin concludes: "*This is a case report in the literature of thrombocytopenia associated with the use of rosuvastatin, and it reinforces the fact that statins may cause thrombocytopenia*".

Paper 266:
Thrombocytopenic purpura during therapy with simvastatin

Possamai G et al Thrombocytopenic purpura during therapy with simvastatin. *Haematologica* 1992 Jul-Aug;77(4):357-8

This paper notes the case of a woman who developed thrombocytopenic purpura after taking statin drugs.

- A very serious thrombocytopenic purpura occurred in a diabetic woman during therapy with simvastatin.

- Stopping the simvastatin drug produced a prompt reversal of the thrombocytic attack.
- One year after stopping the statin, the patient's platelet count remained within the normal range.

Paper 267: Thrombotic thrombocytopenic purpura associated with statin treatment

Sundram F et al Thrombotic thrombocytopenic purpura associated with statin treatment. *Postgraduate Medical Journal* 2004 Sep;80(947):551-2

Thrombotic thrombocytopenic purpura is a rare disorder that involves the blood's tendency to clot. In this disease, tiny clots form throughout the body. These tiny clots have two major consequences. First, the tiny clots can block blood vessels. This stops your blood from being able to reach the organs. This can compromise the functioning of vital organs—such as the heart, brain and kidneys. Second, the tiny clots can use up too many of the blood's platelets. The blood might then be unable to form clots when it actually needs to. For example, if you are injured, you may be unable to stop bleeding.

Researchers from the Leicester Royal Infirmary present the case of a man who developed thrombotic thrombocytopenic purpura after starting statins.

- A 68-year-old man sought medical attention for chest pain.
- He was diagnosed with angina and given simvastatin.
- The next day he experienced nausea and headache.
- He discontinued the statins but over the ensuing 48 hours developed widespread bruising, bleeding in the mouth and pain and swelling in the left knee, left ankle, right elbow, and shoulder joints.
- Tests and examinations led to a diagnosis of thrombotic thrombocytopenic purpura.
- He started to receive treatment but on the third day he sustained an acute coronary syndrome (heart attack or unstable angina).
- After continued treatment he was discharged and advised not to take statins.
- A six month check up revealed he remained symptom free with normal laboratory test results.

The UK researchers concluded: "*Our patient developed symptoms one day after starting simvastatin and thrombotic thrombocytopenic purpura was diagnosed when he was admitted four days later. No other underlying illness was found and there was rapid recovery after discontinuation of the (statin) drug. These features suggested to us the possibility of drug induced thrombotic thrombocytopenic purpura*".

An inspection of the medical literature highlights that statins may potentially trigger or aggravate autoimmune diseases such as lupus and they also have the ability to provoke skin abnormalities.

- Statistics from two databases suggest an association with statins and lupus.
- After starting to take statins, the signs of lupus may appear from as little as a month, to as much as six years.
- Intense immunosuppressive therapy is often needed for patients to recover.
- Despite the aggressive immunosuppressive therapy some patients die from statin induced lupus.
- Symptoms that manifest from lupus caused by statins include: Multiple joint pain, muscle pain, chest pain, fatigue, morning stiffness, swelling in the wrists and hands, and numbness in the hands.
- Statins can induce skin disorders such as:
    - Shingles
    - Dermatomyositis
    - Lichen planus pemphigoides
    - Lichenoid dermatitis
    - Acral cutaneous vesiculobullous
    - Eczema
    - Cheilitis
    - Actinic dermatitis
    - Drug reaction with eosinophilia and systemic symptoms (DRESS)
    - Acute generalized exanthematous pustulosis
    - Eosinophilic fasciitis
    - Hives

- Symptoms from statin induced skin disorders include: Itching, lesions over the body, rashes, thick leathery plaques, spots, itchy pimples, scaly lesions, pus-filled lesions, blisters, swelling in the legs fingers and eyelids, inflammation of the lips, fluid retention in the face, muscle weakness, severe lack of strength, dry skin, malaise, fever, difficulty in talking and swallowing, abdominal pain, and diarrhoea.

Chapter 11

Statins exacerbate asthma and inhibit lung function and exercise

Do statins impair our ability to breathe? Dr Safa Nsouli says that statins may aggravate asthma because they create an imbalance in immune system cells called helper T cells. In 2010, the Food and Drug Administration insisted that the simvastatin (zocor) package insert contained the warning that "interstitial lung disease" be added to the long list of adverse effects caused by the drug and in June 2014, a *Daily Mail* headline read: "Are statins making us lazy? Men who take them are less likely to exercise".

The next 31 papers investigate the accusations that statins aggravate asthma, cause lung disease, and may stop people exercising.

Paper 268: Statins adversely affect asthma

Ostroukhova M et al The effect of statin therapy on allergic patients with asthma. *Annals of Allergy, Asthma and Immunology* 2009 Dec;103(6):463-8

Dr Marina Ostroukhova and her colleagues from Rochester General Hospital conducted a study to ascertain whether statin use adversely affects asthma. The study included 24 patients who were on statin therapy and 26 controls, not on statin therapy.

The study found after six months:

- There was a significant 3% worsening of forced expiratory volume in one second (a worsening of lung function) for the statin group compared with the controls. (Forced expiratory volume in one second is the amount of air which can be forcibly exhaled from the lungs in the first second of a forced exhalation.)

- 40% more patients in the statin group needed increased asthma medication compared with the controls.
- 63% more patients in the statin group used albuterol more frequently compared with the controls. (Albuterol is used to prevent and treat wheezing, difficulty breathing and chest tightness caused by lung diseases.)
- 33% more patients in the statin group had more nocturnal awakenings compared with the controls.
- 34% more patients in the statin group had to see the doctor more frequently for acute asthma.

Paper 269:
Statins can make asthma worse

Nsouli S Statins can make asthma worse. *American College of Allergy, Asthma and Immunology* (ACAAI) 2011 Annual Scientific Meeting: Abstract 30. November 6, 2011.

Dr Safa Nsouli investigated the association of statins with asthma at the Danville Asthma and Allergy Clinic in California. The study, which lasted 12 months, compared 20 patients with asthma who were taking statins with 20 matched patients who were not taking statins.

Dr Nsouli's study revealed:

- In statin patients the forced expiratory volume in one second decreased by an extra 21% compared to patients not taking statins.
- In statin patients the peak expiratory flow decreased by an extra 28% compared to patients not taking statins. (Peak expiratory flow rate is the maximum flow rate generated during a forceful exhalation, starting from full lung inflation. Peak flow rate primarily reflects large airway flow and depends on the voluntary effort and muscular strength of the patient.)
- The use of beta-agonist rescue inhalers was 63% higher in the statin group than in the non-statin group.
- In statin patients the incidence of night time wakening increased by an extra 28% compared to patients not taking statins.
- In statin patients the incidence of daytime asthma symptoms increased by an extra 32% compared to patients not taking statins.

Dr Nsouli concluded: *"Patients with asthma who are prescribed statins should be informed that, because of the adverse immunomodulatory effects that statins produce, their asthma might get worse"*.

Paper 270: Statins worsen lung function in patients with lymphangioleiomyomatosis

El-Chemaly S et al Statins in lymphangioleiomyomatosis: a word of caution. *European Respiratory Journal* 2009 Aug;34(2):513-4

Lymphangioleiomyomatosis is a rare progressive cystic lung disease.

FEV1% (forced expiratory volume) is the volume of air exhaled during the first second. So, the lower the measurement – the lower the lung function. *FEV1% predicted* is defined as FEV1% of the patient divided by the average FEV1% in the population for any person of similar age, sex and body composition.

DL,CO% (diffusing capacity of the lung for carbon monoxide) is the extent to which oxygen passes from the air sacs of the lungs into the blood. The lower the measurement, the less oxygen there is – the lower the lung function. *DL,CO% predicted* is defined as DL,CO% of the patient divided by the average DL,CO% in the population for any person of similar age, sex and body composition.

The lead author of the study was Dr Souheil El-Chemaly, an Assistant Professor of Medicine at Harvard Medical School. Dr El-Chemaly's clinical interest is in interstitial lung disease and lung transplant. This three-year study evaluated the effects of statins on lung function in 335 patients with lymphangioleiomyomatosis.

The study determined:

- Those taking statins had a 1.9% yearly decline in FEV1% predicted levels compared to those not taking statins.
- Those taking statins had a 3.7% yearly decline in DL,CO% predicted levels compared to those not taking statins.

Dr El-Chemaly's study shows that statins worsen lung function in patients with lymphangioleiomyomatosis.

Paper 271: Statin users with pneumonia 10% more likely to die or be admitted to an intensive care unit than non statin users

Majumdar SR et al Statins and outcomes in patients admitted to hospital with community acquired pneumonia: population based prospective cohort study. *British Medical Journal* 2006; 333: 999

This University of Alberta study, published in the prestigious *British Medical Journal,* assessed whether statins reduce mortality or need for admission to intensive care in patients admitted to hospital with community acquired pneumonia.

- The study identified that statin users were 10% more likely to die or be admitted to an intensive care unit than nonusers.

Paper 272: Statin use is associated with a higher incidence of pneumonia

Daniels KR et al The Impact of Statins on the Incidence of Bacteremia and Pneumonia in Military Personnel. 52nd *Interscience Conference on Antimicrobial Agents and Chemotherapy* Sep 09, 2012

Dr Kelly Daniels from the University of Texas was the head researcher in this study. This study sought to determine if statin use is associated with bacteraemia or pneumonia. The study included 14,821 statin-users and 52,787 nonusers.

The study observed:

- There was no difference in the incidence of bacteraemia in statin users and nonusers.
- Statin users had a 15% increased risk of pneumonia compared to nonusers.

Paper 273: Statin use increases severe cases of pneumonia requiring hospitalization by 61%

Dublin S et al Statin use and risk of community acquired pneumonia in older people: population based case-control study. *British Medical Journal* 338:b2137 16 June 2009

The objective of this University of Washington study was to test the effects of statins on pneumonia. It looked at 1,125 cases of pneumonia and matched them against 2,235 controls in people aged 65 to 94.

The study recorded:

- Statin users had a 26% increased risk of pneumonia compared to nonusers.
- Statin users had a 61% increased risk of severe cases of pneumonia requiring hospitalization.

Paper 274:
Statin use is associated with a 60% increased risk of interstitial lung abnormalities in smokers

Xu JF et al Statins and pulmonary fibrosis: the potential role of NLRP3 inflammasome activation. *American Journal of Respiratory and Critical Care* Medicine 2012 Mar 1;185(5):547-56

Dr Jin-Fu Xu (an expert in pulmonary diseases), and his team from Harvard Medical School, evaluated the association between statin use and interstitial lung disease in smokers. The study included 2,115 subjects who were smokers and had had a CT scan. (A CT (computerised tomography) scan uses X-rays and a computer to create detailed images of the inside of the body.)

- Dr Xu's team found that, in people that smoke, statin users have a 60% increased risk of interstitial lung abnormalities compared to those who don't take statins.

Dr Xu concludes: "*Our findings demonstrate that statin use is associated with interstitial lung abnormalities among current and former smokers*".

Paper 275:
Link between statin use and interstitial lung disease

Walker T et al Potential link between HMG-CoA reductase inhibitor (statin) use and interstitial lung disease. *Medical Journal of Australia* 2007 Jan 15;186(2):91-4

Dr Tim Walker from Geelong Hospital Australia describes seven patients who developed interstitial lung disease while on statin treatment. Interstitial lung disease refers to a group of lung diseases affecting the interstitium (the tissue and space around the air sacs of the lungs). (Interstitial pneumonitis is a type of interstitial lung disease.)

Patient 1

- A 78-year-old woman was admitted to hospital with shortness of breath and a dry cough.
- She had been taking atorvastatin 10 mg per day for one year.
- Investigations revealed extensive fibrous connective tissue (fibrosis) in the lungs.
- Atorvastatin was withdrawn.
- Her lung function got slowly worse, and she still had shortness of breath at a three year check up.

Patient 2

- A 78-year-old man sought medical attention at hospital after suffering from shortness of breath for three weeks.
- He had been taking pravastatin 40 mg daily for ten years.
- Investigations revealed extensive emphysema, fibrosis and impaired lung function.
- He initially continued statin treatment and experienced respiratory failure necessitating home oxygen therapy before stopping statins.
- He died 18 months later of respiratory failure.

Patient 3

- A 74-year-old woman was admitted to hospital with a cough and fever of three days duration, (consistent with pneumonia), and a background of worsening shortness of breath.
- She had been taking simvastatin 10 mg daily for two years, then 20 mg daily for one year.
- Investigations found extensive infiltration (fluid, fibrosis) of the lungs and a biopsy led to a diagnosis of interstitial pneumonitis.
- Simvastatin was withdrawn.
- There was a gradual reduction in infiltrate, and her lung function was stable at a nine-month follow up.

Patient 4

- An 83-year-old man arrived at hospital with shortness of breath which had worsened over a six month period.
- He had been taking pravastatin for one year.

- Investigations revealed he had fibrosis.
- He stopped taking pravastatin.
- Despite withdrawal of pravastatin his condition slowly worsened.

Patient 5

- A 67-year-old woman sought medical help after suffering with shortness of breath for nine months and a dry cough for six months.
- She had been taking simvastatin for five years.
- Investigations found patchy infiltration of her lungs and she had a TLCO of 22%. (TLCO is *Transfer factor of the lung for carbon monoxide* and is the extent to which oxygen passes from the air sacs of the lungs into the blood. A low TLCO indicates fibrosis and restrictive lung disease.)
- She stopped taking simvastatin.
- She had a marked improvement: TLCO increased to 51% after one month, and improved further to 65% after one year.

Patient 6

- A 68-year-old man was admitted to hospital with worsening shortness of breath and hypoxia. (Hypoxia is where there is not enough oxygen getting to the tissues of the body.)
- He had been taking simvastatin for two years.
- Investigations revealed he had inflammation and fibrosis in the lungs.
- He continued to take simvastatin.
- He died nine months later from heart disease exacerbated by interstitial lung disease.

Patient 7

- A 64-year-old man sought medical attention for worsening shortness of breath and a dry cough.
- He had been taking atorvastatin 20 mg daily for three years, then 40 mg daily for two years.
- Investigations found the patient had fibrosis. He had a TLCO of 44%.

- Atorvastatin was withdrawn.
- He had an improvement in his condition. His TLCO increased to 52% after two months.

Dr Walker also reviewed some other adverse side effects that statins may cause.

He found:

- The most commonly reported adverse effects include gastrointestinal upset, headache, rash and a dose-dependent elevation in levels of liver transaminases (enzymes).
- The most potentially serious, adverse effects include myopathy (muscle disease) and polyneuropathy (life threatening neurological disorder that occurs when many nerves throughout the body malfunction simultaneously).
- Statins have been associated with lung diseases, lupus-like syndromes and muscle and skin inflammation diseases.
- Many patients take statin therapy for many months or years before these symptoms develop.
- Their clinical features vary in severity from mild dry cough and rash through to severe and progressive respiratory failure.

Dr Walker concluded: "*We hope that our description of our patients and review of the possible role of statins in interstitial lung disease will raise awareness of the potential association between statin therapy and this uncommon and often fatal condition*".

Paper 276:
Statins induce pneumonia

Lantuejoul S et al Statin-induced fibrotic nonspecific interstitial pneumonia. *European Respiratory Journal* 2002; 19:577-580

Professor Sylvie Lantuejoul reports a case of statin-induced lung injury, with a pattern of nonspecific interstitial pneumonia.

- A 51-year-old male was admitted to hospital with fever, polymyalgia, cough and progressive dyspnoea for one month. He was been treated with simvastatin (Zocor) (5 mg·day) for six years.
- Drug-induced pneumonitis (inflammation of the lungs) was highly suspected, so the simvastatin was discontinued and a corticosteroid therapy was added.

- One month later, the patients symptoms had not improved and investigations led to a diagnosis of fibrotic nonspecific interstitial pneumonia.
- Six months later, a progressive response to corticosteroid therapy was observed with improvement of symptoms.
- One month later, pravastatin (pravachol) was inadvertently introduced, and he rapidly deteriorated. He had shortness of breath, muscle pain and tests revealed abnormal substances in his lungs.
- Statins were stopped, which led to progressive improvement.

Paper 277:
Simvastatin induced chylothorax

Volatron AC et al Simvastatin-induced chylothorax.
Revue des Maladies Respiratoires 2003 Apr;20(2 Pt 1):291-3

Chylothorax refers to the presence of lymphatic fluid in the pleural space (the cavity between the lungs and chest wall) resulting from leakage from the thoracic duct or one of its main tributaries.

Loss of lymphatic into pleural space can lead to shock or the patient may exhibit clinical features of severe malnutrition because of the loss of essential proteins, immunoglobulin's, fat, vitamins, electrolytes, and water. Mortality rates are high in patients with untreated chylothorax.

This paper chronicles the case of a man who developed chylothorax while taking statins.

- A 69-year-old male sought medical attention for back pain, fatigue, dry cough and shortness of breath on exertion.
- He had been taking simvastatin for two years.
- Chest examination revealed decreased lung function and lymphatic fluid in the pleural space.
- Laboratory tests showed he had inflammation.
- A biopsy found the existence of a chronic pleural thickening.
- The patient discontinued the simvastatin therapy.
- Within a few weeks, he had a significant improvement in his general condition, with the disappearance of pain and inflammation and his shortness of breath improved.
- It is noted he had no recurrence of chylothorax after several months.

Paper 278:
Statin induced pneumonia

Yoshioka S et al A case of drug-induced pneumonia possibly associated with simvastatin. *Journal of the Japanese Respiratory Society* 2005 Oct;43(10):600-4

Dr Sumako Yoshioka from the Nagasaki University School of Medicine illustrates the case of a woman who developed statin induced pneumonia.

- A 59-year-old woman was admitted to hospital because of general fatigue, cough and progressive dyspnea (shortness of breath) about five months after starting simvastatin.
- Investigations revealed disease in the right middle and lower lung.
- The patient had a high eosinophil count. (A eosinophil is a type of white blood cell. High numbers indicate disease or infection such as lung disease.)
- Simvastatin was discontinued and her condition improved.
- Tests were conducted which led to a diagnosis of statin induced eosinophilic pneumonia.

Dr Yoshioka concluded: *"We should be aware of lung side effects of HMG-CoA reductase inhibitor (statins)"*.

Paper 279:
Simvastatin causes widespread muscle disease which leads to death

Boltan DD et al Fatal and widespread skeletal myopathy confirmed morphologically years after initiation of simvastatin therapy. *American Journal of Cardiology* 2007 Apr 15;99(8):1171-6

This paper, by Dr David Boltan a specialist in internal medicine, outlines the case of a patient who died with widespread muscle disease caused by statin therapy.

- A 59-year-old man had a heart attack (26 months before death). He had been taking simvastatin 20 mg per day for six years.
- He had a coronary artery bypass and his simvastatin was increased to 40 mg per day.

- 22 months later (four months before death), he noticed muscle weakness in both legs and was hospitalised.
- A biopsy revealed muscle damage and the simvastatin was stopped.
- He was transferred to another hospital (46 days before death) because of worsening muscle weakness, swallowing difficulties, difficulty in speaking and shortness of breath.
- Examinations revealed he was frail and chronically ill. His peripheral muscles were severely weak; he had no tendon reflexes and was unable to walk.
- His creatine kinase, alanine aminotransferase and aspartate aminotransferase levels were elevated.
- Because of his worsening health he was placed on a ventilator, a tracheotomy was performed (an operation to open up the windpipe) and haemodialysis was started.
- However, he never improved, and his muscle weakness worsened to the point where he was unable to lift either his arms or legs, or move about in bed, and he died.
- An autopsy revealed he had extensive muscular loss and his lungs contained fluid and abscesses. He had necrotising bronchopneumonia (where the pneumonia causes the death of lung tissue).

Dr Boltan concluded: "*He had widespread acute and chronic myopathy involving apparently all of his striated skeletal muscle and possibly also his cardiac muscle. It appears reasonable to attribute the myopathy in him to simvastatin therapy because other recognised causes of myopathy were ruled out during his extensive clinical evaluation*".

Paper 280:
Statins may induce interstitial lung disease

Fernández AB et al Statins and interstitial lung disease: a systematic review of the literature and of food and drug administration adverse event reports. *Chest* 2008 Oct;134(4):824-30

This study is a review of the scientific literature by Dr Antonio Fernández and his colleagues from Yale University School of Medicine. The review examined the relationship between statins and interstitial lung disease. (Interstitial lung disease is the name for a large group of diseases that inflame or scar the lungs. The inflammation and scarring make it hard to get enough oxygen. The scarring is called pulmonary fibrosis.)

After reviewing evidence from the previous 20 years the researchers reported:

- Interstitial lung disease has been reported with most statins, suggesting that statin-induced interstitial lung disease is a class effect (caused by all statins) and not a specific statin effect.
- The mechanism of injury in possible statin- induced interstitial lung disease, as in most causes of interstitial lung disease, is unknown.
- The time to the onset of symptoms can vary from months to years after initiation of statin therapy.

Dr Fernández concluded: *"Statin-induced interstitial lung disease is a possible newly recognized side effect of statin therapy"*.

Paper 281:
Rosuvastatin leads to worsening fatigue in heart failure patients

Perez AC et al Effect of rosuvastatin on fatigue in patients with heart failure. *Journal of the American College of Cardiology* 2013 Mar 12;61(10):1121-2

This study, based at the University of Glasgow and headed by Dr Ana Cristina Perez, investigated the effects of statins on fatigue in patients with heart failure. The study lasted 7.5 months and included 5,010 patients with chronic systolic heart failure, aged 60 years or over, who received either 10 mg rosuvastatin or placebo daily. The patients were asked to rate their fatigue on a zero to four scale with zero representing no fatigue and four representing the most severe fatigue.

The study pinpointed:

- Compared with placebo patients, 2.8% more statin treated patients reported worsening of fatigue.
- Compared with placebo patients, 1.2% fewer statin treated patients reported improvement in fatigue.
- 39 more patients in the statin group worsened to grade three fatigue compared to the placebo group.

- Five more patients in the statin group worsened to grade four fatigue compared to the placebo group.

Dr Perez concluded: *"In this post hoc analysis of a large randomised, double-blind, placebo-controlled trial, we found some evidence that rosuvastatin leads to worsening fatigue"*.

Paper 282:
Statins cause a drop in energy levels and more fatigue

Golomb BA et al Effects of Statins on Energy and Fatigue With Exertion: Results From a Randomized Controlled Trial. *Archives of Internal Medicine* 2012 Aug 13:1-2

Professor Beatrice Golomb and her team of researchers from the University of California examined the impact of statins on energy or exertional fatigue. The study lasted for six months and included 1,016 subjects, (692 men 20 years or older and 324 nonprocreative women), who were allocated to receive either: 20-mg simvastatin, 40-mg pravastatin or placebo. The subjects rated their energy and fatigue with exertion levels at the start of the study and after six months.

The study ascertained:

- Those taking statins (simvastatin or pravastatin) had a significant drop in energy and more fatigue on exertion. Women were more affected than men especially those taking simvastatin.
- Four in ten women taking simvastatin cited worsening of energy or exertional fatigue compared to women taking placebo.
- Two in ten women taking simvastatin cited worsening of energy and exertional fatigue compared to women taking placebo.
- Two in ten women taking simvastatin rated themselves "much worse" energy or exertional fatigue compared to women taking placebo.
- One in ten women taking simvastatin rated themselves "much worse" energy and exertional fatigue compared to women taking placebo.

Professor Golomb advised: *"Physicians should be alert to patients' reports of exertional fatigue or diminished energy during statin use"*.

Paper 283:
Statins, fibrates and beta blockers increase fatigue during moderate intensity exercise

Eagles CJ et al The effects of combined treatment with beta 1-selective receptor antagonists and lipid-lowering drugs on fat metabolism and measures of fatigue during moderate intensity exercise: a placebo-controlled study in healthy subjects. *British Journal of Clinical Pharmacology* 1997 Mar;43(3):291-300

This Birmingham based study assessed the effects of different combinations of beta blockers (metoprolol and atenolol) and cholesterol-lowering drugs (fluvastatin and bezafibrate) on fatigue, during moderate intensity exercise in healthy young volunteers. The study included 14 healthy men and women, average age 21.9 years, who completed five, 90-minute walks after been treated with either four different combinations of metoprolol or atenolol and fluvastatin or bezafibrate, or placebo.

The study observed:

- Fat oxidation was between 24% to 40 % lower in subjects treated with beta blockers and cholesterol lowering drugs compared to subjects on placebo. (Fat oxidation is the process of breaking down fatty acids, which releases energy.)
- Ammonia levels were between 51% to 170 % higher in subjects treated with beta blockers and cholesterol lowering drugs compared to subjects on placebo. (High ammonia levels can lead to lack of energy and brain damage.)
- Scores on the *Hardy and Rejeski Feeling Scale* (a measure of how good or bad you feel) were significantly lower in subjects treated with beta blockers and cholesterol lowering drugs compared to subjects on placebo. (E.g. subjects treated with beta blockers and cholesterol lowering drugs felt worse compared to subjects on placebo.)
- Subjects treated with beta blockers and cholesterol lowering drugs found it took between: 12% to 40% more perceived cardiorespiratory effort to complete the walks compared to subjects on placebo.
- Subjects treated with beta blockers and cholesterol lowering drugs found it took between: 22% to 40% more perceived

leg effort to complete the walks compared to subjects on placebo.

- Subjects treated with beta blockers and cholesterol lowering drugs suffered 22% to 45% more perceived leg pain compared to subjects on placebo.

In healthy volunteers, this UK study revealed that combinations of beta blockers and cholesterol lowering drugs were associated with increased fatigue during moderate intensity exercise.

Paper 284:
Statins make people less likely to exercise

Lee DS et al Statins and Physical Activity in Older Men: The Osteoporotic Fractures in Men Study. *Journal of the American Medical Association Internal Medicine* 2014 Aug;174(8):1263-70

The objective of the study was to determine the effects of statins on physical activity. The study lasted for nine years and included 4,137 men (989 men (24%) were statin users and 3148 (76%) were nonusers) aged 65 years and older. The Physical Activity Scale for the Elderly (PASE) was used to measure physical activity. (A higher PASE score indicates a higher level of activity.)

The study revealed:

- At the start of the study statin users had a 5.8 points lower PASE score than nonusers.
- PASE score declined by 2.5 points per year for nonusers.
- PASE score declined by 2.8 points per year for prevalent users of statins.
- PASE score declined by 3.4 points per year for new users of statins.
- Statin users engaged in 5.4 fewer minutes in moderate physical activity per day than nonusers.
- Statin users engaged in 0.6 fewer minutes in vigorous physical activity per day than nonusers.
- Statin users engaged in 7.6 more minutes in sedentary behaviour per day than nonusers.

Lead author of the study, David Lee, an Assistant Professor at Orgeon State University and the Oregon Health and Science College of Pharmacy, said: *"Physical activity in older adults helps to maintain a proper weight, prevent cardiovascular disease and helps to maintain physical strength and function. We're trying to find ways to get older adults to exercise more, not less. It's a fairly serious concern if use of statins is doing something that makes people less likely to exercise".*

Paper 285:
Statins block the ability of exercise to improve fitness levels

Mikus CR et al Simvastatin impairs exercise training adaptations. *Journal of the American College of Cardiology* 2013 Apr 10. pii: S0735-1097(13)01403-4

This study sought to determine if simvastatin hindered the positive effects of exercise for obese and overweight adults. The study, which lasted for 12 weeks, included 37 sedentary overweight or obese adults (aged 25-59) with at least two metabolic syndrome risk factors, who completed either:

- 12 weeks of aerobic exercise training.
- 12 weeks of aerobic exercise training in combination with simvastatin (40 mg per day).

The study identified:

- Cardiorespiratory fitness increased by 10% in response to exercise training alone, but was blunted by the addition of simvastatin resulting in only a 1.5% increase.
- Skeletal muscle mitochondrial content (the cells' energy production sites) increased by 13% in the exercise only group (a normal response following exercise training) but decreased by 4.5% in the simvastatin plus exercise group.

One of the study authors, John Thyfault, an Associate Professor of Nutrition and Exercise Physiology at the University of Missouri School of Medicine, concluded: "*Daily physical activity is needed to maintain or improve fitness, and thus improve health outcomes. However, if patients start exercising and taking statins at the same time, it seems that statins block the ability of exercise to improve their fitness levels.*"

Paper 286:
Do statins cause a deterioration in pain-free walking?

Bregar U et al The influence of atorvastatin on walking performance in peripheral arterial disease. *Vasa* 2009 May;38(2):155-9

This study investigated if statins could improve walking performance in patients with peripheral arterial disease. The patients were divided into two groups, the statin group (atorvastatin 20 mg/day), and the control group (placebo), and were asked to practice interval exercise for at least half an hour per day unto a maximum of one hour per day.

The study also measured the Ankle Brachial Pressure Index. The Ankle Brachial Pressure Index (ABPI), known more commonly as an ABI, is the ratio of the blood pressure in the lower legs to the blood pressure in the arms. Compared to the arm, lower blood pressure in the leg is an indication of blocked arteries (peripheral vascular disease). The ABI is calculated by dividing the systolic blood pressure at the ankle by the systolic blood pressures in the arm.

The study found:

- The ankle-brachial pressure index (ABPI) did not change significantly in either group.
- After 3 months, the pain-free walking distance increased 41% in the statin group.
- After 3 months, the pain-free walking distance increased 100% in the placebo group.

To conclude:

- Statins did not improve peripheral arterial disease (no change in the ankle-brachial pressure index).
- The placebo group increased their pain-free walking distance by an extra 59% compared to the statin users.

It may be argued that statins inhibited the expected progress of pain-free walking distance that three months of regular exercise should induce.

Paper 287:
Statins and muscle problems in athletes

Sinzinger H et al Professional athletes suffering from familial hypercholesterolaemia rarely tolerate statin treatment because of muscular problems. *British Journal of Pharmacology* 2004 Apr;57(4):525-8

Dr Helmut Sinzinger analysed the effect of statin treatment on professional athletes. The study included 22 professional athletes who were monitored for eight years.

The study reported:

- Only six out of the 22 finally tolerated at least one member of the statin drugs (atorvastatin, fluvastatin, lovastatin, pravastatin, simvastatin).
- In three of these six the first statin prescribed allowed training performance without any limitation.
- Changing the drug demonstrated that only two out of the 22 tolerated all of the statins examined.

Dr Sinzinger concluded: "*These findings indicate that in top sports performers only about 20% tolerate statin treatment without side-effects*".

Paper 288: Atorvastatin linked to lactic acidosis

Neale R et al Statin precipitated lactic acidosis? *Journal of Clinical Pathology* 2004 Sep;57(9):989-90

Lactic acidosis occurs when the blood becomes too acidic due to the presence of excess lactic acid in the body. As lactic acid builds up, symptoms such as nausea and vomiting, abdominal pain, weakness, rapid breathing, rapid heart rate or irregular heart rhythm, and mental status changes can occur. Lactic acidosis can be a serious condition leading to life-threatening complications such as shock.

This paper reports the case of a woman who developed lactic acidosis following statin treatment.

- An 82-year-old woman was admitted to hospital with worsening shortness of breath.
- She had been taking atorvastatin for at least 18 months.
- She had a deficiency of carbon dioxide in the arterial blood which is known to be a feature of lactic acidosis.
- Her lactic acid levels were raised.
- Her atorvastatin was stopped and she immediately improved.
- Her lactate acid levels returned to normal, and her shortness of breath was moderately improved.

- Subsequently, thiamine (vitamin B1) was also shown to be deficient. (Best sources of vitamin B1 include bacon, pork and organ meats.)

Professor Tim Reynolds, one of the study authors, concluded: "*The acidosis was thought to have been the result of a mitochondrial defect caused by a deficiency of two cofactors, namely: ubiquinone (as a result of inhibition by statin) and thiamine (as a result of dietary deficiency)*".

Paper 289:
Lactic acidosis may develop as a complication of simvastatin therapy

Goli AK et al Simvastatin-induced lactic acidosis: a rare adverse reaction? *Clinical Pharmacology and Therapeutics* 2002 Oct;72(4):461-4

Dr Anil Goli describes the case of a 53-year-old man with lactic acidosis. He had been taking simvastatin, 40 mg, every day for three years.

- o He had nausea, poor appetite, and progressive generalized weakness and malaise of three to four weeks' duration.
- o The man had high levels (1,390 U/L) of creatine kinase. (Normal levels are between 35 – 175 U/L.) An elevated level of creatine kinase is seen in heart attacks, when the heart muscle is damaged, or in conditions that produce damage to the skeletal muscles or brain.
- o He had high levels (2,303 U/L) of aspartate aminotransferase. (Normal levels are between 5 – 40 U/L.) Elevated levels of aspartate aminotransferase indicate damage has occurred in a variety of tissues including liver, heart, muscle, kidney, and brain.
- o He had high levels (1,707 U/L) of alanine aminotransferase. (Normal levels are between 7 – 56 U/L.) High levels of alanine aminotransferase are associated with liver injury.

The patient's simvastatin therapy was discontinued.

- After two days, his symptoms and acidosis was resolved.
- After four days, his creatine kinase level returned to normal.
- After seven days, his aspartate aminotransferase and alanine aminotransferase levels normalised.

Dr Goli concluded: "*We offer evidence that lactic acidosis may develop as a complication of simvastatin therapy*".

Paper 290: Statins impair the ability of muscles to recover from damage

Voermans NC et al Statin-disclosed acid maltase deficiency. *Journal of Internal Medicine* 2005 Aug;258(2):196-7

Acid maltase (an enzyme) deficiency is a genetic disorder affecting muscle tissue. Voermans notes that the absence of the enzyme acid maltase leads to an excessive accumulation of glycogen in many organs including the central nervous system, heart, liver and skeletal muscles. In muscle, this initially results in exercise-induced muscle pain and exercise intolerance.

Neurologist Dr Nicol Voermans chronicles the case of a man who suffered abdominal pain and muscle cramps after starting statins.

- A 34-year-old man had suffered from a stroke, after which he recovered completely. He stopped smoking and was prescribed simvastatin.
- Soon afterwards, he reported severe upper abdominal pain. Moreover, he experienced muscle cramps in his calves.
- Physical examination showed he had an enlarged liver.
- Laboratory investigations revealed increased liver enzymes and creatine kinase (indicating liver and muscle damage).
- Switch of simvastatin to atorvastatin resulted in neither clinical nor biochemical improvement.
- Symptoms completely disappeared after withdrawal of statins.
- Investigations revealed he had acid maltase deficiency.

Dr Voermans concludes: "*Several factors are involved in statin-induced myopathy (muscle disease), for instance reduced cholesterol content of the membrane, which causes membrane instability. More recent work suggests that altered mitochondrial function is involved in statin-associated myopathy. In summary, muscle cells in acid maltase deficiency are probably more susceptible to exercise-induced injury, whereas statins may impair the ability of the muscle to appropriately respond to, and recover from, this damage*".

Paper 291:
Statins, lack of energy and ubiquinone (Coenzyme Q10)

Reidenberg MM Statins, lack of energy and ubiquinone.
British Journal of Clinical Pharmacology
2005 May; 59(5): 606–607

Professor Marcus M Reidenberg is a Professor of Pharmacology at Weill Cornell Medical College. He notes that the painful or tender muscle disease with elevated creatine phosphokinase levels due to statin drugs is well described. Statin muscle disease can also occur without elevated creatine phosphokinase levels or pain. More common is a feeling of lack of energy in people taking these drugs. Since statins block mevalonate synthesis, they lower levels of ubiquinone (coenzyme Q10), an essential compound for mitochondrial energy production. Thus, these people may truly lack energy.

Professor Reidenberg reports:

- A randomised double-blind trial comparing 35 mg coenzyme Q10 with placebo was initiated for patients on statins who felt lack of pep or energy since starting the statins and who did not have muscle pain, tenderness, or elevated creatine phosphokinase.
- By the time this trial started, most patients with these symptoms either stopped the statin or started coenzyme Q10 on their own, thus only three subjects were accrued in 1.5 years and the trial was stopped.
- The three subjects' ages were 68, 69, and 75. Their coenzyme Q10 levels prior to the coenzyme Q10 supplementation were 0.40, 0.35, and 0.36 $\mu g\ ml^{-1}$ (normal values are 0.69 - 1.06).
- Two subjects received placebo and one received coenzyme Q10.
- After two weeks, subjects were asked how they felt. Both subjects taking placebo felt unchanged during the treatment period. The patient receiving coenzyme Q10 stated that several days after starting the study drug, she felt more energetic and could now walk 20 (short New York City) blocks instead of the two blocks that tired her before.
- One of the placebo patients was given coenzyme Q10 for an additional two-week period. After two weeks, he claimed

that he had more energy climbing stairs and was less tired than before.

- Statins lower levels of coenzyme Q10 and our subjects had levels below normal values.
- Statins decrease mitochondrial activity.
- Preliminary data suggests that coenzyme Q10 may reverse the age-related change in skeletal muscle fibre composition.

Professor Reidenberg concludes: "*Whether the level of fatigue and feeling of lack of energy in some people taking statins is related to skeletal muscle effects of these drugs is unknown. The results of this abbreviated randomized double-blind trial suggest it may be due to decreased ubiquinone (coenzyme Q10) levels due to effective statin inhibition of mevalonate synthesis. This would be an unintended adverse effect of the intended pharmacological action of the statin. People taking statins who describe lack of pep or energy may really lack energy because of a deficiency of ubiquinone (coenzyme Q10)*".

Paper 292: Doctor postulates that statins should not be used when exercising

Unnikrishnan D et al Exertion-induced rhabdomyolysis in a patient on statin therapy. *Nephrology, Dialysis, Transplantation* 2005 Jan;20(1):244

This paper illustrates the case of a patient on long-term statin treatment who developed acute renal failure from rhabdomyolysis following severe unaccustomed exertion.

- A 57-year-old male (on atorvastatin 10 mg daily for several years) went trekking and described it as "the most exhausting exercise in recent times".
- Coming downhill, he noticed thigh pain and took two doses of a non-steroidal anti-inflammatory drug (NSAID).
- On day three, his urine output decreased; examination showed blood pressure 160/100 mmHg and clinical evidence of fluid overload.
- Investigations showed: elevated blood urea 141 mg/dl, creatinine 9.4 mg/dl, potassium 6.4 mEq/l, and mildly deranged liver functions.

- Rhabdomyolysis was diagnosed with elevated levels of creatine kinase (CK): 3,389 IU/l (normal 38–174 IU/l), as was lactate dehydrogenase 469 U/l (140–300 U/l) and serum myoglobin 617 μg/l (5–85 μg/l).
- He developed kidney failure.
- Haemodialysis was performed for hyperkalaemia (elevated potassium) and volume overload.
- Atorvastatin was stopped.
- Urine output improved by the fourth day of hospitalization and renal functions started improving in one week.
- At six weeks, urea was 32 mg/dl and creatinine 1.0 mg/dl.

The lead author of the paper, Dr Dilip Unnikrishnan notes: "*It is probable that treatment with statins amplified the muscle damage caused by intense exertion. Statins inhibit GTP (Guanosine-5-triphosphate) activation. (GTP is used as a source of energy for protein synthesis.) Exercise may unmask the effects of statins on skeletal muscle because GTP-dependent protein kinase pathways are important in muscle recovery following exercise*".

Dr Unnikrishnan concluded: "*Based on the association noted, it needs to be considered whether statins should be withheld prior to engaging in 'more than an accustomed range' of physical exertion*".

Paper 293:
Statin use increases muscle damage after exercise

Parker BA et al Effect of Statins on Creatine Kinase Levels Before and After a Marathon Run. *American Journal of Cardiology* 2012 Jan 15;109(2):282-7

Elevation of creatine kinase levels is an indication of damage to muscle. It is therefore indicative of injury, rhabdomyolysis (kidney damage), heart attack, inflammation of the muscles and inflammation of the heart muscle.

The head investigator in this study, Assistant Professor Beth Taylor (formerly Parker), is Director of Exercise Physiology Research at Hartford Hospital. Her research focuses on age and sex differences in vascular function and cardiovascular responses to exercise. This study measured total creatine kinase levels, and the levels of creatine kinase in the heart muscle in 37 subjects treated with statins and 43 non-statin-treated controls running the 2011 Boston Marathon.

The study observed:

- The exercise-related increase in creatine kinase 24 hours after exercise was greater in the statin users than in the controls.
- The increase in creatine kinase in the heart muscle 24 hours after exercise was also greater in the statin users than in the controls.
- Older runners who were statin users had higher increases in creatine kinase.

Professor Taylor finishes: *"In conclusion, our results show that statins increase exercise-related muscle injury"*.

Paper 294:
Statins exacerbate exercise-induced skeletal muscle injury

Thompson PD et al Lovastatin increases exercise-induced skeletal muscle injury. *Metabolism* 1997 Oct;46(10):1206-10

Researchers from the University of Pittsburgh investigated the association between statins, exercise and creatine kinase levels (high levels of creatine kinase are a marker for muscle damage) using a double-blind, placebo-controlled design. The study included 59 healthy men aged 18 to 65 years who were assigned to receive lovastatin (40 mg per day) or placebo for five weeks. The men completed 45 minutes of treadmill walking after four weeks of treatment.

- The study found that the creatine kinase levels of the men who received lovastatin were 62% and 77% higher 24 and 48 hours after the treadmill exercise compared to the men who received placebo.

The researchers finished: "*We conclude that HMG-CoA reductase inhibitors (statins) exacerbate exercise-induced skeletal muscle injury*".

Paper 295:
Statins impair energy production and promote muscle damage

Wu JS et al Evaluation of skeletal muscle during calf exercise by 31-phosphorus magnetic resonance spectroscopy in patients on statin medications. *Muscle and Nerve* 2011 Jan;43(1):76-81

Phosphocreatine is a substance that is fundamental to the ability of the body to produce muscular energy.

Elevated blood levels of creatine kinase are indicative of muscle damage.

The study evaluated the association of statin treatment on recovery from exercise. The study included ten patients, (who were subject to a four-week regimen of statin therapy), who had their phosphocreatine and creatine kinase levels measured pre- and post-statin therapy.

The study ascertained:

- Phosphocreatine levels took 97% longer to recover from exercise after statin therapy.
- Creatine kinase levels rose by 17.7% after statin therapy.

The results of the study suggest that statin therapy may impair energy production and promote muscle damage.

Paper 296: Statin use leads to more falls and a decline in muscle strength

Scott D et al Statin therapy, muscle function and falls risk in community-dwelling older adults. *QJM* 2009 Sep;102(9):625-33

The first author of the study was Dr David Scott, an expert in sarcopenia (sarcopenia can be defined as the age-related loss of muscle mass, strength and function). The aim of this 2.6-year study of 774 older adults was to describe the differences between statin users and nonusers in leg strength, leg muscle quality and fall risk.

The study revealed:

- Statin users had more falls than non-statin users.
- Statin users had decreased leg strength compared to non-statin users.
- Statin users had lower muscle quality compared to non-statin users.
- Statin users had decreased leg strength and lower muscle quality compared to those who had ceased statin use.

Dr Scott commented: "*The results from this longitudinal study suggest that statin therapy may be associated with greater declines in strength and muscle quality, and greater increases in falls risk in the population of community-dwelling older adults".*

Paper 297:
Statin users have poorer leaning balance which may potentially increase their fall risk

Haerer W t al Relationships between HMG-CoA reductase inhibitors (statin) use and strength, balance and falls in older people. *Internal Medicine Journal* 2012 Dec;42(12):1329-34

This Australian study investigated the association between statin use and physical functioning in older people. The study included 500 participants, aged 70-90 years, who were followed for 12 months.

- The study found that statin users had poorer leaning balance which may potentially increase their fall risk.

Paper 298:
Statins increase the risk of falling in the elderly

Lee JS et al Medical illnesses are more important than medications as risk factors of falls in older community dwellers? A cross-sectional study. *Age and Ageing* 2006 May;35(3):246-51

This study investigated the cause of falls in elderly people. The study included 4,000 men and women aged 65 years or over who were followed for 12 months.

Regarding statins, the study found:

- Those using statins had a 19% increased risk of any fall compared to those not using statins.
- Those using statins had a 67% increased risk of recurrent falls compared to those not using statins.

The information gleaned from this chapter points the finger of guilt at statins that they may possibly aggravate asthma, cause lung disease and stop people exercising:

- Asthma symptoms increased by more than 30% in statin users.

- Patients have a decrease in lung function when taking statins.
- Statin drug use leads to an increased risk of lung diseases.
- Fatigue and a drop in energy is experienced with statin use.
- Statins cause the lack of energy by coenzyme Q10 depletion and GTP inhibition.
- The ability to exercise is hampered by statins:
  - Cellular energy production is impaired.
  - Muscles are damaged.
  - Muscles take longer to recover from exercise.
  - Older people are less likely to exercise and cannot walk as far pain free if they do exercise.
  - The capacity of exercise to improve fitness levels is blocked.
  - 80% of athletes don't tolerate statins.
- In older adults statins cause an increase in falls and decline in muscle strength.

To answer the question: Do statins impair our ability to breathe? The atorvastatin (Lipitor) package insert even warns that the drug may have the unwanted side effect of "*difficulty breathing, collapse*". The insert also states that other statins have caused "*breathing problems including persistent cough and/or shortness of breath*".

Chapter 12

The sinister effects of statins on cognition, neurodegenerative diseases, depression and suicide

Dr Marc Micozzi has had a distinguished 40-year career in medicine. He is an Adjunct Professor in the Department of Pharmacology at Georgetown University School of Medicine. In his career Professor Micozzi has won many awards and received numerous honours. He has held editorial positions and is a manuscript reviewer for many peer-reviewed scientific journals.

Dr Micozzi states: "*Without a doubt, statins affect brain function.*"

He explains: "*Statins cripple your liver's ability to make cholesterol. And your brain needs cholesterol. It enables signal transport across the synapses–a critical, ongoing brain function. Longer term, cholesterol encourages the growth of nerve cells. And it keeps the myelin sheath around nerve cells healthy. The myelin sheath is a layer of fatty substance that insulates each and every nerve cell. Without healthy myelin, the nerve cells in your brain can't communicate with each other*".

This chapter reveals the consequences of statins on the brain. The papers look at the effects of statins on cognition, whether they are involved in neurodegenerative diseases, and their influence on mood, depression and suicide.

Paper 299:
Statins impair brain function

Muldoon MF et al Effects of lovastatin on cognitive function and psychological well-being. *American Journal of Medicine* 2000 May;108(7):538-46

Dr Matthew Muldoon, a specialist in clinical pharmacology, and his associates from the University of Pittsburgh School of Medicine, examined the relationship between statins and brain function. Two hundred and nine generally healthy adults with low-density-lipoprotein (LDL) cholesterol level of 160 mg/dL or higher were randomly assigned to six-month treatment with lovastatin (20 mg) or placebo. Subjects were given neuropsychological tests before the treatment and at six months.

Their findings pinpointed:

- After six months, placebo-treated subjects improved on neuropsychological tests in all five performance domains, consistent with the effects of practice on test performance, whereas those treated with lovastatin improved only on tests of memory recall.
- Subjects on statins showed a significant worsening of attention and slowing down of thought compared to subjects on placebo.

Paper 300:
Statins may be detrimental to cognitive functioning

Muldoon MF et al Randomized trial of the effects of simvastatin on cognitive functioning in hypercholesterolemic adults. *The American Journal of Medicine* 2004 Dec 1;117(11):823-9

Dr Muldoon conducted another study that investigated the effects of statin therapy on cognitive functioning. The study, which employed a randomised double-blind design, comprised 308 adults between 35 and 70 years of age who had low density lipoprotein (LDL) cholesterol levels between 160 – 220 mg/dL (4.1 - 5.7 mmol/L).

For six months the participants were assigned to daily treatment of either:

- o Placebo.
- o 10 mg of simvastatin.
- o 40 mg of simvastatin.

Neuropsychological tests were administered to assess cognitive functioning at the start of the study and at the end of the treatment period.

Based on observations from a previous study, the tests were grouped into three categories:

- o Tests previously observed to be sensitive to statins. E.g. planning and drawing time to complete complex lattice-type perceptual mazes.
- o Tests previously observed to be insensitive to statins. E.g. time required to recode numbers into symbols using a key that pairs each of nine digits with a meaningless shape.
- o Tests not previously administered. E.g. number of errors made when tracing over a star pattern that can be seen only in mirror-reversed view.

The investigations indicated:

- In the tests previously observed to be sensitive to statins, patients on placebo improved their perfomance, whilst patients on statins did not.
- In the tests previously observed to be insensitive to statins there was little difference between the placebo and statin groups, although the placebo group improved slightly more than the statin groups.
- In the tests not previously administered, cognition improved more in the placebo group compared to the statin groups.

The results of the study reveal that statins may be detrimental to cognitive functioning.

Paper 301:
Statins can accelerate memory loss in the elderly

Mandas A et al Cognitive decline and depressive symptoms in late-life are associated with statin use: evidence from a population-based study of Sardinian old people living in their own home. *Neurological Research* 2014 Mar;36(3):247-54

The senior researcher in this study was Antonella Mandas from the department of medical sciences at the University of Cagliari. This study investigated the effects of statins on cognitive functions and mood in older people. The study included 329 subjects aged over 65 years. The participants were assessed using the mini mental state examination (where low scores indicate cognitive impairment) and the geriatric depression scale (where higher scores indicate more severe levels of depression).

- The study found statin users had significantly lower mini mental state examination scores and significantly higher geriatric depression scale scores than nonusers.

Mandas concluded that the study: *"Provides substantial indications that caution should be exercised in the provision of statins in elderly subjects to avoid accelerated memory loss"*.

Paper 302: Statins related to memory dysfunction

Okeahialam BN et al Statin related memory dysfunction in a Nigerian woman: a case report. *Current Drug Safety* 2012 Feb;7(1):33-4

Professor Basil Okeahialam, a consultant physician and cardiologist, describes the case of a woman who with simvastatin developed memory deficits which adversely affected activities of her daily living.

- The woman was first observed in 2005, at 41 years of age, for sensation of weight in the chest.
- She was put on atorvastatin (Lipitor) 10 mg daily.
- Levels of her high density lipoprotein (HDL) cholesterol fell and since low HDL cholesterol increases heart disease risk, the drug was withheld.
- In 2008, she restarted statin treatment, this time she took simvastatin (simvor) 10 mg daily.
- While on this, she complained of feeling ill and cramped up each morning.
- She stopped taking simvastatin.
- In time simvastatin was re-introduced at 20mg daily.
- She started to experience muscle cramps, incoherence in thought and speech as well as memory impairment.
- She reduced the dose to 10 mg daily with some respite in the short term.
- With time and still on 10mg of simvastatin she once again started to have rising muscle pains. Lapses in memory were also observed. She was not remembering things and to her embarrassment, kept repeating instructions which she had

earlier given. The urge to read vanished and if she forced herself to read, she could not absorb.
- She totally discontinued Simvastatin which led to recovery.

Professor Okeahialam also notes that low levels of cholesterol and low levels of low density lipoprotein (LDL) cholesterol may be associated with cognitive dysfunction and concludes: *"It is suggested that patients on statins be monitored for side effects especially memory deficits which can adversely effect quality of life... It may also be unwise to reduce the lipid (cholesterol) sub fractions to very low levels"*.

Paper 303:
Statin therapy causes memory complaints and mood changes

Parker BA et al Changes in Memory Function and Neuronal Activation Associated with Atorvastatin Therapy. *Pharmacotherapy* 2010;30(6):236e–240e

This paper, headed by Dr Beth Parker from the Hartford Hospital, describes a 65-year-old man who reported cognitive complaints (memory complaints and mood changes) after taking atorvastatin 10 mg/day for one year. He had no history of alcohol consumption, major head trauma, psychiatric problems, or memory impairment.

- After one year of taking the statin, the patient described his complaints as "fuzzy thinking" and "brain fog." His wife also noted that the patient demonstrated a progressive decline in cognitive function and memory accompanied by increasing mood changes.
- Cognitive testing and assessment of neuronal activation using functional magnetic resonance imaging (fMRI) (procedure that measures brain activity) were performed during a working memory task while he was receiving atorvastatin therapy.
- The patient demonstrated altered neuronal activation and reduced performance on the cognitive tests, which was consistent with his cognitive symptoms.
- He stopped taking atorvastatin. The cognitive tests were repeated two months after discontinuation of the drug and the patient exhibited improved cognitive test performance

and fMRI patterns similar to those expected in a healthy individual.

- The patient also reported subjective improvement of his cognitive complaints within days of cessation of atorvastatin.

Dr Parker concludes that a: *"growing number of reports suggest that statins evoke adverse cognitive effects"*.

Paper 304: Statins induce a decline in cognition

Padala KP et al Simvastatin-induced decline in cognition. *Annals of Pharmacotherapy* 2006 Oct;40(10):1880-3

This Nebraska Medical Centre paper chronicles a case of new-onset cognitive difficulties in an older patient after initiation of simvastatin therapy.

- A 64-year-old man developed cognitive difficulties (short-term memory loss, long-term memory loss, and item misplacement) within one week after starting simvastatin 40 mg/day.
- Simvastatin was discontinued, and the patient's cognition improved to normal within six weeks.
- He again tried simvastatin, this time at half the original dose and his cognition deteriorated over a two-week period.
- Simvastatin was stopped, and his normal cognition returned within four weeks.

Paper 305: Clinicians should be aware of possible adverse cognitive reactions during statin therapy

Galatti L et al Short-term memory loss associated with rosuvastatin. *Pharmacotherapy* 2006 Aug;26(8):1190-2

This paper reports the case of rosuvastatin-related short-term memory loss.

- A 53-year-old man experienced memory loss after being treated with rosuvastatin at 10 mg per day.
- After discontinuation of rosuvastatin, the neuropsychiatric adverse reaction resolved gradually, suggesting a probable drug association.

- During the following year, the patient remained free from neuropsychiatric disturbances.

The lead researcher of the paper, Dr Laura Galatti a specialist in pharmacology, concluded: "*Clinicians should be aware of possible adverse cognitive reactions during statin therapy*".

Paper 306:
Statins can impair brain functioning

Davies GR Reversible dysphasia and statins. *Journal of Korean Medical Science* 2012 Apr;27(4):458-9

Dysphasia is a partial or complete impairment of the ability to communicate resulting from brain injury.

This paper, authored by Dr Gordon Davies a consultant psychiatrist, presents a case of reversible dysphasia occurring in a patient prescribed atorvastatin.

- A 58-year-old woman was presented for medicolegal examination with regard to a compensation claim involving allegations of harassment at work producing anxiety and depression. At the time of her initial presentation for treatment her general practitioner had noted that her blood pressure was higher than usual and had prescribed the statin Lipitor (atorvastatin) 10 mg per day together with indapamide 2.5 mg per day.
- A few days later, the patient reported that she had developed problems in "word finding" in that her speech would be interrupted because she would be unable to find a word to describe an object.
- The patient ceased the Lipitor and said that her symptoms had resolved quite quickly.
- The patient then commenced on crestor (rosuvastatin) 5 mg daily while continuing on indapamide and four weeks later, at her medico-legal assessment, she was noted to have clear but intermittent difficulty in word finding. She was also tense and tearful at times.
- She was reviewed two weeks later. At this point she had stopped the rosuvastatin and her speech was fluent and clear. She was continuing to take indapamide 2.5 mg per day.

This case highlights the possibility that statins can impair brain functioning. Dr Davies concludes: "*The immediate inference from the above observations is that the patient had developed dysphasia as a direct side effect of the use of simvastatin. That this is likely to have been a generic statin effect is supported by the recurrence of milder symptoms on rosuvastatin and their remission on its cessation*".

Paper 307: Transient global amnesia associated with statin intake

Healy D et al Transient global amnesia associated with statin intake. *British Medical Journal Case Reports* 2009;2009. pii: bcr06.2008.0033

Transient global amnesia is a syndrome where there is a temporary but almost total disruption of short-term memory with a range of problems accessing older memories.

This paper illustrates the case of a man who developed Transient global amnesia after taking statin drugs.

- A 57-year-old man was referred with end-stage renal failure. In 2001, he was started on dialysis for renal failure and was prescribed 40 mg simvastatin.
- His worsening condition in 2004 led to unhappiness and his simvastatin was changed to 10 mg rosuvastatin in December 2004.
- In February 2005, two confusion episodes were noted. In one, he had made 40 cups of tea but could later give no reason for this other than he must have been dreaming of having guests to the house. In the other, during home dialysis he had cut the lines into the dialysis machine with a pair of scissors. He vaguely remembered freeing himself from the lines and retiring to bed.
- This latter incident and concerns that he might be drinking more water than advised led to a referral to the psychiatric liaison service in August 2005 because of possible self-harm. He denied thoughts of self-harm. But he described feeling that there were further episodes of behaviours for which he had no recall. Psychiatric assessment found no evidence of psychotic or delirious phenomena. He was not depressed.
- In September 2005, the patient's wife reported that he was having episodes when he was uncertain where he was or

what he was supposed to be doing. He complained of feeling disorganised at these times.

- Physical investigations returned no evidence of triggers to these episodes.
- In May 2006, he reported that he was completely unable to remember anything for a full day after his previous dialysis session.
- Statin-induced global amnesia was diagnosed.
- He discontinued his statin.
- His difficulties cleared on discontinuation of treatment and he remained symptom free thereafter.

Paper 308:
The use of statins is associated with a significantly increased risk of postoperative delirium among elderly patients undergoing elective surgery

Redelmeier DA et al Delirium after elective surgery among elderly patients taking statins. *Canadian Medical Association Journal* 2008 Sep 23;179(7):645-52

Delirium is a condition of severe confusion and disorientation. Medical problems, surgery and medications can all cause delirium. Postoperative delirium after elective surgery (non emergency surgery) is frequent and potentially serious.

This study sought to determine whether the use of statin medications was associated with a higher risk of postoperative delirium. The study included 284,158 patients aged 65 years and older who were admitted for elective surgery.

- The study found that patients taking statins had a 28% higher rate of delirium compared to patients not taking statins.

Paper 309:
Statins may adversely affect cognition in patients with dementia

Padala KP et al The Effect of HMG: CoA Reductase Inhibitors on Cognition in Patients With Alzheimer's Dementia: A Prospective Withdrawal and Rechallenge Pilot Study. *American Journal of Geriatric Pharmacotherapy* 2012 Oct;10(5):296-302

The aim of this study was to evaluate the impact statins have on cognition. The study included 18 older subjects with Alzheimer's dementia who were on statin therapy who underwent a six-week withdrawal phase of statins followed by a six-week rechallenge with the drug. The primary outcome measure was cognition, measured by the Mini-Mental State Examination (MMSE).

The mini–mental state examination (MMSE) or Folstein test is a brief 30-point questionnaire test that is used to screen for cognitive impairment. It is commonly used in medicine to screen for dementia. Any score greater than or equal to 25 points (out of 30) indicates a normal cognition. Below this, scores can indicate severe (less than 9 points), moderate (10-20 points) or mild (21-24 points) cognitive impairment.

The study indicated:

- The subjects had an improvement in MMSE scores with discontinuation of statins and a decrease in MMSE scores after rechallenge.
- Cholesterol levels increased with statin discontinuation and decreased with rechallenge.

The head investigator of the study, Dr Kalpana P. Padala from the University of Arkansas, concluded that: "*The study found an improvement in cognition with discontinuation of statins and worsening with rechallenge. Statins may adversely affect cognition in patients with dementia*".

Paper 310:
Statins increase the risk of dementia by 19% in the elderly

Li G et al Statin therapy and risk of dementia in the elderly: a community-based prospective cohort study. *Neurology* 2004 Nov 9;63(9):1624-8

This University of Washington study assessed the association between statin therapy and risk of dementia. The study included 2,356 cognitively intact persons, aged 65 and older, who were assessed biennially for dementia.

- The study revealed that statin users had a 19% increased risk of all-cause dementia compared to nonusers.

Paper 311:
Statins increase the risk of Alzheimer's by 21%

Rea TD et al Statin use and the risk of incident dementia: the Cardiovascular Health Study. *Archives of Neurology* 2005 Jul;62(7):1047-51

The study investigated the association of statin use and the risk of dementia. Over an average period of 5.3 years, the study analysed 2,798 adults, aged 65 years and older, who were free of dementia at the start of the study.

The study ascertained:

- Those who used statins had an 8% increased risk of dementia compared to those who had never used cholesterol lowering drugs.
- Those who used statins had a 21% increased risk of Alzheimer's compared to those who had never used cholesterol lowering drugs.

Paper 312:
Statins have a significant negative impact on quality-of-life

Evans MA et al Statin-associated adverse cognitive effects: survey results from 171 patients. *Pharmacotherapy* 2009 Jul;29(7):800-11

The objective of the study, headed by Dr Marcella Evans from the University of California-San Diego, was to characterize the adverse cognitive effects of statins. In the study, a survey was completed by 171 patients (age range 34-86 yrs) who had self-reported memory or other cognitive problems associated with statin therapy.

The study unearthed:

- Of 143 patients who reported stopping statin therapy, 128 (90%) reported improvement in cognitive problems, sometimes within days of statin discontinuation.
- In some patients, a diagnosis of dementia or Alzheimer's disease reportedly was reversed.
- 19 patients whose symptoms improved or resolved after they discontinued statin therapy, and who underwent rechallenge with a statin, exhibited cognitive problems again (multiple times in some).

- Higher potency statins led to higher rates of cognitive-specific adverse drug reaction.
- Quality of life was significantly adversely affected.

Dr Evans concludes: "*Findings from the survey suggest that cognitive problems associated with statin therapy have variable onset and recovery courses, a clear relation to statin potency, and significant negative impact on quality-of-life*".

Paper 313:
Medical researchers conclude that simvastatin should not be used as treatment for multiple sclerosis

Sorensen PS et al Simvastatin as add-on therapy to interferon β-1a for relapsing-remitting multiple sclerosis (SIMCOMBIN study): a placebo-controlled randomised phase 4 trial. *Lancet Neurology* 2011 Aug;10(8):691-701

Medical researchers from the Copenhagen University Hospital investigated the effects of statins in patients relapsing-remitting multiple sclerosis who were receiving the multiple sclerosis drug interferon beta. The three-year study was a placebo-controlled, double-blind, randomised, parallel-group trial and included 307 patients who received either simvastatin or placebo.

The study recorded:

- Patients in the simvastatin group had a 39% higher risk of relapse compared to patients in the placebo group.
- Patients in the simvastatin group had their first relapse 3.4 months earlier than patients in the placebo group.
- Patients in the simvastatin group had a 17% higher risk of new or enlarging lesions compared to patients in the placebo group.
- Patients in the simvastatin group had a 58% reduced chance of having no disease activity.

The researchers concluded: "*The combination of interferon beta and simvastatin should not be used as treatment for relapsing-remitting multiple sclerosis*".

Paper 314:
Statins increase disease activity in multiple sclerosis

Birnbaum G et al Combining beta interferon and atorvastatin

may increase disease activity in multiple sclerosis. *Neurology* 2008 Oct 28;71(18):1390-5

The objective of this randomised double-blind study was to explore the effects of atorvastatin to persons with relapsing-remitting multiple sclerosis taking the multiple sclerosis drug interferon beta-1a. The study included 26 patients with clinically stable, relapsing-remitting MS, on standard high-dose subcutaneous interferon beta-1a. 17 patients received atorvastatin and nine had placebo for six months.

The study pinpointed:

- Ten of the 17 patients on atorvastatin had either new or enhancing lesions or clinical relapses.
- Only one of the nine patients on placebo had a relapse.

The subjects receiving atorvastatin were at greater risk for disease activity compared to placebo.

Paper 315: Strong association between statins and an increased rate of functional decline and muscle cramping in patients with amyotrophic lateral sclerosis

Zinman L et al Are statin medications safe in patients with ALS? *Amyotrophic Lateral Sclerosis* 2008 Aug;9(4):223-8

Amyotrophic lateral sclerosis (the most common motor neurone disease) is a nervous system disease that attacks nerve cells called neurons in your brain and spinal cord which is characterized by rapidly progressive weakness, muscle wasting, and difficulty speaking, difficulty swallowing, and difficulty breathing.

Dr Lorne Zinman, whose research focus is amyotrophic lateral sclerosis and neuromuscular diseases, was the lead scientist in this study. The aim of this study was to determine how statin medications affect patients with amyotrophic lateral sclerosis. The study included 164 patients with amyotrophic lateral sclerosis who were followed for 21 months.

The study found:

- Patients taking statins had a 63% increase in the rate of functional decline compared to patients not taking statins.
- Patients on statin therapy also reported a significant increase in muscle cramp frequency and severity.

Dr Zinman concluded: "*This study has demonstrated a strong association between statin medications and an increased rate of functional decline and muscle cramping in patients with amyotrophic lateral sclerosis*".

Paper 316:
A possible relationship between statins and amyotrophic lateral sclerosis

Edwards IR et al Statins, neuromuscular degenerative disease and an amyotrophic lateral sclerosis-like syndrome: an analysis of individual case safety reports from vigibase. *Drug Safety* 2007;30(6):515-25

The Uppsala Monitoring Centre (UMC) is the name for the World Health Organization Collaborating Centre for International Drug Monitoring.

Professor Ivor Ralph Edwards from the Uppsala Monitoring Centre analysed the UMC data concerning reports of amyotrophic lateral sclerosis (ALS)-like syndrome and statin use.

Edwards reports:

- There is disproportionally high reporting of statin use and amyotrophic lateral sclerosis.
- The disproportionally high reporting of the connection between statins and amyotrophic lateral sclerosis is an important signal since amyotrophic lateral sclerosis is serious clinically and statins are so widely used.

Professor Edwards concluded: "*We do advocate that trial discontinuation of a statin should be considered in patients with serious neuromuscular disease such as the ALS-like syndrome, given the poor prognosis and a possibility that progression of the disease may be halted or even reversed*".

Paper 317:
Statins may be associated with amyotrophic lateral sclerosis

Golomb BA et al Amyotrophic lateral sclerosis-like conditions in possible association with cholesterol-lowering drugs: an analysis of patient reports to the University of California, San Diego (UCSD) Statin Effects Study. *Drug Safety* 2009;32(8):649-61

The study leader, Dr Beatrice Golomb, notes that cases of amyotrophic lateral sclerosis (ALS) or ALS-like conditions have arisen in apparent association with statins (and other cholesterol-lowering drugs). This study sought to find evidence whether the connection may be causal.

The study included ten patients, with either a formal or probable diagnosis of amyotrophic lateral sclerosis arising in association with statin drug therapy.

The study unearthed:

- All patients reported improvement of symptoms with drug discontinuation.
- All patients reported onset or exacerbation of symptoms with drug change, rechallenge or dose increase.

The results from the study suggest that statins (and other cholesterol-lowering drugs) may be associated with amyotrophic lateral sclerosis.

Paper 318: Statin drugs might be harmful for amyotrophic lateral sclerosis patients

Samson K High Cholesterol Levels May Benefit ALS Patients, Study Suggests. *Neurology Today* 17 April 2008 – Volume 8 – Issue 8 – pp 1,9

In the *American Academy of Neurology* publication *Neurology Today,* Kurt Samson reviews a study that investigates the association of cholesterol levels with survival rates in patients with amyotrophic lateral sclerosis. The study included 369 amyotrophic lateral sclerosis patients and 286 healthy individuals.

Samson's review found:

- Amyotrophic lateral patients with considerably higher cholesterol ratios lived, on average, one year longer than patients with lower levels.
- Higher cholesterol levels may help prolong survival in patients with amyotrophic lateral sclerosis by warding off malnutrition and muscle wasting.
- The finding that high cholesterol is a prognostic factor for survival in amyotrophic lateral sclerosis patients, is of great significance, and calls into question the use of cholesterol-lowering medications (statins) in these patients.

- Statin therapy might increase the risk of amyotrophic lateral sclerosis or an amyotrophic lateral sclerosis-like syndrome.
- Raising the cholesterol levels of amyotrophic lateral sclerosis patients by dietary means might be beneficial.
- Doctors have noted the possible worsening effect of statins in amyotrophic lateral sclerosis patients and systematically stop statin drugs in patients.
- By reducing low density lipoprotein (LDL) cholesterol, statins decrease nutrient availability to muscle, which might contribute to neuromuscular junction damage and motor neuron death.
- Multiple pathways activated by statins might be deleterious in amyotrophic lateral sclerosis patients.

Dr Hiroshi Mitsumoto, the Wesley J. Howe Professor of Neurology at Columbia University and Medical Director of the Eleanor and Lou Gehrig MDA/ALS Centre at Columbia Presbyterian Medical Centre in New York City, commented: *"Many patients are taking statin drugs, and other experts have said the drugs might be harmful for amyotrophic lateral sclerosis patients, so we need to look into this immediately"* and *"it seems to me that amyotrophic lateral sclerosis patients benefit more from having higher blood fat levels"*.

Paper 319:
Statins and fibrates increase the risk of Parkinson's

Becker C et al Use of statins and the risk of Parkinson's disease: a retrospective case-control study in the UK. *Drug Safety* 2008;31(5):399-407

This Swiss study set out to explore the risk of the development of Parkinson's disease in people with untreated high cholesterol and with people treated with statins and fibrates. 3,637 people with Parkinson's were compared with the same number of controls.

The study identified:

- Those people with high cholesterol who did not take statins had a 2% lower risk of Parkinson's compared to those with lower cholesterol.
- Those who took statins had a 6% higher risk of Parkinson's.
- Those who took fibrates had a 25% higher risk of Parkinson's.

Paper 320:
Elderly man develops Parkinson's after taking statins

Müller T Statin-induced Parkinson's-syndrome.
Der Nervenarzt 2003 Aug;74(8):726-7

Professor Thomas Müller is the Head of the Department of Neurology and Consultant in Neurology/Psychiatry at St. Joseph Hospital Berlin-Weissensee, Germany. In this paper Professor Muller describes the case of an elderly man who developed Parkinson's after starting statin treatment.

- In 1996, a 60-year-old man started to take Fluvastatin.
- By 1997, he had increasing weakness with shoulder and hip pain on the right.
- In 1999, he was given a diagnosis of right sided Parkinson syndrome of akinetic (impaired muscle movement) dominance type.
- He was prescribed the Parkinson drugs, pergolid with daily doses of 3 mg and selegiline 7.5 mgm.
- By 2000, he was complaining about increasing edema development in legs, loss of hair. He increased Pergolid medication from 4.5 mg in June 2000 to 6 mgm in December and started a potassium sparing diuretic.
- He stopped taking Fluvastatin in March 2001.
- His edema had improved by September 2001.
- By March 2002, he had stopped taking Pergolid, Selegiline and the diuretic.

Professor Muller Comments: "*Long-term use of statins, especially Lovastatin, leads to the reduction of coenzyme Q10 and can cause damage of the mitochondrial breathing chain. Dysfunction of various parts of the mitochondrial breathing chain is also considered in the pathophysiological mechaism of idiopathic Parkinson's disease*".

The mitochondrial breathing chain is part of cellular respiration which is the process of creating cell energy. Most of the chemical reactions involved in cellular respiration happen in the mitochondria.

Paper 321:
Severe irritability associated with statin cholesterol-lowering drugs

Golomb BA et al Severe irritability associated with statin cholesterol-lowering drugs. *QJM* 2004 Apr;97(4):229-35

The aim of this paper, conducted by Professor Beatrice Golomb and her team from the University of California San Diego, was to assess the possible connection of statin usage to severe irritability. The study included six patients referred or self-referred with irritability and short temper on statin drugs who completed a survey providing information on character of behavioural effect, time-course of onset and recovery, and factors relevant to drug adverse effect causality.

Patient 1

- A 63-year-old single male initiated statins (including simvastatin and pravastatin) five times over five years.
- Statins were discontinued after a maximum of five months on each occasion, due to adverse effects including significant irritability.
- All symptoms resolved on discontinuation. Most recently, he initiated atorvastatin and within two weeks again noted extreme irritability, violence, and anger (similar to but more extreme than in prior statin usages), citing as his chief complaint: 'I wanted to kill someone'.
- The episodes worsened with statin use over the ensuing week. On several occasions he awoke with rage, 'uncontrollable pent up tension' and a desire 'to kill someone' and 'smash things'.
- He damaged property, and stated that he believes had he been married he would be a widower.
- He stated that these behaviours constituted a marked departure from his usual personality, which he reports is even-tempered and mild.
- He had no prior history of aggression off lipid-lowering drugs.
- After three weeks on atorvastatin, he advised his doctor of his perceived marked personality change with the desire to kill.
- He was instructed to discontinue atorvastatin immediately. Anger, irritability and homicidal impulses resolved completely within two days.

Patient 2

- A 59-year-old married male was over three years successively placed on fenofibrate, gemfibrozil, pravastatin, niaspan, cerivastatin, and simvastatin, discontinuing each agent within six weeks (as little as one week on cerivastatin), due to side-effects deemed intolerable, including irritability or 'crabbiness.'

- Irritability resolved with discontinuation in each instance.
- Most recently he initiated simvastatin (5 mg); he developed severe irritability, which he described as entailing 'short fuse' and 'quick temper', becoming 'furious' at minor things.
- He twice developed homicidal impulses toward his wife, and in one instance chased her with intent to act upon them but was able to restrain himself.
- He recalled the similar (though less severe) reaction on prior lipid-lowering agents and discontinued treatment with prompt resolution.
- Irritability was barely perceptible at two weeks, and had resolved completely by six weeks.
- He had no prior history of aggression off cholesterol-lowering drugs. He remains off lipid-lowering drugs.

Patient 3

- A 76-year-old female commenced simvastatin and after some months on treatment, became aware that a significant change in her personality and psychological state had occurred.
- She experienced extreme irritability, impatience, a 'short fuse' and short temper. She found herself becoming increasingly confrontational about little things, and reacting unreasonably when annoyed.
- She states she had never previously been easily angered or had an irritable personality, stating that she was 'a different person than I had been in my life'.
- She began to avoid social encounters to avoid alienating others with her problematic personality.
- She discontinued simvastatin, and states the irritability and other effects resolved after three days.
- One month later, she commenced atorvastatin; in three days she again began to re-experience personality change, and discontinued treatment.

Patient 4

- A 46-year-old female experienced extreme irritability while taking atorvastatin 20 mg for nine months.

- She was placed on atorvastatin and within six weeks began experiencing side-effects.
- She reports mild pre-existing irritability due to a recent back injury, and was initially not conscious of its amplification, but became aware when 'anything' irritated and upset her to the 'exploding' point.
- She was very 'short' with her husband, and when responding to his requests that she speak louder or repeat herself she would 'blow up' at him.
- She states she treated her husband very badly. This reportedly contrasted with her normal even-tempered personality, in which only major complications bothered her. 'Suddenly any minor inconvenience made me mad instantly. I wasn't a nice person at all'.
- She identified a new physician, who discontinued atorvastatin immediately.
- The irritability dissipated progressively from the time of discontinuation and by the sixth week, she noticed it had gone.

Patient 5

- A 59-year-old male with diabetes enrolled in a major atorvastatin research study in 3/98, receiving either 10 mg or 80 mg atorvastatin (he remains blinded to which he received).
- His wife noted progressive changes in his temperament: He became angry and 'explosive' with people, developing 'road rage' and becoming angry with his family.
- Following one road rage instance that led him to return home without reaching his destination, he kept his family away, stating 'if someone had said something to me I would have put them in the hospital'.
- His wife states she became 'afraid to be around him' noting he became 'violent for no reason,' and had, in the time on the drug (totalling three years) 'become a completely different person,' with violent episodes increasingly frequent and severe.
- He discontinued driving due to road rage, but still had angry episodes directed at other drivers while a passenger.
- The study physician was approached by patient and wife about the major personality change with timing of study

participation. The physician reportedly stated the problems could not be related to atorvastatin, noting that others in the study had not reported similar problems.

- The patient became very angry and persisted in extreme anger after returning home. His wife states 'he turned into a raging person, even when nothing provoked him.'
- He discontinued atorvastatin. The anger dissipated over two weeks at which point he was back to his normal temperament.
- He states that while on atorvastatin, 'I was very angry around people, even loved ones. I wasn't like that before atorvastatin...I was very hard on everyone, especially my wife'.

Patient 6

- A 45-year-old married male commenced lovastatin.
- He developed what he described as a 'quick temper,' which led him to exhibit temper with his wife and daughter and to experience road rage.
- He noticed that each time he ran out of medication and failed to refill it for several days, the quick temper resolved.
- He discontinued medication, with full resolution of irritability.
- Over the ensuing eight years, he was tried successively on niacin, simvastatin several times, and atorvastatin twice.
- Each time he instituted treatment he experienced recurrence of irritability. He describes the irritability by noting that it is characterized by a hypersensitivity to little things, ready susceptibility to provocation, and a feeling 'not of paranoia but as though one is under attack, under external threat'; that one 'reacts with fight or flight', and 'doesn't have enough calm.'
- After the final rechallenge with atorvastatin, he stated he would never resume statins, noting that there was a 'huge difference' when he stopped it.
- As an example, he states that on the day the (re)interview occurred he was nearly run into by another car. 'Before, I would have pursued them down the road. Now, off cholesterol drugs, I no longer follow other cars'.

Professor Golomb concluded: *"These case reports suggest that severe irritability may occur in some statin users"*.

Paper 322:
Statins increase aggression in women

Olson MB et al Lipid-lowering medication use and aggression scores in women: a report from the NHLBI-sponsored WISE study. *Journal of Womens Health* 2008 Mar;17(2):187-94

The aim of this study was to examine the association between the use of cholesterol lowering medication and aggression. The study measured aggression levels in 498 women who had suspected heart disease.

- The study revealed that women on cholesterol lowering medication (88% were on statins) had higher aggression levels than those not on medication.

Marian Olson, research associate from the University of Pittsburgh and first author of the paper finished: "*In summary, cholesterol-lowering medications are being prescribed to increasingly large numbers of patients worldwide, and this report finds that such treatment in women is associated with increased self-reported aggression*".

Paper 323:
Statins increase the risk of depression

Hyyppä MT et al Does simvastatin affect mood and steroid hormone levels in hypercholesterolemic men? A randomized double-blind trial. *Psychoneuroendocrinology* 2003 Feb;28(2):181-94

This Finnish study investigated the effects of statins on mood changes. It consisted of a randomised double-blind placebo-controlled trial of 120 healthy middle-aged men that analysed the separate and combined effects of a Mediterranean-type diet and treatment with simvastatin 20 mg per day for 12 weeks.

The study revealed:

- Treatment with simvastatin resulted in a significant decline in serum testosterone levels.
- Treatment with simvastatin resulted in a significant increase of depression and somatisation. (Somatisation is where a patient frequently complains about the existence of physical bodily adverse symptoms in the absence of a known medical condition.)

Paper 324: Cholesterol lowering medication is linked to higher depression rates

Steffens DC et al Cholesterol-lowering medication and relapse of depression. *Psychopharmacology Bulletin* 2003;37(4):92-8.

The head of the study, Dr David Steffens, is the president of the American Association for Geriatric Psychiatry, has authored more than 250 peer-reviewed papers and is the co-editor of the leading textbook in geriatric psychiatry. This study examined the effects of taking cholesterol-lowering medication on outcomes of depression among 167 older depressed adults over six years of duration.

Dr Steffens observed:

- Those taking cholesterol lowering medication were 21.6% more likely to relapse into depression compared to those not taking cholesterol lowering medication.
- Those taking cholesterol lowering medication relapsed more quickly into depression compared to those not taking cholesterol lowering medication.

Paper 325: Statins lead to negative thoughts and depression in older people

Morales K et al Simvastatin causes changes in affective processes in elderly volunteers. *Journal of the American Geriatric Society* 2006 Jan;54(1):70-6

Dr Knashawn Morales and her colleagues from the University of Pennsylvania investigated the effect of statins on depression and positive or negative mood of elderly people. The study included 80 older volunteers, average age 70, who received either simvastatin 20 mg per day or placebo for 15 weeks.

Positive or negative mood was measured by the Lawton positive and negative affect scales. The Lawton Positive and Negative Affect scale contains 10 items rated from 1–5 each. The positive items are energetic, warmth toward others, interested, happy, and content. The negative items are annoyed, irritated, depressed, worried, and sad/blue.

The study identified:

- Statin users had over a 400% increased risk of experiencing depressive symptoms compared to nonusers.
- For positive mood effects, simvastatin significantly decreased positive mood in a medication-by-time interaction. This was particularly so in those patients whose final total cholesterol levels were below 148 mg/dL (3.8 mmol/L).
- For negative mood effects, simvastatin significantly increased negative mood in a medication-by-event, and medication-by-event-by-time interaction.

Dr Morales concludes: "*The decrease in positive affect may be significant clinically and relevant to the quality of life of many patients*".

Paper 326:
Paranoia may be an adverse effect due to statin therapy

Peters JT et al Behavioral changes with paranoia in an elderly woman taking atorvastatin. *American Journal of Geriatric Pharmacotherapy* 2008 Mar;6(1):28-32

Dr Jessica Peters from Wayne State University, reports of behavioural changes in a patient taking atorvastatin.

- A 79-year-old woman developed paranoia, anxiety, and behavioural changes approximately 2.5 weeks after starting atorvastatin at 10 mg per day.
- After two months of therapy, the patient discontinued atorvastatin, and her symptoms fully resolved after four days.

Dr Peters concluded: "*This report emphasizes the possibility of paranoia as a central nervous system adverse effect due to statin therapy*".

Paper 327:
Statins may cause nightmares

Gregoor PJ et al Atorvastatin may cause nightmares. *British Medical Journal* 2006 Apr 22;332(7547):950

This case report relates atorvastatin to the occurrence of nightmares.

- A 72-year-old woman was prescribed 10 mg atorvastatin once a day.

- Five days after starting atorvastatin, she had extreme nightmares each night for two and a half weeks.
- She stopped taking the statins for five days and no nightmares occurred.
- She restarted the atorvastatin again, which promptly resulted in nightmares; these dreams again disappeared after discontinuation.

The author of this paper, Dr Peter Gregoor an internist-nephrologist at the Albert Schweitzer Hospital in Holland, speculates that: "*The nightmares could be a direct effect of atorvastatin on the central nervous system*".

Paper 328:
Statins could lead to depression by lowering cholesterol

You H et al The relationship between statins and depression: a review of the literature. *Expert Opinion on Pharmacotherapy* 2013 Aug;14(11):1467-76

This paper examined the relationship between statins and depression with an extensive literature search from 1972 to 2012.

- After reviewing 40 years of evidence the authors concluded: "*This article shows that statins could lead to depression by lowering cholesterol and that we should draw attention to this in clinical application, especially for patients complicated with depressive symptoms or low serum cholesterol levels*".

Paper 329:
Statins put patients at risk from depression and chronic fatigue syndrome

Maes M et al Lower plasma Coenzyme Q10 in depression: a marker for treatment resistance and chronic fatigue in depression and a risk factor to cardiovascular disorder in that illness. *Neuroendocrinology Letters* 2009;30(4):462-9

The author of the paper, Dr Michael Maes, holds over 12 appointments worldwide across Schools of Medicine, Psychiatry, Hospitals and Research Clinics for his work with the phenomenological and epidemiological aspects of mood disorders (e.g. depression, panic disorder, post-traumatic stress disorder, myalgic encephalopathy/

chronic fatigue syndrome). He has published more than 550 scientific papers worldwide.

Dr Maes states there is now evidence that major depression is accompanied by an induction of inflammation, stress and by a lowered antioxidant status. Coenzyme Q10 is a strong antioxidant that has anti-inflammatory effects.

This study examines the relationship between coenzyme Q10 levels, treatment resistant depression and chronic fatigue syndrome. The study included 35 depressed patients and 22 normal volunteers.

The study found:

- Coenzyme Q10 levels were significantly lower in depressed patients than in normal volunteers.
- Coenzyme Q10 levels were significantly lower in patients with treatment resistant depression and with chronic fatigue syndrome than in the other depressed patients.

The results show that lower coenzyme Q10 levels play a role in depression and in particular in treatment resistant depression and with chronic fatigue accompanying depression.

Dr Maes notes: "*The findings that lower coenzyme Q10 is a risk factor to coronary artery disease and chronic heart failure and mortality due to chronic heart failure suggest that low coenzyme Q10 is another factor explaining the risk to cardiovascular disorder in depression*".

He concludes: "*Since statins significantly lower plasma coenzyme Q10, depressed patients and in particular those with treatment resistant depression and with chronic fatigue syndrome represent populations at risk to statin treatment*".

Paper 330:
Cardiovascular drugs increase the risk of suicide

Callréus T et al Cardiovascular drugs and the risk of suicide: a nested case-control study. *European Journal of Clinical Pharmacology* 2007 Jun;63(6):591-6

This study investigated the possible association between the use of cardiovascular drugs and suicide. 743 cases of suicide were matched with 14,860 age- and sex-matched controls and their previous cardiovascular drug use was compared.

- Regarding statins, the study reported that taking statins increased the risk of suicide by 21%.

Paper 331: Statins increase the risk of suicidal thoughts by 159%

Davison KM et al Lipophilic statin use and suicidal ideation in a sample of adults with mood disorders. *Crisis* 2014 Jan 1;35(4):278-82

This study investigated the relationship between statins and suicidal ideation (suicidal thoughts) in adults with mood disorders. The study included 97 patients, aged over 18 years.

- The study found those taking statins had a 159% increased prevalence of suicidal ideation compared to those not taking statins.

One of the study authors, Dr Bonnie Kaplan, from the University of Calgary commented: "*Individuals with mood disorders may be susceptible to neuropsychiatric effects of cholesterol-lowering drugs*".

The testimony from the papers in this chapter demonstrates that statins do indeed adversely affect brain function:

- A battery of neuropsychological tests found that statins have an adverse effect on cognition.
- Memory may be impaired whilst taking statins, sometimes to such an extent as to result episodes of a total disruption of memory.
- Statins have been shown to confer an increased risk of neurodegenerative diseases such as Alzheimer's, dementia, Parkinson's, multiple sclerosis and amyotrophic lateral sclerosis.
- Increases, in irritability, anger, aggression and violence are associated with the use of statins.
- People taking statins have more risk of suffering nightmare's and paranoia.
- Statin use is linked to an elevated danger of depression and suicidal thoughts.

In 2012, the USA Food and Drug Administration issued a statement that all statins must carry warnings about increased risks of possible memory and cognition problems.

Chapter 13

Damaged eyes and other detrimental side effects around the head

The last chapter detected that statins may have harmful effects to the workings of the brain. But, what about the rest of the head?

Do statins adversely affect the eyes, and what about the ears, nose and throat? Can they also contribute to baldness, trigger headaches, and could they damage facial muscles?

The next 21 papers will take you on a journey around the head to observe the toxic effects that statins can have on this region of your body.

Paper 332:
Statins increase the risk of cataract
Smeeth L Cataract and the use of statins: a case-control study. *QJM* 2003 May;96(5):337-43

A cataract is a clouding of the lens inside the eye which leads to a decrease in vision. It is the most common cause of blindness.

The aim of the study was to assess the risk of cataracts associated with the use of statins. The study included 15,479 people with cataract and 15,479 controls without cataract.

- The study identified that those who were exposed to statins had a 4% increased risk of cataract compared to those who had never used statins.

Paper 333:
Statin users have an increased risk of cataract
Leuschen J et al Association of Statin Use With Cataracts: A Propensity Score-Matched Analysis. *Journal of the American Medical Association Ophthalmology* 2013 Nov;131(11):1427-34

The Charlson Comorbidity Index predicts the ten-year mortality for a patient who may have a range of comorbid conditions, such as heart disease, AIDS, or cancer (a total of 22 conditions).

Dr Jessica Leuschen an expert in ophthalmology, led this study which compared the risks for development of cataracts between statin users and nonusers. The study included 6,972 statin users who were compared with 6,972 nonusers.

The study pinpointed:

- The risk for cataract was 9% higher among statin users in comparison with nonusers.
- In patients with no comorbidities according to the Charlson Comorbidity Index, the risk for cataract was 27% higher among statin users in comparison with nonusers.

Dr Leuschen concludes: *"The risk for cataract is increased among statin users as compared with nonusers"*.

Paper 334:
Statins increase the risk of cataracts by 20%

Lai CL et al Statin Use and Cataract Surgery: A Nationwide Retrospective Cohort Study in Elderly Ethnic Chinese Patients. *Drug Safety* 2013 Oct;36(10):1017-24

This study investigated the relationship between statin therapy and cataracts. The study included 50,165 adults aged between 65 and 90 years who were followed for an average of 10.7 years.

- The study revealed that statin users had a 20% increased risk of cataract surgery compared to statin nonusers.

Paper 335:
Statin use is associated with a 57% increased risk of age-related cataract

Machan CM et al Age-related cataract is associated with type 2 diabetes and statin use. *Optometry and Vision Science* 2012 Aug;89(8):1165-71

Optometrist Dr Carolyn Machan and colleagues of University of Waterloo, examined the associations between age-related cataract, type two diabetes, and statin use. The study included 6,397 patients aged 1-93 years.

The study recorded:

- Statin users had a 57% increased risk of age-related cataract compared to nonusers.
- The 50% probability of cataract in statin users occurred at age 51.7 and 54.9 years in patients with type 2 diabetes and without diabetes, respectively. In non-statin users, it was significantly later at age 55.1 and 57.3 years for patients with type two diabetes and without diabetes, respectively.

Dr Machan concludes: "*Statin use was significantly associated with age-related cataract such that the probability of cataract for patients with type 2 diabetes who did not use statins was similar to patients without diabetes who did use statins*".

Paper 336:
Stains increase the risk of age-related macular degeneration by 19%

Maguire MG et al Statin use and the incidence of advanced age-related macular degeneration in the Complications of Age-related Macular Degeneration Prevention Trial. *Ophthalmology* 2009 Dec;116(12):2381-5

Age-related macular degeneration is the most common cause of vision loss in those aged over 50. It causes a gradual loss of central (but not peripheral) vision. Central vision is needed for detailed work and for things like reading and driving.

Drusen are yellow deposits under the retina. While drusen likely do not cause age-related macular degeneration, their presence increases a person's risk of developing age-related macular degeneration. In the expression, 20/40 vision, the 20 is the distance in feet between the subject and the chart. The 40 means that the subject can read the chart (from 20 feet away) as well as a normal person could read the same chart from 40 feet away.

The aim of the study was to evaluate the impact of statin use on the incidence of advanced age-related macular degeneration among patients with large drusen. The study included 744 patients, aged 50 years or more, who were followed for at least five years. Eligibility criteria for the clinical trial required that the participants have more than ten large drusen and visual acuity no better than 20/40 in each eye.

- The study found that patients taking statins had a 19% increased risk of developing advanced age-related macular degeneration compared to patients not taking statins.

Paper 337:
Statins may be associated with an increase in the risk of age-related macular degeneration

Etminan M et al Use of statins and angiotensin converting enzyme inhibitors (ACE-Is) and the risk of age-related macular degeneration: nested case-control study. *Current Drug Safety* 2008 Jan;3(1):24-6

Angiotensin-converting enzyme inhibitors (ACE inhibitors) are drugs that are used to treat high blood pressure and heart failure.

Dr Mahyar Etminan, whose research focus is drug safety, sought to explore the association between statins, angiotensin-converting enzyme inhibitors and the development of age-related macular degeneration. The study included 2,867 patients, aged 65 years or older, with age-related macular degeneration who were compared with 11,468 controls who were free from age-related macular degeneration.

The study findings indicated:

- Those using statin drugs had a 30% increased risk of developing age-related macular degeneration compared to those not using statins.
- Those using angiotensin-converting enzyme inhibitor drugs had a 19% increased risk of developing age-related macular degeneration compared to those not using angiotensin-converting enzyme inhibitors.

Dr Etminan concludes: *"Based on the results of our study, statin and angiotensin-converting enzyme inhibitor use may be associated with an increase in the risk of age-related macular degeneration"*.

Paper 338:
Statin use might increase the risk of age-related macular degeneration

McGwin G et al 3-hydroxy-3-methylglutaryl coenzyme a reductase inhibitors and the presence of age-related macular degeneration in the Cardiovascular Health Study. *Archives of Ophthalmology* 2006 Jan;124(1):33-7

The objective of the study was to evaluate both the use of cholesterol-lowering medications as a group and the use of statins specifically with regard to the risk of age-related macular degeneration. The study included 2,755 men and women aged over 65 years.

The study detected:

- Those taking cholesterol-lowering medications had a 35% increased risk of age-related macular degeneration compared to those not taking cholesterol-lowering medications.
- Those taking statins had a 40% increased risk of age-related macular degeneration compared to those not taking statins.

The first author of the study, Dr Gerald McGwin, a Professor and Vice Chairman in the Department of Epidemiology in the School of Public Health at the University of Alabama at Birmingham, concluded: "*Statin use might increase the risk of age-related macular degeneration*".

Paper 339: Statins, double vision and other eye problems

Fraunfelder FW et al Diplopia, blepharoptosis, and ophthalmoplegia and 3-hydroxy-3-methyl-glutaryl-CoA reductase inhibitor use. *Ophthalmology* 2008 Dec;115(12):2282-5

This study, based in the Department of Ophthalmology at the Oregon Health and Science University, investigated the association of statins with ptosis (droopy eyelids), diplopia (double vision), and ophthalmoplegia (ophthalmoplegia refers to weakness or paralysis of the extraocular muscles which are responsible for eye movements).

The study, headed by Dr Fredrick Fraunfelder, examined the scientific data from 256 case reports submitted to the National Registry of Drug-Induced Ocular Side Effects, the World Health Organization, and the Food and Drug Administration.

- After examining the data Dr Fraunfelder concluded: "*According to World Health Organization criteria, the relationship between statin therapy and diplopia, ptosis, or ophthalmoplegia is possible. This causality assessment is based on the time relationship of drug administration and adverse drug reaction development, the multiple positive dechallenge and rechallenge reports, and the plausible mechanism by which diplopia, ptosis, or ophthalmoplegia may occur: myositis (muscle inflammation) of the extraocular muscles, the levator palpebrae superioris (upper eyelid) muscles, or both".*

Paper 340:
Statins damage the eyelid muscle

Ertas FS et al Unrecognized side effect of statin treatment: unilateral blepharoptosis. *Ophthalmic Plastic and Reconstructive Surgery* 2006 May-Jun;22(3):222-4

The levator eye muscle is responsible for elevating the upper eyelid. Blepharoptosis is drooping of the upper eyelid. Myositis is a disease in which the immune system chronically inflames the body's own healthy muscle tissue. Persistent inflammation progressively weakens the muscles.

A 43-year-old man, receiving 10 mg atorvastatin daily, developed myositis of the levator muscle which resulted in unilateral blepharoptosis (drooping of one eyelid).

- This case reveals that statins may damage the eyelid muscle and study author Dr Faith Ertas (a Professor of Cardiology) concludes: *"Statin-induced myositis in the levator muscle should be considered in the differential diagnosis of acquired unilateral blepharoptosis of unknown cause".*

Paper 341:
Atorvastatin associated with double vision and pins and needles

Negevesky GJ et al Reversible atorvastatin-associated external ophthalmoplegia, anti-acetylcholine receptor antibodies, and ataxia. *Archives of Ophthalmology* 2000 Mar;118(3):427-8

External ophthalmoplegia is a paralysis or weakness of one or more of the muscles that control eye movement.

Dr Gerald Negvesky, a specialist in ophthalmology, reports the case of a woman who developed external ophthalmoplegia after starting statins.

- A 60-year-old woman experienced double vision, vertigo, blurry vision, and pins and needles of both upper extremities for one week.

- She had been taking atorvastatin 10 mg daily for 2 1/2 months.
- Neurological abnormalities included generalized overactive reflexes, lack of coordination of muscle movements and gait instability.
- She had droopy upper eyelids.
- Examination revealed upgaze and outward gaze eye limitation.
- Anti-acetylcholine receptor antibodies were ten times the upper limit of the normal range. (Anti-acetylcholine receptor antibodies are associated with neuromuscular disorders.)
- The patient stopped taking atorvastatin.
- Neurological improvement began within two days.
- At ten weeks from the discontinuation of atorvastatin therapy, the patient had complete resolution of the gait instability, pins and needles, droopy eyelids and double vision.
- Gaze range of the eyes was remarkably improved.
- Anti-acetylcholine receptor antibodies returned to normal levels.

Dr Negevesky concluded: *"It is important that they (statins) be considered as a possible cause for unexplained external ophthalmoplegia"*.

Paper 342:
Statins associated with muscle and eye fatigue

Parmar B et al Statins, fibrates, and ocular myasthenia.
Lancet 2002 Aug 31;360(9334):717

Ocular myasthenia gravis is where the muscles that move the eyes and control the eyelids are easily fatigued and weakened.

This paper, published in the eminent UK journal *The Lancet*, describes the case of a woman who developed muscle weakness and ocular myasthenia after starting statin drugs.

- A 67-year-old woman started to take atorvastatin.
- Within three months, she began to experience eye fatigue and generalised muscle weakness.
- The atorvastatin was discontinued, and after six weeks her muscle weakness resolved.
- She was started sequentially on fluvastatin, simvastatin, and benzafibrate. With each cholesterol lowering drug the muscle weakness recurred after two to three months of treatment.

- She again restarted atorvastatin.
- She soon was suffering with ptosis (droopy eyelids), double vision and muscle weakness.
- Examination revealed she had a strikingly fatigable myogenic ptosis and shoulder weakness.
- She was diagnosed with ocular myasthenia.
- Discontinuation of atorvastatin led to a brisk clinical improvement. Two months later, she had residual mild ptosis and slight weakness of the shoulder girdle.

Paper 343:
Atorvastatin inflames and destroy blood vessels

Haroon M et al A case of ANCA-associated systemic vasculitis induced by atorvastatin. *Clinical Rheumatology* 2008 Dec;27 Suppl 2:S75-7

Vasculitis is a group of disorders that destroy blood vessels by inflammation. ANCA-associated vasculitides are diseases caused by vasculitis in which antineutrophil cytoplasmic antibodies (ANCAs) can be detected in the blood.

Dr Muhammad Haroon from Waterford Regional Hospital chronicles a case of statin induced ANCA-associated vasculitides.

- A 45-year-old male patient reported to an Accident and Emergency department with a six-week history of pain and stiffness involving his legs. Both calves were markedly tender, and he was not able to bear weight.
- He also complained of numbness involving his left big toe for a few days, which later spread to involve his arms, and tinnitus and hearing loss in his left ear.
- He had been taking atorvastatin 10 mg for six months.
- Investigations showed markedly increased inflammatory markers, markedly increased antineutrophil cytoplasmic antibody (ANCA) levels and muscle damage.
- A diagnosis of statin-induced ANCA-associated vasculitis and statin-induced distal myopathy (muscle disease) was made.
- The patients symptoms and laboratory abnormalities resolved rapidly after cessation of the statin drug and implementation of treatment.

Paper 344:
Doctor recommend that clinicians and patients be aware of the risk of atorvastatin-associated tinnitus and permanent hearing loss

Liu M et al Irreversible atorvastatin-associated hearing loss. *Pharmacotherapy* 2012 Feb;32(2):e27-34

The case of a man who suffered hearing loss after starting statins is illustrated by Dr Michael Liu, a Clinical Assistant Professor of Pharmacy Practice at Long Island University.

- A 32-year-old man started to take atorvastatin.
- Six months later, he complained of occasional episodes of tinnitus.
- By 18 months, the tinnitus became continuous. An audiogram revealed middle-frequency hearing loss.
- Atorvastatin was immediately discontinued, and the patient was fitted with hearing aids.
- Four years after drug discontinuation, his hearing loss had neither progressed nor regressed.
- The manufacturer of atorvastatin has received other unpublished cases of deafness.

Dr Liu concluded: "*Based on this case report, we recommend that clinicians and patients be aware of the risk of atorvastatin-associated tinnitus and permanent hearing loss*".

Paper 345:
Statins and nasal polyps

Bucca C et al Statins and nasal polyps. *Annals of Internal Medicine* 2005 Feb 15;142(4):310-1

This paper outlines the case of a woman who developed nasal polyps (warty growths) after taking statins.

- A 57-year-old woman with rhinosinusitis (rhinosinusitis is inflammation of the nasal passage and sinuses) and asthma sought medical attention for the recent onset of rhinosinusitis associated with asthma.
- With treatment the patient's condition nearly normalised.
- She started to take atorvastatin.

- One month later, the patient returned because of severe persistent nasal obstruction with extensive polyp growth.
- Tests found she had abnormally high amounts of eosinophil's (white blood cells) and her sinuses were completely stuffed with polyps.
- The polyps were removed, but returned within one month of surgery.
- She stopped taking atorvastatin, and within three weeks her condition had dramatically improved, with her nasal polyps disappearing.
- She restarted atorvastatin and her nasal symptoms and polyps returned shortly afterwards, together with nasal eosinophilia.
- The patient improved after again stopping atorvastatin.
- She later started to take simvastatin and again the polyps recurred.

Paper 346:
Statins cause adverse side effects in the oral cavity

Cruz MP et al Adverse side effects of statins in the oral cavity.
Medicina Oral, Patologia Oral y Cirugia Bucal
2008 Feb 1;13(2):E98-101

The objective of this Spanish study was to analyze the side effects of statins in the mouth cavity, and to analyze the symptoms after interruption of the treatment. The study included 26 patients aged 50-70 undergoing treatment with statins.

Patients were initially assessed for side effects of statins in the mouth cavity, statin treatment was then discontinued for two weeks and the patients response was observed.

The study ascertained:

- Of those patients with dryness, 73.9% showed improvement after discontinuing statins for two weeks.
- Of those patients with itch, 86.7% showed improvement or had complete recovery after discontinuing statins for two weeks.
- Of those patients with bitterness, 92.8% had complete recovery after discontinuing statins for two weeks.
- Of those patients with a cough, 91.7% showed improvement after discontinuing statins for two weeks.

- Additionally, of those patients who had insomnia, 94.1% showed improvement after discontinuing statins for two weeks.

This study shows that there is a marked improvement of mouth cavity ailments after statin treatment is discontinued.

Paper 347:
Chronic cough as a complication of treatment with statins

Psaila M et al Chronic cough as a complication of treatment with statins: a case report. *Therapeutic Advances in Respiratory Disease* 2012 Aug;6(4):243-6

Dr Matthew Psaila from Mater Dei Hospital portrays the case of an elderly man who developed a dry cough on being treated with statins.

- An 80-year-old gentleman was referred to a respiratory clinic with a history of cough.
- He complained of a persistent cough after being started on simvastatin.
- His cough came in bouts with increasing frequency as worsening from one to two bouts of coughing per day at symptom onset to five to six bouts per day after approximately ten days from onset. Each bout lasted from one to five minutes.
- Of his own accord he stopped the simvastatin in view of the dry cough two months later.
- A decrease in frequency of symptoms occurred after stopping simvastatin with eventual complete resolution eight days later.
- He switched over to fluvastatin. Two months into treatment, however, his cough started again and increased in frequency after onset only to resolve one week after stopping fluvastatin.
- He again started simvastatin and again his cough returned and he stopped taking the statin.
- He had stopped and resumed his treatment for three times (twice with simvastatin and once with fluvastatin) with resolution and recurrence of his symptoms, respectively, before being referred to the respiratory clinic.
- Examinations revealed he had a clear chest and normal lung function.

- A further attempt at introducing statin therapy was undertaken. The patient was advised to continue taking simvastatin at his usual dose until symptoms occur. He was then advised to change over to another formulation (vitamin C tablets), the nature of which was not revealed to the patient thus acting as a placebo drug to monitor symptoms.
- His cough recurred after eight weeks of statin treatment, with resolution on stopping simvastatin and changing over to placebo.
- In a follow up visit after stopping the statin treatment the patient's cough had not returned.

Dr Psaila hypothesised that: "*Statin therapy could lead to an increase in bronchial or cough reflex hypersensitivity thus resulting in an increased incidence of cough. This hypothesis is supported by the fact that the symptoms diminish when statin therapy is terminated*".

Paper 348:
Statins linked to alopecia

Segal AS Alopecia associated with atorvastatin. *American Journal of Medicine* 2002 Aug 1;113(2):171

The case of a woman who suffered alopecia after atorvastatin treatment is presented by Dr Alan Segal from the Division of Nephrology and Hypertension at the University of Vermont.

- A 38-year-old woman was admitted to hospital because of a six-week history of progressive swelling.
- Physical examination found severe edema around her eyes and pitting edema around her extremities.
- Tests revealed the patient had nephrotic syndrome. Nephrotic syndrome occurs when the kidneys do not work properly and leak large amounts of protein into the urine.
- She was given various drugs including prednisone, benazepril and atorvastatin.
- She improved over the next four weeks and the prednisone dosage was gradually reduced.
- Two weeks later, the patient complained of progressive hair loss.
- She continued to take benazepril but discontinued atorvastatin.

- Several weeks later, the patient reported that new hair growth had begun.
- Nephrotic syndrome recurred five months later. Prednisone and atorvastatin were restarted.
- Within two weeks, the patient complained again of excessive hair loss.
- Atorvastatin, but not prednisone, was stopped, and normal hair growth returned as the patients symptoms improved.
- Three months later, while still been treated with benazepril, nephrotic syndrome again recurred and prednisone was restarted, but atorvastatin was not restarted.
- Hair loss did not occur during this episode of nephrotic syndrome.
- On two more recurrences of nephrotic syndrome in the next seven months, the patient did not restart atorvastatin and hair loss did not occur.

The above events show that hair loss was not due to prednisone, benazepril or the nephrotic syndrome itself.

Dr Segal concludes: *"The pattern of our patient's hair loss strongly suggest a relation between atorvastatin and alopecia"*.

Paper 349:
Statins linked to headaches:
Doctor says patients should purchase book on drug side effects as they have more time to read this information than physicians

Rapoport D Unrecognized adverse drug reactions. *Canadian Medical Association Journal* 1993 Nov 1;149(9):1233

Dr David Rapoport depicts the case of a female who developed severe headaches after starting statin treatment.

- A female was been monitored by her physician (Dr Rapoport) for several chronic illnesses.
- She was prescribed lovastatin.
- Severe headaches developed after 21 months of increasing doses of lovastatin.
- She was admitted to hospital.
- After three days, she was given pain killers and discharged.

- Two weeks later, Dr Rapoport again had to refer her to hospital where she was prescribed various pain relief medicines with no success.
- Finally, Dr Rapoport read information about lovastatin in the *Compendium of Pharmaceuticals and Specialities* which revealed, in the section on adverse reactions, that lovastatin was the source of the patients headaches.
- Discontinuation of lovastatin led to the patients rapid recovery.

Dr Rapoport suggested two solutions to prevent adverse drug reactions: *"Educate patients: provide them with the monographs for drugs they receive or encourage the purchase of a book on medications. Patients likely have more time to read this information than physicians"* and *"Physicians should suspect any new symptom as an adverse drug reaction until proven otherwise"*.

Paper 350:
Pravastatin triggers migraine-type headache in airline captain at altitude

Ramsey CS et al Altitude-induced migraine headache secondary to pravastatin: case report. *Aviation, Space and Environmental Medicine* 1998 Jun;69(6):603-6

This paper describes the case of a man who developed headaches at altitude after starting pravastatin treatment.

- Within days of starting pravastatin, a 46-year-old airline captain with many exposures to altitude chamber, fighter, and airliner flight developed migraine-type headaches after exposure to cabin altitudes above 6,000 feet.
- He had no prior history of chronic headaches or migraine.

The case highlights that pravastatin has the potential to trigger migraine-type headaches at altitude.

Paper 351:
Myasthenic weakness is a potential adverse effect of statins

Pasutharnchat N et al Statin-associated myasthenic weakness. *Journal of the Medical Association of Thailand* 2011 Feb;94(2):256-8

Dr Nath Pasutharnchat reports the case of a woman who developed bulbar myasthenia gravis (facial weakness, difficulties in chewing, swallowing, articulation, and breathing, and weakness of the neck muscles) a few weeks after starting statin treatment.

- A 50-year-old woman with generalized, limb predominated, myasthenia gravis, whose myasthenia gravis status has been "minimal manifestation" for several years, developed moderately severe fluctuating bulbar myasthenia gravis weakness a few weeks after starting simvastatin of 20 mg per day.
- Simvastatin was discontinued and the symptoms resolved and she was back to her previous status in one month.
- She again started simvastatin, this time at 10 mg per day, and within two weeks bulbar weakness re-occurred.
- The symptoms were again resolved after discontinuation of the statin and she was back to her previous status in two months.

Dr Pasutharnchat concludes: "*Because of the wide use of statins in clinical practice, physicians should be aware of this potential adverse effect. Furthermore, patients should also be informed of the potential adverse effect*".

Paper 352:
Statins increase the risk of Bell's palsy by 47%

Hung SH et al Association Between Statin Use and Bell's Palsy: A Population-Based Study. *Drug Safety* 2014 Sep;37(9):735-42

Bell's palsy is a weakness (paralysis) that affects the muscles of the face. It is due to a problem with the facial nerve. The weakness usually affects one side of the face.

This study aimed to evaluate the association between statin use and Bell's palsy. This case-control study identified 1,977 subjects with Bell's palsy as cases and 5,931 sex- and age-matched subjects without Bell's palsy.

- The study found that statin users had a 47% increased risk of Bell's palsy compared to nonusers.

This information exposes statins noxious effects on areas on and around the head.

- Statins increase the likelihood of cataracts and macular degeneration.
- Double vision and blurry vision have been found to be statin side effects.
- Muscle weakness in the eyelids and eye fatigue are other abnormalities linked to statins.
- Statin use has been recorded to be associated with tinnitus and hearing loss.
- Nasal polyps have been known to be formed by taking statins.
- Coughing has been exacerbated and areas of the mouth cavity have been aggravated when prescribed statin drugs.
- Statin usage has been linked to hair loss and headaches.
- Weakness and paralysis of the face is also known in people that have taken statins.

Chapter 14

Statins increase impotence in men and birth defects in babies

The Food and Drink Administration classifies statins as pregnancy category X, which means they are not supposed to be taken by pregnant women. Category X drugs have been linked to fetal abnormalities in studies.

However, how do statins affect men in the process of reproduction?

As well as documenting the well-known dangers of statins causing birth defects, this chapter assesses the scientific literature to determine statins effects on mens' ability to reproduce healthy offspring.

Paper 353:
Lipitor significantly worsens erectile dysfunction

Nurkalem Z et al The effect of rosuvastatin and atorvastatin on erectile dysfunction in hypercholesterolemic patients. *Kardiologia Polska* 2014;72(3):275-9

The IIEF-5 (International Index of Erectile Function-5) is an international questionnaire for identifying erectile dysfunction. A low score represents severe erectile dysfunction, whereas higher scores indicate better erectile function.

The aim of this study was to evaluate effect of different statin types on erectile dysfunction in "patients" with "high" cholesterol. The study lasted for six months and included 90 healthy men, (average age 50 years), with low density lipoprotein (LDL) cholesterol levels above 160mg/dL (4.1 mmol/l). Patients were divided into two different groups. One group received rosuvastatin while the other group was given atorvastatin.

The study found:

- The IIEF-5 scores of men taking rosuvastatin (Crestor) decreased by .4%.
- The IIEF-5 scores of men taking atorvastatin (Lipitor) decreased significantly by 8.5%.

The results of the study reveal Lipitor significantly worsens erectile dysfunction.

Paper 354: Statins are associated with erectile dysfunction

Solomon H et al Erectile dysfunction and statin treatment in high cardiovascular risk patients. *International Journal of Clinical Practice* 2006 Feb;60(2):141-5

Expert cardiologist Dr Hemant Solomon and his associates, investigated the relationship between statins and erectile dysfunction. In this study, International Index of Erectile Function IIEF scores were measured in 93 men attending cardiovascular risk clinics.

The study observed:

- Prior to statin therapy, the average IIEF score was 21.
- After statin therapy, IIEF scores were reduced to 6.5.
- After statin therapy 22% of the men experienced new onset erectile dysfunction.

Dr Solomon concludes: "*Statin-induced erectile dysfunction is common in patients with high cardiovascular risk*".

Paper 355: Statins increase the risk of erectile dysfunction by 51%

Bruckert E et al Men treated with hypolipidaemic drugs complain more frequently of erectile dysfunction. *Journal of Clinical Pharmacy and Therapeutics* 1996 Apr;21(2):89-94

The objective of this study was to assess whether there is an association between impotence and treatment with cholesterol lowering drugs. The study included 339 men taking cholesterol lowering drugs and 339 controls.

The study pinpointed:

- Men taking statins had a 51% increased risk of erectile dysfunction compared to men not taking cholesterol lowering drugs.
- Men taking fibrates had a 46% increased risk of erectile dysfunction compared to men not taking cholesterol lowering drugs.

Paper 356:
Statins associated with erectile dysfunction

Hall SA et al Is hyperlipidemia or its treatment associated with erectile dysfunction?: Results from the Boston Area Community Health (BACH) Survey. *Journal of Sexual Medicine* 2009 May;6(5):1402-13

The objectives of the study, which included data from 1,899 men aged 30-79, were to examine the association between:

- o Cholesterol lowering drugs and erectile dysfunction.
- o Cholesterol levels and erectile dysfunction.

In the study, high cholesterol was classified as over 240 mg/dL (6.2 mmol/L), whilst normal cholesterol was classified as under 240 mg/dL (6.2 mmol/L). 84% of the men on cholesterol lowering drugs were taking statins.

The study ascertained:

- In men under 55: Compared to men with normal cholesterol, men taking cholesterol lowering drugs had an 180% increased risk of erectile dysfunction.
- In men over 55: Compared to men with normal cholesterol, men taking cholesterol lowering drugs had a 48% increased risk of erectile dysfunction.
- In men under 55: Compared to men with normal cholesterol, men with high cholesterol had a 73% reduced risk of erectile dysfunction.
- In men over 55: Compared to men with normal cholesterol, men with high cholesterol had a 4% reduced risk of erectile dysfunction.

In this study, cholesterol lowering drugs (mainly statins) were associated with erectile dysfunction.

Paper 357:
Statins may induce or worsen erectile dysfunction

Do C et al Statins and erectile dysfunction: results of a case/ non-case study using the French Pharmacovigilance System Database. *Drug Safety* 2009;32(7):591-7

Dr Catherine Do, and her colleagues from the University of Toulouse, investigated the relationship between exposure to drugs such as statins and the occurrence of erectile dysfunction. Over a 20-year period the researchers extracted data about 110,685 men aged 13 – 80 years old from the French Pharmacovigilance System Database who had reported an incidence of erectile dysfunction to see if they had being taking statins, fibrates or other drugs.

Dr Do used the case/non-case method was to measure the disproportionality of combination between a statin and erectile dysfunction. Cases were defined as those reports corresponding to the adverse drug report of interest (i.e. erectile dysfunction) and non-cases are all reports of other adverse drug reports.

The French researchers discovered:

- Statins users had a 140% increase in erectile dysfunction compared to users of other drugs.
- Erectile dysfunction usually started to occur within one month.
- Just over half of these men recovered if they stopped taking the statins.
- Erectile dysfunction happened no matter what the dose or duration of the statin therapy.
- Fibrate users had a 260% increase in erectile dysfunction compared to users of other drugs.

Dr Do concluded: *"The present study suggests that statins may induce or worsen erectile dysfunction"*.

Paper 358:
Review finds that statins and fibrates may cause erectile dysfunction

Rizvi K et al Do lipid-lowering drugs cause erectile dysfunction? A systematic review. *Family Practice* 2002 Feb;19(1):95-8

The aim of this study was to clarify the relationship between cholesterol lowering drugs and erectile dysfunction. To achieve this aim a systematic review of the scientific literature was carried out by Dr Kash Rizvi from the University of Wales College of Medicine.

The review indicated:

- Information from review articles, clinical trials and from regulatory agencies identified fibrates as a source of erectile dysfunction.
- A substantial number of cases of erectile dysfunction associated with statin usage have been reported to regulatory agencies.
- Case reports and clinical trial evidence supported the suggestion that statins can also cause erectile dysfunction.

Dr Rizvi concluded: "*The systematic review procedure was applied successfully to collect evidence suggesting that both statins and fibrates may cause erectile dysfunction*".

Paper 359:
Testosterone levels decline in men on statin therapy

Tobert JA et al Cholesterol-lowering effect of mevinolin, an inhibitor of 3-hydroxy-3-methylglutaryl-coenzyme a reductase, in healthy volunteers. *Journal of Clinical Investigation* 1982 Apr;69(4):913-9

Cholesterol is the precursor to testosterone. Low levels of testosterone may lead to hypogonadism. (Hypogonadism occurs when the body's sex glands produce little or no hormones and may lead to loss of body hair, muscle loss, low libido and erectile dysfunction.)

The effects of mevinolin (lovastatin) were evaluated in a double-blind, placebo-controlled study in 59 healthy men. The men received doses of either 6.25, 12.5, 25, 50 mg or placebo twice daily for four weeks.

- Regarding testosterone, the study found the testosterone levels in men receiving statins declined by 8% compared to men on placebo.

Paper 360:
Statins and hypogonadism

Stanworth RD et al Statin therapy is associated with lower

total but not bioavailable or free testosterone in men with type 2 diabetes. *Diabetes Care* 2009 Apr;32(4):541-6

This study compared testosterone levels with statin use in a study of 355 men with type two diabetes.

The study reported:

- Men taking statins had 11% lower levels of total testosterone compared to men not taking statins.
- Men taking statins had 7% lower levels of free testosterone compared to men not taking statins.
- Men taking statins had 6% lower levels of bioavailable testosterone compared to men not taking statins.
- Further analysis revealed an apparent dose-response relationship, with the lowest testosterone levels seen in men taking higher doses of atorvastatin.

This study shows that men with type two diabetes taking statins have lower levels of testosterone than those not taking statins.

Paper 361:
Statin therapy results in a decline in testosterone levels

Dobs AS et al Effects of high-dose simvastatin on adrenal and gonadal steroidogenesis in men with hypercholesterolemia. *Metabolism* 2000 Sep;49(9):1234-8

This study evaluated the effect of statin therapy on hormone levels. This randomised, placebo-controlled study lasted 12 weeks and included 81 men with low-density lipoprotein (LDL) cholesterol levels more than 145 mg/dL (3.74 mmol/L) who received either 80 mg simvastatin daily or placebo.

Regarding testosterone levels, the study found after 12 weeks:

- Total testosterone levels declined by 13.6% in the simvastatin group, and declined by only 1.5% in the placebo group.
- The pooled free testosterone declined by 6.3% in the simvastatin group, versus a 4.9% increase in the placebo group.
- The pooled bioavailable testosterone declined 10.2% in the simvastatin group and increased 1.4% in the placebo group.

Paper 362:
Statins might induce hypogonadism

Corona G et al The effect of statin therapy on testosterone levels in subjects consulting for erectile dysfunction. *Journal of Sexual Medicine* 2010 Apr;7(4 Pt 1):1547-56

A group led by Dr Giovanni Corona from the University of Florence, carried out a study to examine the association between statin therapy and hormone levels in erectile dysfunction. The study included 3,484 men with erectile dysfunction, average age 51.6 years.

The study revealed:

- Both total and calculated free testosterone levels were significantly lower in subjects taking statins.
- Statin use was associated with a reduced testis volume.
- Statin use was associated with a higher prevalence of hypogonadism-related symptoms. (Hypogonadism is where the sex glands produce little or no hormones.)

Dr Corona Concludes: "*Our data demonstrated that statin therapy might induce an overt primary hypogonadism*".

Paper 363:
Statins associated with decreased libido

de Graaf L et al Is decreased libido associated with the use of HMG-CoA-reductase inhibitors? *British Journal of Clinical Pharmacology* 2004 September; 58(3): 326–328

The aims of this study, headed by Dr Linda de Graff, were to describe patients with decreased libido during use of statin drugs, and to discuss causality and pharmacological hypotheses for this association. In this Dutch study, eight patients were identified as having decreased libido during use of statins.

The study reported:

- In two of these cases testosterone levels were determined and appeared to be decreased.
- Patient A is a 46-year-old male.
  - o The patient started treatment with fluvastatin, initially 20 mg daily, increased to 40 mg daily.
  - o Shortly after initiation of therapy, the patient noticed a decrease in libido. His testosterone value was measured

  and determined at 7.2 nmol l^{-1} (morning value, normal range for adult men 12–35 nmol l^{-1}).
  - o Fluvastatin was withdrawn and five days later, testosterone had increased to 13.2 nmol l^{-1} (morning value). The patient's libido had also returned to normal.
- Patient B, a 54-year-old male, started treatment with pravastatin.
  - o Within days after initiation of this therapy, he experienced a decrease in his libido. His testosterone level was determined at 5.8 nmol l^{-1} (morning value).
  - o Pravastatin was discontinued seven months later, and after a few days his libido returned to normal.
  - o Four months later, testosterone level was determined again and had risen to 22.8 nmol l^{-1} (morning value).
- Testosterone levels were not determined in the other six patients (including one woman) although it is known two patients recovered after withdrawal of the statin drugs.
- Libido is related to testosterone levels: lower testosterone levels decrease male libido. Testosterone in males is produced mainly from cholesterol in the Leydig cells (found in the testes). Statins may interfere with the synthesis of testosterone in three ways.
  - o By decreasing levels of low density lipoprotein (LDL) cholesterol, statins lower the total amount of cholesterol offered to the Leydig cell.
  - o Statins are found in the testes and can inhibit the synthesis of cholesterol.
  - o Statins also interfere with the process that converts two intermediate products, dehydroepiandrosterone (DHEA) and dehydroandrostenedione, into androstenediol and testosterone, respectively. DHEA, dehydroandrostenedione, androstenediol, and testosterone are not just important in men's sexual desire, they are also important in women's sexual desire. This is why some women may also suffer loss of libido when they take statins.

Dr de Graff concluded: "*Our reports on fluvastatin, pravastatin, simvastatin and atorvastatin and the suggested pharmacological explanation generate the hypothesis that decreased libido may be associated with the use of statins*".

Paper 364: Statins deplete important hormones

Kanat M et al A multicenter, open label, crossover designed prospective study evaluating the effects of lipid lowering treatment on steroid synthesis in patients with Type 2 diabetes (MODEST Study). *Journal of Endocrinological Investigation* 2009 Nov;32(10):852-6

Steroid hormones are crucial substances for the proper function of the body. They mediate a wide variety of vital physiological functions ranging from anti-inflammatory agents to regulating events during pregnancy. They are synthesized and secreted into the bloodstream by endocrine glands such as the adrenal cortex and the gonads (ovary and testis). Vital steroid hormones include:

Dehydroepiandrosterone (DHEA)

Dehydroepiandrosterone is the most abundant circulating steroid hormone in humans. It is produced in the adrenal glands, the gonads, and the brain. Dehydroepiandrosterone is used for slowing or reversing aging, improving thinking skills in older people, and slowing the progress of Alzheimer's disease. Athletes and other people use dehydroepiandrosterone to increase muscle mass, strength, and energy. It is also used by men for erectile dysfunction, and by healthy women, and women who have low levels of certain hormones to improve well-being and sexuality. Some people try dehydroepiandrosterone to treat systemic lupus erythematosus, osteoporosis, multiple sclerosis, low levels of steroid hormones (Addison's disease), depression, schizophrenia, chronic fatigue syndrome, and to slow the progression of Parkinson's disease. It is also used for preventing heart disease, breast cancer, diabetes, and metabolic syndrome. Dehydroepiandrosterone is used for weight loss, for decreasing the symptoms of menopause, and for boosting the immune system. People with HIV sometimes use dehydroepiandrosterone to ease depression and fatigue.

Testosterone

Signs and symptoms associated with low testosterone include poor erectile function, low libido, weaker and fewer erections, and reduced sexual activity. Other symptoms include increased body fat, decreased energy and fatigue, reduced muscle mass, and depression.

Estradiol

Estradiol is a type of estrogen. Low levels can indicate polycystic ovary syndrome or hypopituitarism. (Hypopituitarism is the decreased secretion of one or more of the eight hormones normally produced by the pituitary gland at the base of the brain.) In hypopituitarism women may experience infertility. Men lose facial, scrotal and trunk hair, as well as suffering decreased muscle mass and anaemia. Both sexes may experience a decrease in libido and loss of sexual function, and have an increased risk of osteoporosis.

This study investigated the effect of statins on steroid hormones in patients with type two diabetes. The study was a randomised, multicentre trial involving 98 patients. The patients were randomised into two groups: group I received 10 mg of atorvastatin plus 10 mg of ezetimibe, and group II 80 mg of atorvastatin for the first three months. Then, the first group received 80 mg of atorvastatin, and the second group 10 mg of atorvastatin plus 10 mg of ezetimibe for the following three months.

- The study found the levels of the vital adrenal and gonadal steroid hormones, dehydroepiandrosterone, testosterone and estradiol decreased in both groups of patients when they were taking either 80 mg of atorvastatin or 10 mg of atorvastatin plus 10 mg of ezetimibe.

Paper 365:
Statins cause testicular pain

Linnebur SA et al Probable Statin-Induced Testicular Pain. *Annals of Pharmacotherapy* Vol. 41, No. 1, pp. 138-142

Assistant Professor Sunny A Linnebur describes a case of a patient experiencing testicular pain on three occasions after taking three different statins.

- A 54-year-old man was started on lovastatin therapy.
- Seven months after starting lovastatin, the patient experienced testicular discomfort that resolved upon discontinuation of the drug.
- Afterward, he started simvastatin and again experienced testicular discomfort.
- The simvastatin was changed to atorvastatin, and the pain resolved. However, three months after starting atorvastatin,

the patient developed testicular pain, which resolved after the drug was stopped.

To conclude: A 54-year-old man tried three different types of statins and each time he developed testicular pain, which disappeared after the drugs were stopped.

Paper 366:
Statins reduce male fertility

Pons-Rejraji H et al Effects of atorvastatin on male fertility. *Endocrine Abstracts* 2010 22 P526

High levels of the enzyme Alpha-glucosidase are associated with higher percentages of sperm that have good motility.

The Acrosome is the "cap" on the head of the sperm that contains enzymes that make it possible for the sperm to penetrate the egg.

The epididymis is a tightly coiled mass of thin tubes that carries sperm from the testes to the ductus deferens in the male reproductive system. Sperm matures as it passes through the epididymis so that it is ready to fertilize ova by the time it enters the ductus deferens.

The aim of the study, headed by Dr Hanae Pons-Rejraji from the University of Clermont, was to analyze the consequences on sperm parameters with atorvastatin (Lipitor) intake. The study included 17 men who were administered 10 mg/day of atorvastatin for five months. Various sperm parameters were measured before taking the treatment, after five months of treatment, and three months after its withdrawal.

The study observed:

- Live spermatozoa percentage was reduced by atorvastatin by 8%.
- Concentrations of alpha-glucosidase were significantly decreased three months after ending the atorvastatin treatment.
- Significantly high concentrations of spermatozoa had spontaneously lost their acrosome three months after ending the atorvastatin treatment.

Dr Pons-Rejraji concluded: "*The intake of atorvastatin, in secondary prevention conditions, significantly affects epididymal functional marker and live spermatozoa proportion*".

Paper 367:
Statins significantly increase sperm abnormalities

Pons-Rejraji H et al Evaluation of atorvastatin efficacy and toxicity on spermatozoa, accessory glands and gonadal hormones of healthy men: a pilot prospective clinical trial. *Reproductive Biology and Endocrinology* 2014 Jul 12;12(1):65

This paper (published in 2014), contains additional information from Dr Pons-Rejraji's study from 2010 *(see paper 366)*. The study investigated the effect of statins on male fertility. In the study, semen parameters were measured in 17 healthy young men (average age 24 years) who were given atorvastatin for five months.

The additional information is as follows:

- Semen volume decreased by 10%.
- Sperm concentration decreased by 25%.
- The number of sperm decreased by 31%.
- The vitality of the sperm decreased by 9.5%
- Sperm head abnormalities increased by 11%.
- Sperm neck and midpiece abnormalities increased by 33%.
- Sperm tail abnormalities increased by 4.5%.
- Excess residual cytoplasm (which can impair overall sperm function and produce higher levels of reactive oxygen species, potentially leading to male infertility) increased by 68%.

Dr Pons-Rejraji concluded that atorvastatin: *"affected significantly sperm parameters of young and healthy men and was considered as deleterious... in view of our results in this young population, it may be considered that the effects could be more pronounced among older men specifically if less healthy"*.

Paper 368:
Prenatal exposure to statin drugs results in 27% increased risk of spontaneous abortions

Taguchi N et al Prenatal exposure to HMG-CoA reductase inhibitors: effects on fetal and neonatal outcomes. *Reproductive Toxicology* 2008 Oct;26(2):175-7

This study examined the effects of statins on foetuses. The study included 64 pregnant women taking statins during the first trimester, and 64 pregnant women without exposure to statins.

The study identified:

- The women taking statins had an 11.5% increased risk of not having a live birth compared to the women not taking statins.
- The women taking statins had a 27.3% increased risk of spontaneous abortions compared to the women not taking statins.
- The gestational age at birth was reduced by one week in the women taking statins compared to the women not taking statins.
- The child's birth weight was 9% lower in the women taking statins compared to the women not taking statins.

Paper 369: Simvastatin and lovastatin should not be taken during pregnancy

Pollack PS et al Pregnancy outcomes after maternal exposure to simvastatin and lovastatin. *Birth Defects Research Part A Clinical Molecular Teratology* 2005 Nov;73(11):888-96

The objective of the study was to determine the frequency of adverse outcomes after maternal exposure to simvastatin and/or lovastatin during pregnancy. Dr Pia Pollack led a team that carried out a review of the Merck & Co pharmacovigilance database for reports of exposure to simvastatin or lovastatin during pregnancy

The review found:

- The rate of congenital anomalies was 21% higher after maternal exposure to simvastatin and/or lovastatin during pregnancy compared to background population rates.
- Congenital anomalies included; chromosomal abnormalities, genetic disorders, abnormality of the urethra and penis, part of the small bowel (the duodenum) had not developed properly, cleft lip, and brown growths on the skin.

Dr Pollack concluded: "*Simvastatin and lovastatin remain contraindicated during pregnancy*".

Paper 370: Statins increase the risk of birth defects, miscarriage and premature birth

Winterfeld U et al Pregnancy outcome following maternal exposure to statins: a multicentre prospective study. *British Journal of Obstetrics and Gynaecology* 2013 Mar;120(4):463-71

The aim of the study was to investigate the risk associated with exposure to statins during pregnancy. The study collected observations from 249 statin-exposed pregnancies and 249 women not taking statins.

The study revealed:

- The statin-exposed women had a 50% increased risk of having a child with a major birth defect compared to the women not taking statins.
- The statin-exposed women had a 36% increased risk of having a miscarriage compared to the women not taking statins.
- The statin-exposed women had a 110% increased risk of having a premature birth compared to the women not taking statins.

Paper 371:
Antiphospholipid antibodies (indicate an increased risk of blood clots or pregnancy loss) are associated with statin use

Broder A et al High antiphospholipid antibody levels are associated with statin use and may reflect chronic endothelial damage in non-autoimmune thrombosis: cross-sectional study. *Journal of Clinical Pathology* 2012 Jun;65(6):551-6

Persistently elevated antiphospholipid antibodies and positive lupus anticoagulant are associated with an increased risk of pregnancy complications, including preeclampsia, thrombosis, autoimmune thrombocytopenia, fetal growth restriction, and fetal loss.

The study explored whether antiphospholipid antibodies and positive lupus anticoagulant were associated with statin use in 270 patients without autoimmune diseases hospitalised with arterial or venous thrombosis (blood clots).

- The study found that statin users were 220% more likely to have antiphospholipid antibody positivity.

Paper 372: Congenital abnormalities in baby born to mother using lovastatin

Ghidini A et al Congenital abnormalities (VATER) in baby born to mother using lovastatin. *Lancet* 1992 Jun 6;339(8806):1416-7

Dr Alessandro Ghidini, a Maternal-Fetal Medicine Specialist, reports the case of an infant born with many malformations after the mother used a statin during pregnancy.

- A woman was treated for five weeks with lovastatin, starting approximately six weeks from her last menstrual period.
- The statin was discontinued when her pregnancy was diagnosed at 11 weeks' gestation.
- A female infant was delivered by caesarean section at 39 weeks' gestation. The infant had a constellation of malformations termed the VATER association (vertebral anomalies, anus not developed properly, an abnormal connection between the oesophagus and the trachea with part of the oesophagus missing, and kidney, forearm and wrist abnormalities).
- Her anomalies included a deformed chest, spinal deformity, absent left thumb, foreshortened left forearm, shortened left elbow, fusion of the ribs on the left, anomalies in the spine, deformed left forearm, and a narrow lower oesophagus.

Paper 373: Statin exposure causes birth abnormalities

Edison RJ et al Central Nervous System and Limb Anomalies in Case Reports of First-Trimester Statin Exposure. *New England Journal of Medicine* 350, 1579-82 2004

Dr Robin Edison reviewed 52 cases of first-trimester statin exposure reported to the Food and Drug Administration.

The review found:

- Among these cases, there were 20 reports of malformation, including five severe defects of the central nervous system (two of which were holoprosencephaly) and five unilateral limb deficiencies.

- One patient had both of these malformations. The two simvastatin-exposed cases of limb deficiency were complex lower-limb anomalies including both long-bone shortening and aplasia or hypoplasia of the foot structures. The infant in one of these cases and a lovastatin-exposed infant also had rare forms of the VACTERL association (i.e., three or more of the following findings: vertebral, anal, cardiac, tracheal, oesophageal, renal, and limb defects).
- It is thought that only a small proportion of statin adverse events are reported to the FDA.
- There would be no expected cases of most of the malformations listed in the paper; yet three rare anomalies are each observed twice.

Paper 374:
Birth defects have been associated with statins

Girardin F et al The selection of a drug in a defined therapeutic class: the case of the HMG-CoA reductase inhibitors. *Revue Medicale Suisse* 2005 Apr 6;1(14):949-53

Category X drugs are drugs which have such a high risk of causing permanent damage to the foetus that they should not be used in pregnancy or when there is a possibility of pregnancy.

Dr Francois Girardin from the University of Geneva conducted a review of the scientific literature concerning the side effects of statins.

Regarding birth defect, his review revealed:

- Statins are categorised category X in pregnancy and are therefore contraindicated during the entire gestation period and in patients of reproductive age when contraception is not guaranteed.
- Statins such as simvastatin and atorvastatin have a well-documented teratogenic (birth defects) risk.
- Cases of severe multiple malformations have been reported including:
    - o Holoprosencephaly (Holoprosencephaly is a birth defect of the brain, which often can also affect facial features, including closely spaced eyes, small head size, and sometimes clefts of the lip and roof of the mouth, as well as other birth defects.)

- o Hypoplasia of the digestive tract and the respiratory system. (Hypoplasia is underdevelopment or incomplete development of a tissue or organ.)
- o Vertebral aplasia (where a vertebrae is missing).

Paper 375:
Statin use during pregnancy could lead to birth defects and malformations

No authors listed Statins: beware during pregnancy.
Prescrire international 2006 Feb;15(81):18-9

This paper is a review of the scientific literature regarding statins and pregnancy.

- Central nervous system and limb defects have been reported in newborns exposed to statins in the uterus. Several case reports describe malformations that are very rare in the general population.
- Animal toxicity studies also suggest that statins cause malformations of an embryo or fetus.
- The data suggests that statins should be avoided during pregnancy and that pregnant women exposed to cholesterol-lowering drugs should be monitored very closely.

This chapter documents the potential disastrous effects of statins for couples wanting to produce a healthy baby:

- Men taking statins have an increased risk of erectile dysfunction, a lower libido and a lack of testosterone and other vital hormones. These factors increase the chances of men been unable to father a child.
- Statin use is linked to a decreased sperm volume and sperm abnormalities. These factors increase the chances of men fathering a child with birth defects.
- Women taking statin drugs have more miscarriages and premature births. Their babies also have an increased risk of birth defects and congenital abnormalities.

Chapter 15

Some other toxic effects of statins

The papers in this chapter of the book document some of the other toxic side effects of statin drugs.

Paper 376: Statin use increases the risk of osteoarthritis and joint pain by 26%

Mansi IA et al Incidence of musculoskeletal and neoplastic diseases in patients on statin therapy: results of a retrospective cohort analysis. *American Journal of Medical Sciences* 2013 May;345(5):343-8

Osteoarthritis and rheumatoid arthritis are different types of arthritis. The main difference between osteoarthritis and rheumatoid arthritis is the cause behind the joint symptoms. Osteoarthritis is caused by mechanical wear and tear on joints. Rheumatoid arthritis is an autoimmune disease in which the body's own immune system attacks the body's joints.

This study was led by Dr Ishak Mansi from the University of Texas Health Science Centre. The study was conducted to investigate the incidence of various musculoskeletal diseases in statin users and nonusers. The study included 12,980 statin users and 45,997 nonusers who were followed for four years.

The study found:

- Statin users had a 26% increased risk of osteoarthritis and arthropathy (joint pain) compared to nonusers.
- Statin users had a 20% increased risk of dorsopathies (back or spinal pain), rheumatism (joint and connective tissue problems) and chondropathies (cartilage disease) compared to nonusers.

Dr Mansi concluded: "*Statin use was associated with an increased incidence of musculoskeletal diseases, including arthropathy*".

Paper 377:
Statins significantly associated with worsening in knee pain and physical function in patients with osteoarthritis

Riddle DL et al Associations between Statin use and changes in pain, function and structural progression: a longitudinal study of persons with knee osteoarthritis. *Annals of the Rheumatic Diseases* 2013 Feb;72(2):196-203

The Western Ontario and McMaster Universities Osteoarthritis Index (WOMAC) is a tested questionnaire to assess pain and physical functional disability in patients osteoarthritis with of the knee and the hip.

The first author of this study was Dr Daniel Riddle. His research interests are in the areas of recovery following knee arthroplasty. (Arthroplasty is a surgical procedure to restore the integrity and function of a joint. A joint can be restored by resurfacing the bones or artificially.) The study set out to determine if statin usage was associated with changes in knee pain and physical function in persons with knee osteoarthritis. Changes in the WOMAC score were assessed over four years in 2,207 patients with knee osteoarthritis.

- A significant finding of the study, Dr Riddle concluded was that: "*Increased duration of statin use was associated with worsening in WOMAC Physical Function scores over the study period*".

Paper 378:
Statins are associated with a 71% increased risk of rheumatoid arthritis

de Jong HJ et al Use of statins is associated with an increased risk of rheumatoid arthritis. *Annals of the Rheumatic Diseases* 2012 May;71(5):648-54

This Dutch study investigated whether statin use was associated with an increased risk of developing rheumatoid arthritis. The study included 508 patients aged 40 years or older with a first-time diagnosis of rheumatoid arthritis who were compared with 2,540 subjects without rheumatoid arthritis.

- The study identified that statin users had a 71% increased risk of rheumatoid arthritis compared to nonusers.

Paper 379: Possible association between statin use and bowel dysmotility

Fernandes R et al Possible association between statin use and bowel dysmotility. *British Medical Journal Case Reports* 2012 Feb 25;2012. pii: bcr1020114918

Roland Fernandes from the Vascular Surgery Department at the Medway Maritime Hospital in Kent, reports the case of a patient taking statins who developed impaired bowel motility.

- A 70-year-old man was admitted to hospital 14 times in six years following recurrent episodes of abdominal discomfort and a persistent sensation that he was unable to open his bowels fully.
- He had started to take simvastatin eight years previously, approximately six months prior to the onset of his symptoms.
- Test revealed he had colonic dilation and volvulus. (Colonic dilation is an abnormal dilation (enlargement) of the colon. The dilation is often accompanied by a paralysis in bowel movements. A volvulus is a complete twisting of a loop of intestine causing a blockage.)
- The colonic dilation and volvulus was treated with a sigmoid colectomy. (A sigmoid colectomy is an operation to remove part of the left side of the colon known as the sigmoid colon.)
- His symptoms initially improved but returned two years later.
- The patient stopped taking statins and his symptoms markedly improved and he was able to open his bowels daily with no discomfort.
- Statins were inadvertently restarted which caused the symptoms to reoccur.
- He again stopped the statin.
- The patient was reviewed several months later, at which time he continued to report a beneficial effect from the discontinuation of the statins. He reported that both the frequency and ease with which he opened his bowels to have improved.

Paper 380:
Statins cause a massive rise in constipation

Gau JT et al Risk factors associated with stool retention assessed by abdominal radiography for constipation. *Journal of the American Medical Directors Association* 2010 Oct;11(8):572-8

One of the aims of the study, headed by Dr Jen-Tzer Gau a specialist in geriatric Medicine, was to identify risk factors associated with constipation. 122 adults aged 65 or over with constipation were included in the study.

The study found:

- The use of statins was significantly associated with constipation, with statin users having a 286% increased risk of clinical constipation.
- Statin users had a greater severity of stool retention.

Paper 381:
Rising diarrhoea rates linked to statins

McGuire T et al Clinically important interaction between statin drugs and Clostridium difficile toxin? *Medical Hypotheses* 2009 Dec;73(6):1045-7

Clostridium difficile is a type of bacterial infection that can affect the digestive system and can lead to diarrhoea.

Clostridium difficile associated disease, a common type of antibiotic associated diarrhoea, is increasing in frequency and is now occurring more commonly in younger patients who are relatively healthy and may not be receiving antibiotics.

Dr Timothy McGuire and a team of researchers from the University of Nebraska Medical Centre investigated the factors which may have caused the rise in Clostridium difficile associated disease.

The investigations observed:

- Clostridium difficile toxin comes as two major forms that are closely related, toxin A and toxin B and both are able to produce Clostridium difficile associated disease.
- Clostridium difficile produces these toxic effects by inactivating a protein called Rho which is involved in multiple cellular signalling pathways.

- Statins also inhibit Rho.
- Statins could heighten Clostridium difficile toxin effects in the colon which leads to an increased risk of Clostridium difficile associated disease.
- A statin trial demonstrated an increased rate of Clostridium difficile associated disease in patients receiving statins compared to non-statin controls.

McGuire concludes: "*The weight of the evidence leads to our hypothesis that statins interact with Clostridium difficile toxin A and B causing an increase in the rate and severity of Clostridium difficile associated disease (diarrhoea)*".

Paper 382:
Statin consumption increases the risk of microscopic colitis

Fernández-Bañares F et al Drug consumption and the risk of microscopic colitis. *American Journal of Gastroenterology* 2007 Feb;102(2):324-30

The aim of this Spanish study was to investigate the possible association of chronic drug consumption with microscopic colitis. Microscopic colitis is a type of inflammatory bowel disease that is only visible using a microscope. Microscopic colitis has two main forms: collagenous colitis and lymphocytic colitis. The symptoms of both are identical in which chronic watery and nonbloody diarrhoea is the main symptom.

The study included 130 patients with microscopic colitis or chronic watery diarrhoea who were compared with 103 control subjects.

Regarding statins, the study found:

- Statin users had a 360% increased risk of lymphocytic colitis compared to nonusers.
- Statin users had a 440% increased risk of chronic watery diarrhoea compared to nonusers.

Paper 383:
Statins linked to colitis

Mukhopadhya A et al Pravastatin-induced colitis. *European Journal of Gastroenterology and Hepatology* 2008 Aug;20(8):810-2

Dr Ashis Mukhopadhya, specialist in gastroenterology, describes the case of an elderly lady who developed colitis (inflammation of the colon) after starting pravastatin therapy.

- Within 48 hours of starting pravastatin therapy, an 80-year-old woman developed symptoms of colitis.
- Examination revealed ulceration and inflammation throughout the colon.
- She stopped taking pravastatin, and five months later there was complete resolution of the colonic lesions.

Paper 384: Ulcerative colitis and statins

Rea WE et al Ulcerative colitis after statin treatment. *Postgraduate Medical Journal* 2002 May;78(919):286-7

This paper illustrates the case of a man who developed ulcerative colitis as an adverse reaction to simvastatin. (Ulcerative colitis is a form of inflammatory bowel disease.)

- A 65-year-old man was admitted to hospital with a one month history of diarrhoea, passing between five and ten loose, watery motions per day, occasionally with blood.
- The patient had had one similar episode, approximately one year before admission. On that occasion, it was felt by his general practitioner that the episode coincided with the patient starting pravastatin.
- The pravastatin was discontinued and the patient's symptoms resolved.
- At the time of the present admission, the patient was taking simvastatin 20 mg once a day. He had been started on simvastatin 10 mg once a day, six months before admission, and this had been increased to simvastatin 20 mg once a day one month before admission.
- Shortly afterwards, the symptoms had started.
- Examination revealed he was dehydrated and had generalised rectal tenderness with a small amount of fresh blood.
- Investigations showed: A raised serum urea concentration. Reduced haemoglobin. Low albumin. Partial blockage of the small intestine.

- Tests found inflammation of the colon and the lining of the rectum.
- A biopsy confirmed a diagnosis of simvastatin induced ulcerative colitis.
- The simvastatin was discontinued.
- The patient received treatment but by day five had significantly more abdominal pain.
- Investigations revealed severe ulcerative colitis with ulceration and polyp formation throughout.
- The patient had an operation to remove all of the colon, rectum and anus.
- Despite treatment in an intensive care unit the patient developed multiple organ failure and died.

The authors note that reports have also been received about:

- o Ulcerative colitis and colitis associated with pravastatin.
- o Colitis with atorvastatin.
- o Inflammatory bowel disease for fluvastatin.

One of the authors of the paper, Dr David Boldy a Consultant Physician in respiratory medicine, comments that this side effect of statin treatment "*is almost certainly subject to under-reporting*".

He concludes that one of the learning points of the paper is that: "*Colitis may be an effect of all statins*".

Paper 385: Statin users have a 45% increased risk of acute large bowel ischemia

Longstreth GF et al Diseases and drugs that increase risk of acute large bowel ischemia. *Clinical Gastroenterology and Hepatology* 2010 Jan;8(1):49-54

Acute large bowel ischemia is damage to the large intestine due to a decrease in its blood supply. It is a common cause of hospitalisation for acute abdominal pain, rectal bleeding, or diarrhoea that increases markedly with age.

This study investigated factors that may be associated with acute large bowel ischemia. The study included 379 patients with acute large bowel ischemia and 1,516 controls (average age, 69 years; range, 25-97 years).

- Regarding statins, the study found that statin users had a 45% increased risk of acute large bowel ischemia compared to nonusers.

Paper 386:
Use of statins and risk of fractures

van Staa TP et al Use of statins and risk of fractures.
Journal of the American Medical Association
2001 Apr 11;285(14):1850-5

This study was led by Dr Tjeerd-Pieter van Staa, who has more than 15 years of significant research experience in pharmaco-vigilance and epidemiology. The objective of the study was to investigate risk of fracture among statin users. The study included 81,880 patients aged 50 years or older who had had a fracture who were compared with 81,880 participants with no fractures.

The study pinpointed:

- Those who had used statins for six to 12 months had a 14% increased risk of a fracture compared to those who did not use statins.
- Those who had used statins for over 12 months had a 17% increased risk of a fracture compared to those who did not use statins.
- Those who had a cumulative dose of statins of up to 2.4 grams had a 2% increased risk of a fracture compared to those who did not use statins.
- Those who had a cumulative dose of statins of over 7.5 grams had a 29% increased risk of a fracture compared to those who did not use statins.

Paper 387:
Statins increase the risk of bone fracture in postmenopausal women

LaCroix AZ et al Statin use, clinical fracture, and bone density in postmenopausal women: results from the Women's Health Initiative Observational Study.
Annals of Internal Medicine 2003 Jul 15;139(2):97-104

The aim of the study was to examine the association of statin use with the incidence of hip, lower arm or wrist, and other fractures.

The study included 93,716 postmenopausal women, aged 50 to 79 years who were followed for an average of 3.9 years.

The study indicated:

- Women using statins had a 22% increased risk of hip fracture compared to women not using statins.
- Women using statins had a 4% increased risk of lower arm or wrist fracture compared to women not using statins.
- Women using statins had an 11% increased risk of other fractures compared to women not using statins.

Paper 388: Statins associated with increased bone loss in early postmenopausal women

Sirola J et al Relation of statin use and bone loss: a prospective population-based cohort study in early postmenopausal women. *Osteoporosis International* 2002 Jul;13(7):537-41

This University of Kuopio study assessed the effects of statin use on the change in bone mineral density in early postmenopausal women. The study measured annual change in spine and thigh bone mineral density in 620 women aged 53-64 years who were divided into four groups:

- Group 1: 55 who had continuous use of statins
- Group 2: 63 who had occasional statin use.
- Group 3: 142 nonusers of statins who had "high" cholesterol.
- Group 4: 360 nonusers of statins who did not have "high" cholesterol.

The Finnish investigators found:

- In all groups spine bone mineral density increased whereas thigh bone mineral density decreased.
- Both groups of nonusers had higher increases in spine bone mineral density compared to the groups of statin users. (High cholesterol nonusers had highest increase.)
- Both groups of nonusers had smaller decreases in thigh bone mineral density compared to the groups of statin users. (High cholesterol nonusers had smallest decrease.)
- The nonusers of statins who had "high" cholesterol had a 79% higher increase in spine bone mineral density compared to the continuous statin users.

- The nonusers of statins who had "high" cholesterol had a 34% smaller decrease in thigh bone mineral density compared to the continuous statin users.

The results from the study suggest statin use is associated with increased bone loss in early postmenopausal women.

An interesting finding noted by the researchers is the potential for "high" cholesterol itself to be protective against osteoporosis and fractures, as the smallest annual bone loss and greatest gain of lumbar bone were seen in those with "high" cholesterol.

Paper 389:
Statins increase the risk of tendon rupture

Beri A et al Association between statin therapy and tendon rupture: a case-control study. *Journal of Cardiovascular Pharmacology* 2009 May;53(5):401-4

This study investigated the relationship between statins and tendon rupture. The study included 93 patients with tendon rupture who were compared with 279 control subjects.

- The study revealed statin users had a 10% increased risk of tendon rupture compared to nonusers.

Paper 390:
Orthopaedic surgeon finds an association of spontaneous distal biceps tendon ruptures with statin administration

Savvidou C et al Spontaneous distal biceps tendon ruptures: are they related to statin administration? *Hand Surgery* 2012;17(2):167-71

A distal biceps rupture occurs when the tendon attaching the biceps muscle to the elbow is torn from the bone.

The purpose of the study, headed by orthopaedic surgeon Dr Christiana Savvidou, was to identify a possible correlation between statin administration and incidence of spontaneous distal biceps tendon ruptures. The study included 104 patients with distal biceps tendon rupture average age 47 years (range, 22-78).

- The study detected it was nearly two times more likely to have spontaneous distal biceps tendon rupture with use of statins.

Dr Savvidou concluded: "*Based on the results of our study we conclude that there is a trend of association of spontaneous distal biceps tendon ruptures with statin administration*".

Paper 391:
Doctor says statins may increase the risk of tendon rupture

Pullatt RC et al Tendon rupture associated with simvastatin/ ezetimibe therapy. *American Journal of Cardiology* 2007 Jul 1;100(1):152-3

Cardiologist Dr Raja Pullatt outlines the case of a man who suffered a tendon rupture while on simvastatin and ezetimibe.

- A 46-year-old man had been taking simvastatin and ezetimibe for four months.
- He ruptured his left biceps tendon while lifting a box out of his car.
- He stopped taking simvastatin and ezetimibe and the rupture was surgically repaired.
- Two months after the repair he restarted the drug and promptly developed pain in the biceps.
- The pain abated two weeks after discontinuing the medication.

Dr Pullatt notes that: "*Physiological repair of an injured tendon requires degradation and remodelling of the extracellular matrix through matrix metalloproteinases*", (matrix metalloproteinases are enzymes that play an important part in wound healing) and "*Statins are known to inhibit matrix metalloproteinases*".

Dr Pullat concluded: "*Statins may increase the risk of tendon rupture by altering matrix metalloproteinases activity*".

Paper 392:
Rupture of the quadriceps tendons associated with simvastatin

Rubin G et al Bilateral, simultaneous rupture of the quadriceps tendon associated with simvastatin. *Israel Medical Association Journal* 2011 Mar;13(3):185-6

This paper portrays the case of a man who simultaneously ruptured both quadricep tendons while on simvastatin therapy.

- A 58-year-old man sought treatment at a hospital emergency department with an "electric shock" type pain while walking in both of his legs.
- He had been taking simvastatin for four years (the last two years with 80 mg per day).
- Examination revealed complete rupture in both quadricep tendons.
- Simvastatin treatment was discontinued.
- Investigations found that statin-related tendon complications were the cause of the rupture.

Paper 393: Statins increase the risk of haemorrhage in hernia patients by 60%

Hauer-Jensen M et al Influence of statins on postoperative wound complications after inguinal or ventral herniorrhaphy. *Hernia* 2006 Mar;10(1):48-52

This study investigated the relationship between statins and postoperative wound complications in patients undergoing hernia repair. The study included 10,782 patients who had undergone herniorrhaphy (surgical repair of a hernia).

- The study found that patients taking statins had a 60% increased risk of postoperative wound hematoma (where blood collects and pools) or haemorrhage.

Paper 394: Database reveals an association between statins and urinary tract symptoms

Fujimoto M et al Association of statin use with storage lower urinary tract symptoms (LUTS): data mining of prescription database. *International Journal of Clinical Pharmacology and Therapeutics* 2014 Sep;52(9):762-9

The objective of this study, conducted by a group led by Dr Mai Fujimoto, was to examine the association between statin use and the risk of lower urinary tract symptoms. The study analysed a large database of prescriptions of statin use in combination with drugs administered for storage lower urinary tract symptoms. (Storage lower urinary tract symptoms include increased frequency and urgency of passing urine, urge incontinence and needing to get up to pass urine at night.)

- The study observed that after one year of starting statins, 17% of statin users had to be prescribed drugs to combat storage lower urinary tract symptoms.

Dr Fujimoto concluded: *"Analysis of the prescription database showed significant association for storage LUTS (lower urinary tract symptoms) in statin users"*.

Paper 395:
Statins associated with lower urinary tract infections

Fujimoto M et al Statin-associated lower urinary tract symptoms: data mining of the public version of the FDA adverse event reporting system, FAERS. *International Journal of Clinical Pharmacology and Therapeutics* 2014 Apr;52(4):259-66

Dr Fujimoto carried out another study regarding urinary tract symptoms. The aim of this study was to examine the association between statin use and the risk of lower urinary tract symptoms in reports submitted to the US Food and Drug Administration Adverse Event Reporting System. The risk was calculated using the case/non-case method. Cases were identified by the presence of reports of an adverse drug reaction in which statins were the suspected drug. Non-cases were all the reports of the same reactions induced by drugs other than statins. A total of 44,959,104 drug-reaction pairs were found in 2,681,739 reports.

The study revealed:

- Statin users had a 16% increased risk of lower urinary tract voiding symptoms (poor stream, hesitancy, intermittent flow and straining when passing urine) compared to users of all other drugs.
- Statin users had a 25% increased risk of lower urinary tract storage symptoms (increased frequency and urgency of passing urine, urge incontinence and needing to get up to pass urine at night) compared to users of all other drugs.

Dr Fujimoto concluded: *"Analysis of the FAERS (US Food and Drug Administration Adverse Event Reporting System) database showed small but reliable signals for LUTS (lower urinary tract symptoms) in statin users. The mechanism responsible for these reactions is unknown. However, these adverse events should be monitored closely".*

Paper 396:
Atorvastatin can induce hemorrhagic cystitis

Martinez-Suarez HJ et al Atorvastatin-induced hemorrhagic cystitis: a case report. *Urology* 2009 Mar;73(3):681.e5-6

Urologist Dr Humberto Joseph Martinez-Suarez depicts the case of a woman who developed hemorrhagic cystitis after starting atorvastatin therapy. (Hemorrhagic cystitis is bleeding in the lower urinary tract. It results from damage to the bladder's blood vessels by toxins, pathogens, radiation, drugs, or disease.)

- A 77-year-old woman sought medical help for persistent haematuria of four weeks duration. (Hematuria is blood in the urine.)
- She had started taking atorvastatin one week before the onset of her hematuria.
- She also complained of some mild muscle pain since starting atorvastatin.
- Investigations revealed grossly bloody urine, inflammation and oozing lesions in the bladder.
- She was diagnosed with atorvastatin induced hemorrhagic cystitis.
- She discontinued atorvastatin.
- Her hematuria resolved within one week of discontinuation of atorvastatin.
- She restarted atorvastatin with a rapid recurrence of her hematuria.
- Investigations reconfirmed the previous findings.
- She again discontinued atorvastatin and her hematuria rapidly resolved.

Paper 397:
Statin users have a 13% increased incidence of common infections

Magulick JP et al The effect of statin therapy on the incidence of infections: a retrospective cohort analysis. *American Journal of the Medical Sciences* 2014 Mar;347(3):211-6

The goal of the study was to compare the incidence of infections in statin users to that in nonusers. The six-year study included 45,247 subjects.

The study identified:

- Statin users had a 13% increased incidence of common infections compared to nonusers.
- Statin users had a 6% increased incidence of influenza and fungal infections compared to nonusers.

Paper 398:
MRSA: a link to statin therapy?

Goldstein MR et al Methicillin-resistant Staphylococcus aureus: a link to statin therapy? *Cleveland Clinic Journal of Medicine* 2008 May;75(5):328-9

Dr Mark Goldstein, a specialist in internal medicine, comments on a possible link between statins and an increase in the incidence of methicillin-resistant *Staphylococcus aureus* (MRSA) bacteraemia.

- There is an increasing incidence of methicillin-resistant *Staphylococcus aureus* (MRSA) bacteraemia which may be related in part to the increasing use of statin therapy in both outpatient and hospital settings.
- A study revealed that skin and soft tissue infections as the source of bacteraemia were significantly more prevalent among patients treated with statins compared with patients not receiving statins and there have been reports of recurrent community-acquired MRSA skin infections in subjects on statin therapy.
- The epidermis (outer skin) is a very active site of cholesterol synthesis and acts as a barrier to infection. It has been shown that if the barrier of the skin is disrupted, there is a brisk increase in epidermal cholesterol synthesis to repair the damage. So if the cholesterol synthesis in the epidermis is inhibited by statins, the barrier function of the skin will be impaired.

To conclude: It is possible that statin therapy alters the cholesterol content of the epidermis which results in an inadequate barrier and impaired immune function of the skin which may leave it vulnerable to external pathogens and resulting bacteraemia such as MRSA.

Paper 399:
The risk of statins for contracting norovirus disease may have considerable consequences for the Western world

Rondy M et al Norovirus disease associated with excess mortality and use of statins: a retrospective cohort study of an outbreak following a pilgrimage to Lourdes. *Epidemiology and Infection* 2011 Mar;139(3):453-63

Noroviruses are a group of viruses that can cause gastroenteritis. Gastroenteritis is an infection of the gut (intestines) which usually causes vomiting and diarrhoea.

The lead author of the study is epidemiologist Dr Marc Rondy. His work includes coordinating a European network of hospitals aimed at estimating influenza vaccine effectiveness. This study examined the association of statins with norovirus. The study examined a group of psychiatric patients returning from Lourdes (France).

The study reported:

- Statin users had a 290% increased risk of contracting norovirus compared to nonusers.
- Death rates were 1,990% higher in patients infected with norovirus.

Dr Rondy concluded: *"The newly identified risk of statins for contracting norovirus disease may have considerable consequences for the Western world"*.

Paper 400:
Doctor says physicians should be aware of hyperthermia as a possible side effect of lovastatin use

von Pohle WR Recurrent hyperthermia due to lovastatin. *Western Journal of Medicine* 1994 Oct;161(4):427-8

Dr William von Pohle from Loma Linda University highlights the case of a woman who developed hyperthermia (very high body temperature) whilst on lovastatin.

- A 55-year-old woman was admitted to hospital with hyperthermia (40.5 degrees).
- She was taking lovastatin.
- She had suffered two weeks of low grade fever, was sleepy and drowsy and had cogwheel rigidity. (Cogwheel rigidity is

abnormal shaking during fever in muscle tissue characterized by jerky movements when the muscle is passively stretched. The condition is often found in cases of Parkinson's disease.)

- Laboratory tests revealed that her sodium, potassium and chloride levels were low.
- Lovastatin was discontinued and she was treated with potassium chloride and a saline solution.
- After two days her fever resolved, her mental state was normal and her sodium, potassium and chloride levels returned to normal.
- She restarted lovastatin.
- Three months later, she again had hyperthermia, low grade fever, was sleepy and drowsy and had cogwheel rigidity.
- She again stopped lovastatin, her mental state returned to normal and her fever resolved.
- She again restarted lovastatin.
- A month later, she was again in hospital with the same findings.
- The lovastatin therapy was again discontinued.
- After three days, her fever again resolved and her mental state became normal.
- She was seen 12 months after the discontinuation of lovastatin and has had no further episodes of hyperthermia.

Dr von Pohle concludes: "*Physicians should be aware of hyperthermia as a possible side effect of lovastatin use*".

Paper 401: Statins cause flu-like symptoms

Sinzinger H Flu-like response on statins.
Medical Science Monitor 2002 May;8(5):CR384-8

This paper describes five patients who developed flu-like symptoms after starting statin therapy.

- The patients reported a flu-like response on statins with very severe symptoms of exhaustion, weakness, aching muscles and joints and raised body temperature.
- These symptoms started within three weeks of starting statin therapy.

- The symptoms appeared even in the lowest available dose of statins.
- Only three of the patients had elevated creatine kinase levels.
- Four of the patients had elevated 8-epi-prostaglandin-F(2 alpha) levels, (an indication of muscle damage).
- The patients discontinued the statins, and within five weeks their symptoms completely disappeared.

Paper 402: Doctor says statin drug hypersensitivity reactions are potentially life-threatening

Liebhaber MI et al Polymyalgia, hypersensitivity pneumonitis and other reactions in patients receiving HMG-CoA reductase inhibitors: a report of ten cases. *Chest* 1999 Mar;115(3):886-9

This paper, headed by Dr Myron Liebhaber from the University of California Los Angeles School of Medicine, describes ten patients who developed hypersensitivity-type reactions after taking statin medications. (A hypersensitivity reaction is an exaggerated inflammatory response by the immune system to a drug or other foreign substance.)

Patient 1

- Nine months after starting lovastatin, 20 mg daily, a 54-year-old man developed urticaria over his entire body and angioedema of his upper lip. (Urticaria also known as hives, is a kind of skin rash with pale red, raised, itchy bumps. Angioedema is swelling under the skin.)
- Tests revealed an autoimmune disorder (where the body attacks its own tissues).
- Lovastatin was discontinued, and his symptoms gradually resolved over seven days.

Patient 2

- A 69-year-old woman was referred for medical attention for an evaluation of a cough.
- She had been taking pravastatin, 20 mg to 40 mg daily, for six years.
- She was given medication and her condition improved although tests revealed impaired lung function.

- Over the next six weeks her symptoms became much worse and she was given additional medication.
- Despite the treatment her cough continued.
- A scan found inflammation in the lungs.
- A lung biopsy led to a diagnosis of pravastatin induced hypersensitivity pneumonitis. (Hypersensitivity pneumonitis is a disease in which your lungs become inflamed when they are exposed to substances to which you are allergic.)
- The pravastatin was stopped, and her cough resolved two weeks later.
- A follow-up scan seven weeks after the first one showed complete resolution of the inflammation in her lungs.

Patient 3

- Three years after starting pravastatin 20 mg daily, a 77-year-old man developed gradually increasing inflammation, with symptoms of polymyalgia. (Polymyalgia is pain, stiffness and tenderness in many muscles.)
- In addition, three years after starting pravastatin, the patient had retinal vein thrombosis. (Retinal vein thrombosis is when one of the tiny retinal veins becomes blocked by a blood clot.)
- The patient then developed a sudden worsening of his heart function.
- After discontinuing the pravastatin his heart function normalized, and resolution of the polymyalgia syndrome occurred over one month.

Patient 4

- A 66-year-old man started taking lovastatin, 20 mg daily.
- Four years later, the patient complained of fatigability, drowsiness, shortness of breath and joint pain.
- Tests revealed inflammation and an autoimmune disorder.
- He stopped taking lovastatin.
- His symptoms gradually resolved over two months.

Patient 5

- A 76-year-old woman was started on lovastatin, 20 mg daily.
- One year later, she began to complain of muscle aches.

- Two years later, she developed shortness of breath, joint pain and psoriasis. (Psoriasis is inflammation of the skin and develops as patches of red, scaly skin.)
- She then had a small heart attack and a failed artery graft.
- Lovastatin was discontinued, and she had a gradual improvement of her shortness of breath, joint pain, muscle pain and back pain over a two month period.

Patient 6

- An 80-year-old woman had been taking simvastatin, 10 mg daily, for three years.
- She began having shortness of breath on exertion.
- Investigations revealed she had inflammation.
- Simvastatin was discontinued.
- Her shortness of breath improved and inflammation decreased over the next three weeks.

Patient 7

- A 49-year-old man had been taking pravastatin, 40 mg daily, for four years.
- During this period, he had generalised itching and urticaria, along with swelling of his fingers and feet.
- Test revealed an autoimmune disorder.
- Pravastatin was discontinued, and the itching and swelling gradually resolved over the subsequent month.

Patient 8

- A 77-year-old woman was treated with pravastatin, 10 mg daily, for three years.
- During this period, she had generalised itching with urticaria.
- Investigations revealed she had inflammation and an autoimmune disorder.
- Her symptoms cleared one month after discontinuing the pravastatin.

Patient 9

- A 53-year-old man started to take pravastatin 40 mg daily.
- Within six months, he developed angioedema (swelling) of the eyelids and a sensation of his airway closing.

- He discontinued pravastatin.
- His symptoms gradually resolved 30 days later.

Patient 10

- A 73-year-old man developed intense itching and urticaria after taking pravastatin 20 mg daily for three years.
- Tests revealed she had an autoimmune disorder.
- He discontinued pravastatin and 12 days later, his symptoms resolved.

Dr Liebhaber concluded: "*We feel it is important for clinicians to recognize early symptoms of statin drug hypersensitivity because they are potentially life-threatening*".

The papers in this chapter show that statins may increase the risk of the following conditions:

- Osteoarthritis, joint pain, back or spinal pain, rheumatism, cartilage disease, rheumatoid arthritis, constipation, diarrhoea, bowel disease, bone fracture, tendon rupture, urinary tract infections, common infections, meticillin-resistant staphylococcus aureusis (MRSA), gastroenteritis an influenza.

These are not the only conditions that may be triggered or exacerbated by statins. On the simvastatin (zocor) package insert, the following conditions are listed as adverse reactions. (The package inserts from the other statin drugs also give similar warnings.):

- Gastrointestinal disorders, myalgia, arthralgia, upper respiratory infections, headache, abdominal pain, constipation, nausea, edema/swelling, atrial fibrillation, diabetes, insomnia, vertigo, bronchitis, sinusitis, eczema, urinary tract infection, myopathy, rhabdomyolysis, diarrhoea, rash, dyspepsia, flatulence, asthenia, pruritus, alopecia, a variety of skin changes (e.g. nodules, discoloration, dryness of skin/mucous membranes, changes to hair/nails), dizziness, muscle cramps, pancreatitis, paresthesia, peripheral neuropathy, vomiting, anaemia, erectile dysfunction, interstitial lung disease, hepatitis/jaundice, fatal and non-fatal hepatic failure, depression, immune-mediated necrotizing myopathy, anaphylaxis, angioedema, lupus erythematous-like syndrome, polymyalgia rheumatica, dermatomyositis, vasculitis, purpura, thrombocytopenia, leukopenia, hemolytic anaemia, positive ANA, ESR increase, eosinophilia, arthritis, arthralgia, urticaria, asthenia, photosensitivity, fever, chills, flushing, malaise, dyspnea, toxic epidermal necrolysis, erythema multiforme, including Stevens- Johnson syndrome, cognitive impairment, memory loss, forgetfulness, amnesia, memory impairment and confusion).

Chapter 16

How many people suffer from statin induced toxic side effects?

Rory Collins is co-director of the Clinical Trial Service Unit (who have a huge influence on UK health policy) at Oxford. He says statin side effects affect less than 1% of patients.

However, his organisation has received multi-million pound funding from the manufacturers of statins *(see paper 490).*

Concerns about the pharmaceutical industry funding the Clinical Trials Service Unit were raised in an open letter, signed by nine doctors and academics, including the president of the Royal College of Physicians, Sir Richard Thompson *(see paper 491).*

The letter notes: "*The Clinical Trials Service Unit (CTSU) in Oxford, which has carried out many very large studies on statins, and other lipid modification agents with pharmaceutical company support, has received hundreds of millions in funding over the years*".

Sir Richard warns: "*We fear that the CTSU could be perceived as having a major conflict of interest in the area of cardiovascular disease prevention/lipid modification*".

The objective of this chapter is to ascertain the realistic figures of statin toxic effect victims by analysing the scientific literature.

Paper 403:
17% of statin users suffer side-effects
Zhang H et al Discontinuation of statins in routine care settings: a cohort study. *Annals of Internal Medicine* 2013 Apr 2;158(7):526-34

The objective of the study was to investigate statin discontinuation rates. The study included 107,835 adults who received a statin prescription between 1 January 2000 and 31 December 2008.

The study found:

- Statins were discontinued at least temporarily by 53% of patients.
- Statin-related events were documented for 17.4% patients.

Paper 404:
After only six months of therapy with a statin (Zocor), nearly a quarter of the patients suffered from side effects

Scott RS et al Simvastatin and side effects. *New Zealand Medical Journal* 1991 Nov 27;104(924):493-5

The aim of this New Zealand study was to investigate the side effects of simvastatin (Zocor). The study included 110 patients newly commenced on simvastatin who completed a side effects questionnaire after six months of therapy.

The study reported:

- 23.6% of patients suffered side effects.
- 13.6% of patients suffered muscle aches.
- 4.5% of patients suffered gastrointestinal symptoms.

After only six months of therapy with a statin (Zocor), nearly a quarter of the patients suffered from side effects.

Paper 405:
One third of all statin users report side effects

Cohen JD et al Understanding Statin Use in America and Gaps in Patient Education (USAGE): an internet-based survey of 10,138 current and former statin users. *Journal of Clinical Lipidology* 2012 May-Jun;6(3):208-15

This study, authored by Dr Jerome Cohen from St. Louis University School of Medicine, assessed the effects of statins on current and former users. The study included 10,138 participants, average age 61 years.

The study revealed:

- 28% of current statin users reported side effects.
- 33% of all statin users reported side effects.
- 65% of former statin users reported side effects.
- 62% of former statin users stopped taking statins because of the side effects.

Paper 406: With only 12 weeks of statin therapy, 36% of the patients have side effects

Wierzbicki AS et al Atorvastatin compared with simvastatin-based therapies in the management of severe familial hyperlipidaemias. *QJM* 1999 Jul;92(7):387-94

This UK based study analysed the side effects caused by statin therapy (Lipitor). Patients unable to tolerate previous statin therapy were excluded from the study. The trial lasted for 12 weeks and included 201 "patients" with alleged high cholesterol.

The study ascertained:

- 36% of patients had to withdraw from the trial because of side effects.
- 7% of patients suffered from diarrhoea.
- 5% of patients developed an erythematous rash (An erythematous rash is characterized by redness resulting from skin inflammation surrounding a patch of skin where a rash is located.)
- 4% of patients suffered from joint pains.

Paper 407: Statins side effects

Serruys PW et al Fluvastatin for prevention of cardiac events following successful first percutaneous coronary intervention: a randomized controlled trial. *Journal of the American Medical Association* 2002 Jun 26;287(24):3215-22

The objective of the study, (named the Lescol Intervention Prevention Study or LIPS), was to determine the effects of fluvastatin (Lescol) in patients who have undergone percutaneous coronary intervention. (Percutaneous Coronary Intervention, commonly known as a coronary angioplasty, is a procedure used to treat the narrowed or obstructed coronary arteries of the heart found in coronary heart disease.) The study was a randomised, double-blind, placebo-controlled trial, and included 1,677 patients (aged 18-80 years) who were followed for up to four years. The patients were randomly assigned to receive either fluvastatin, 80 mg per day or placebo.

Regarding side effects, the study found:

- Patients in the fluvastatin group had a 20% increased risk of atrial fibrillation compared with patients in the placebo group.
- Patients in the fluvastatin group had a 40% increased risk of abdominal pain compared with patients in the placebo group.
- Patients in the fluvastatin group had a 57% increased risk of constipation compared with patients in the placebo group.
- Patients in the fluvastatin group had a 12% increased risk of indigestion compared with patients in the placebo group.
- Patients in the fluvastatin group had a 28% increased risk of a gastric disorder compared with patients in the placebo group.
- Patients in the fluvastatin group had a 17% increased risk of nausea compared with patients in the placebo group.
- Patients in the fluvastatin group had a 30% increased risk of fatigue compared with patients in the placebo group.
- Patients in the fluvastatin group had a 51% increased risk of peripheral edema compared with patients in the placebo group.
- Patients in the fluvastatin group had a 15% increased risk of bronchitis compared with patients in the placebo group.
- Patients in the fluvastatin group had a 33% increased risk of the common cold compared with patients in the placebo group.
- Patients in the fluvastatin group had a 16% increased risk of joint pain compared with patients in the placebo group.
- Patients in the fluvastatin group had a 37% increased risk of muscle pain compared with patients in the placebo group.
- Patients in the fluvastatin group had a 51% increased risk of pain in the extremities compared with patients in the placebo group.
- Patients in the fluvastatin group had a 11% increased risk of dizziness compared with patients in the placebo group.
- Patients in the fluvastatin group had a 9% increased risk of fainting compared with patients in the placebo group.
- Patients in the fluvastatin group had a 16% increased risk of shortness of breath compared with patients in the placebo group.

- Patients in the fluvastatin group had a 38% increased risk of high blood pressure compared with patients in the placebo group.
- Patients in the fluvastatin group had a 9% increased risk of intermittent claudication compared with patients in the placebo group.

Paper 408:
Elderly patients do not like taking statin drugs

Jackevicius CA et al Adherence with statin therapy in elderly patients with and without acute coronary syndromes. *Journal of the American Medical Association* 2002 Jul 24-31;288(4):462-7

This Canadian study compared adherence rates in diverse groups of elderly patients taking statins. The two-year study included 22,379 patients with acute coronary syndrome, 36,106 patients with coronary artery disease and 85,020 without any coronary disease. Patients were aged 66 years and older.

The study ascertained, after two years:

- 59.9% of the patients with acute coronary syndrome had discontinued their statin drugs.
- 63.9% of the patients with coronary artery disease had discontinued their statin drugs.
- 74.6% of the patients without any coronary disease had discontinued their statin drugs.

The very high dropout rate of these diverse groups of patients taking statins, suggests that a large percentage of them would have suffered from some of the myriad side effects of statins.

Paper 409:
63.5% of patients report experiencing side-effects due to statins

Mashayekhi SO et al Patients' report of statins use and side-effects in a sample of hospitalized cardiac patients in the Islamic Republic of Iran. *Eastern Mediterranean health Journal* 2011 May;17(5):460-4

Dr Simin-Ozar Mashayekhi, an Assistant Professor of Clinical Pharmacology at Tabriz University of Medical Sciences, was the first author of this study. The aim of the study was to ascertain the prevalence of the side-effects of statins among patients admitted to a cardiac-specialized hospital who had taken statins prior to hospitalization. Data was collected on 200 patients, average age 61.5 years.

The findings of the study were:

- 63.5% of patients reported experiencing side-effects due to statins. The side-effects included:
  - Gastrointestinal 18.5%
  - Headache 16.5%
  - Elevated transaminase levels 12.5% (elevated transaminase levels indicate liver damage).
  - Muscle problems 9.5%
  - Allergic reactions 5%
  - Respiratory problems 4%
  - Rash 0.5%
- Muscle pain was observed in 100% of patients receiving 80 mg per day of atorvastatin.

Dr Mashayekhi concludes that: *"Clinicians should be aware of the adverse effects of statins"*.

Paper 410:
Statin side effects

Langsjoen PH et al Treatment of statin adverse effects with supplemental Coenzyme Q10 and statin drug discontinuation. *Biofactors* 2005;25(1-4):147-52

This study was conducted by Dr Peter Langsjoen and his team from the East Texas Medical Centre. The study investigated the effects of discontinuing statin drugs and beginning Coenzyme Q10 supplementation in cardiology (heart disorder) clinic patients. The study included 50 new cardiology clinic patients who were on statin drug therapy (for an average of 28 months), who on their initial visit were evaluated for possible adverse statin effects (muscle pain, fatigue, shortness of breath, memory loss, and peripheral neuropathy). All patients discontinued statin therapy due to side effects and began supplemental Coenzyme Q10. The patients were followed for an average of 22 months.

The study found that after stopping statins and starting Coenzyme Q10:

- Fatigue decreased from 84% to 16%.
- Muscle pain decreased from 64% to 6%.
- Shortness of breath decreased 58% to 12%.
- Memory loss decreased from 8% to 4%.
- Peripheral neuropathy decreased from 10% to 2%.
- Measurements of heart function either improved or remained stable in the majority of patients.
- There were no adverse consequences from statin discontinuation.

Dr Langsjoen concluded: "*Statin-related side effects, including statin cardiomyopathy, are far more common than previously published and are reversible with the combination of statin discontinuation and supplemental Coenzyme Q10. We saw no adverse consequences from statin discontinuation*".

Paper 411:
The unintended adverse effects of statins in men and women

Hippisley-Cox J et al Unintended effects of statins in men and women in England and Wales: population based cohort study using the QResearch database. *British Medical Journal* 2010 May 20;340:c2197

The objective of the study, published in the prestigious *British Medical Journal,* was to quantify the unintended effects of statins. The study included 2,004 692 patients aged 30-84 years.

The study revealed after five years:

- Women who used statins had a 56% increased risk of acute renal (kidney) failure compared to women who did not use statins.
- Women who used statins had a 30% increased risk of cataracts compared to women who did not use statins.
- Women who used statins had a 53% increased risk of liver disease compared to women who did not use statins.
- Women who used statins had a 197% increased risk of myopathy (muscle disease) compared to women who did not use statins.
- Men who used statins had a 61% increased risk of acute renal (kidney) failure compared to men who did not use statins.

- Men who used statins had a 32% increased risk of cataracts compared to men who did not use statins.
- Men who used statins had a 53% increased risk of liver disease compared to men who did not use statins.
- Men who used statins had a 515% increased risk of myopathy (muscle disease) compared to men who did not use statins.

Paper 412: Professor says that data from Adverse Event Reports submitted to the US Food and Drug Administration strongly suggests the necessity of well-organized clinical studies with respect to statin-associated adverse events.

Sakaeda T et al Statin-associated muscular and renal adverse events: data mining of the public version of the FDA adverse event reporting system. *PLoS One* 2011;6(12):e28124

The objective of the study, led by Professor Toshiyuki Sakaeda of Kyoto University, was to analyse the Adverse Event Reports submitted to the US Food and Drug Administration to assess the muscular and renal adverse events induced by the administration of statins compared to other drugs. Adverse Event Reports involving pravastatin, simvastatin, atorvastatin, or rosuvastatin were analysed. Myalgia (muscle pain), rhabdomyolysis and an increase in creatine phosphokinase level were focused on as the muscular adverse events, and acute renal failure, non-acute renal failure, and an increase in blood creatinine level as the renal adverse events. The study was based on 1,644,220 Adverse Event Reports.

The study indicated:

- Rosuvastatin users had a 864% increased risk of myalgia compared to other drug users.
- Atorvastatin users had a 259% increased risk of myalgia compared to other drug users.
- Simvastatin users had a 252% increased risk of myalgia compared to other drug users.
- Pravastatin users had a 206% increased risk of myalgia compared to other drug users.
- Simvastatin users had a 659% increased risk of rhabdomyolysis compared to other drug users.

- Rosuvastatin users had a 507% increased risk of rhabdomyolysis compared to other drug users.
- Atorvastatin users had a 191% increased risk of rhabdomyolysis compared to other drug users.
- Pravastatin users had a 125% increased risk of rhabdomyolysis compared to other drug users.
- Rosuvastatin users had a 470% increased risk of an increase in creatine phosphokinase levels compared to other drug users.
- Simvastatin users had a 275% increased risk of an increase in creatine phosphokinase levels compared to other drug users.
- Atorvastatin users had a 194% increased risk of an increase in creatine phosphokinase levels compared to other drug users.
- Pravastatin users had a 147% increased risk of an increase in creatine phosphokinase levels compared to other drug users.
- Other muscular adverse events found commonly for these four statins included asthenia, chest pain, pain in the extremities, muscle spasms, muscular weakness, myositis, and myopathy, and a stronger association was found for rosuvastatin.
- Simvastatin users had a 72% increased risk of acute renal failure compared to other drug users.
- Pravastatin users had a 42% increased risk of acute renal failure compared to other drug users.
- Rosuvastatin users had a 33% increased risk of acute renal failure compared to other drug users.
- Atorvastatin users had a 13% increased risk of acute renal failure compared to other drug users.
- Rosuvastatin users had a 36% increased risk of non-acute renal failure compared to other drug users.
- Simvastatin users had a 18% increased risk of non-acute renal failure compared to other drug users.
- Pravastatin users had a 16% increased risk of non-acute renal failure compared to other drug users.
- Pravastatin users had a 63% increased risk of an increase in blood creatinine levels compared to other drug users.
- Simvastatin users had a 26% increased risk of an increase in blood creatinine levels compared to other drug users.
- Rosuvastatin users had a 23% increased risk of an increase in blood creatinine levels compared to other drug users.

Professor Sakaeda concluded: *"That the adverse events, including myalgia, rhabdomyolysis, an increase in creatine phosphokinase level and other muscular events, were associated with pravastatin, simvastatin, atorvastatin, and rosuvastatin, and these events were more noteworthy for rosuvastatin than pravastatin and atorvastatin. Acute renal failure was also associated with four statins, but the association was marginal for atorvastatin. These data strongly suggest the necessity of well-organized clinical studies with respect to statin-associated adverse events".*

Paper 413:
Over 94% of statin users report adverse side effects

Pedersen TR et al High-dose atorvastatin vs. usual-dose simvastatin for secondary prevention after myocardial infarction: the IDEAL study: a randomized controlled trial.
Journal of the American Medical Association
2005 Nov 16;294(19):2437-45

This Oslo study compared the effects of atorvastatin or simvastatin on the risk of cardiovascular disease among patients with a previous heart attack. The study included 8,888 heart attack patients aged 80 years or younger who were followed for 4.8 years. This study included data on the number of adverse events the patients suffered throughout the trial.

The Norwegian researchers unearthed:

- 94.7% of the patients in the atorvastatin group suffered an adverse event. 46.5% of these adverse events were considered a serious adverse event.
- 94.4% of the patients in the simvastatin group suffered an adverse event. 47.4% of these adverse events were considered a serious adverse event.

This analysis of the scientific literature reveals that Rory Collins has grossly underestimated the extent of side effects of statin drugs.

The data reveals that the President of he Royal College of Physicians, Sir Richard Thompson, has good reason to be concerned about the potential for a major conflict of interest regarding the figures emanating from Collins, as the amount and breadth of statins toxic effects is many-fold more than Collins' estimate.

Chapter 17

Statins deplete vital nutrients

The next two chapters look at why statins are toxic and how they cause their plethora of toxic effects.

Chapter 17 is a quick probe into the evidence regarding a few of the vitamins, minerals and other vital nutrients that are depleted when taking statin drugs.

Paper 414: Statins deplete levels of vitamin A, vitamin E and coenzyme Q10

Jula A et al Effects of diet and simvastatin on serum lipids, insulin, and antioxidants in hypercholesterolemic men: a randomized controlled trial. *Journal of the American Medical Association* 2002 Feb 6;287 (5):598-605

The head researcher of this study was Dr Antti Jula a specialist in internal medicine. The study investigated the effects of statins on men with cholesterol levels of at least 232 mg/dL (6.0 mmol/L). The study included 120 men, aged 35 to 64 years, who were randomly allocated to a habitual diet, or dietary treatment group, and each of these groups was further randomised to receive simvastatin or placebo, each for 12 weeks.

The study observed:

- The alpha-tocopherol (vitamin E) levels of men taking simvastatin decreased by 16.2%.
- The beta-carotene (a precursor of vitamin A) levels of men taking simvastatin decreased by 19.5%.
- The ubiquinol-10 (ubiquinol-10 is the active form of coenzyme Q10) levels of men taking simvastatin decreased by 22%.

Paper 415:
Statins deplete vitamin E and coenzyme Q10 levels in type two diabetic patients

Oranje WA et al Effect of atorvastatin on LDL oxidation and antioxidants in normocholesterolemic type 2 diabetic patients. *Clinica Chimica Acta* 2001 Sep 25;311(2):91-4

This study investigated the effects of statins in type two diabetic patients. The three month study included 19 patients who received either atorvastatin or placebo.

Regarding nutrient levels the study found:

- The alpha-tocopherol (vitamin E) levels of patients receiving atorvastatin reduced by 38%.
- The ubiquinol (ubiquinol is the active form of coenzyme Q10) levels of patients receiving atorvastatin reduced by 37%.

Paper 416:
Decrease of Coenzyme Q10 during treatment with statins

Mortensen SA et al Dose-related decrease of serum coenzyme Q10 during treatment with HMG-CoA reductase inhibitors. *Molecular Aspects of Medicine* 1997;18 Suppl:S137 41

Dr Svend Aage Mortensen, a Professor at the Copenhagen University Hospital, notes that coenzyme Q10 (ubiquinone) is an antioxidant, a molecule that is essential in the chemical reactions of the mitochondria (for energy production) and may help to prevent clogged arteries.

This randomised in a double-blind trial investigated the effect of statin drugs on coenzyme Q10 levels. The trial included 45 patients with "high" cholesterol who were treated with increasing dosages of either lovastatin (20-80 mg per day) or pravastatin (10-40 mg per day) over a period of 18 weeks.

The study revealed after 18 weeks of statin therapy:

- The coenzyme Q10 levels of patients taking lovastatin decreased by 29%.
- The coenzyme Q10 levels of patients taking pravastatin decreased by 20%.

Professor Mortensen concludes that: "*Continued vigilance of a possible adverse consequence from coenzyme Q10 lowering seems important during long-term (statin) therapy*".

Paper 417: Statins reduce Coenzyme Q10 by 25%

Laaksonen R et al Serum ubiquinone concentrations after short- and long-term treatment with HMG-CoA reductase inhibitors. *European Journal of Clinical Pharmacology* 1994;46(4):313-7

This study analysed the effect of long- and short-term statin treatment on the levels of ubiquinone (coenzyme Q10). The study included 17 men with "high" cholesterol who had their coenzyme Q10 levels were measured:

- After they had received simvastatin (20-40 mg per day) for 4.7 years.
- After a four-week treatment pause.
- Again after they had resumed treatment with lovastatin (20-40 mg per day) for 12 weeks.

The study ascertained:

- During the statin treatment pause the average coenzyme Q10 levels increased by 32%.
- Resumption of statin treatment caused a reduction of 25% in coenzyme Q10 levels.

Paper 418: Atorvastatin reduces coenzyme Q10 levels in all patients

Mabuchi H et al Reduction of serum ubiquinol-10 and ubiquinone-10 levels by atorvastatin in hypercholesterolemic patients. *Journal of Atherosclerosis and Thrombosis* 2005;12(2):111-9

This study, headed by Dr Hiroshi Mabuchi from the Kanazawa University Graduate School of Medical Science, analysed the effect of atorvastatin on ubiquinol-10 and ubiquinone-10 (coenzyme Q10) levels. (Ubiquinol is the reduced and active form of coenzyme Q10.) Ubiquinol is a potent antioxidant present in nearly all human tissue and coenzyme Q10 is vital for cellular energy production. In the study, 14 patients with cholesterol levels above 220 mg/dL (5.7 mmol/L), were treated with 10 mg per day of atorvastatin for eight weeks.

The study identified:

- All patients showed definite reductions of ubiquinol-10 and ubiquinone-10 levels.
- Levels of ubiquinol-10 decreased significantly by 43%.
- Levels of ubiquinone-10 decreased significantly by 40%.

Dr Mabuchi concludes: *"As atorvastatin reduces serum ubiquinol-10 in all patients, it is imperative that physicians are forewarned about the risks associated with ubiquinol-10 depletion"*.

Paper 419:
Statins significantly reduce zinc and copper levels

Ghayour-Mobarhan M et al Effect of statin therapy on serum trace element status in dyslipidaemic subjects. *Journal of the Trace Elements in Medicine and Biology* 2005;19(1):61-7

This study examined the effects of statins on trace element levels. The study included 20 patients, average age 49 years, who were given either simvastatin or atorvastatin for four months.

- The study found that statin treatment was associated with a significant 9% reduction in the levels of the vital minerals zinc and copper.

Paper 420:
Selenoprotein synthesis inhibited by statins

Moosmann B et al Selenoprotein synthesis and side-effects of statins. *Lancet* 2004 Mar 13;363(9412):892-4

A selenoprotein is any protein that includes a selenocysteine amino acid. Selenium is incorporated as selenocysteine in a wide range of selenoproteins. Selenium is of fundamental importance to human health. Selenium is important for a healthy immune system, it is protective effect against some forms of cancer and may enhance male fertility. Selenium may reduce cardiovascular disease and give protection from asthma and Alzheimer's.

Assistant Professor Dr Bernd Moosmann discusses the effects of statins on the synthesis of selenoprotein.

- Statins cause some unusual side-effects with potentially severe consequences, most prominently myopathy or rhabdomyolysis and polyneuropathy.

- Moosmann notes that the pattern of side-effects associated with statins resembles the pathology of selenium deficiency, and postulates that the mechanism is because statins inhibit the enzymatic reactions required for the synthesis of selenoproteins.

Dr Moosmann concludes: "*A negative effect of statins on selenoprotein synthesis does seem to explain many of the enigmatic effects and side-effects of statins, in particular, statin-induced myopathy*".

Paper 421:
Statins significantly reduce dolichol levels

Atil B et al Statins reduce endogenous dolichol levels in the neuroblastoma cell line SH-SY5Y. *BMC Pharmacology and Toxicology* 2012, 13(Suppl 1):A51

Dolichols play an important role in cell vitality, immune system health and in helping the body build proteins and other important compounds. Dolichols exist in the cells of all living creatures. Low dolichol levels can cause such health problems as: decrease in energy, compromised immune system, hormone imbalance or deficiency, low sperm count, cell damage or cell death, poor brain function, nervous disorders, depression, neurodegenerative diseases such as Alzheimer's.

This study assessed the effects of simvastatin on dolichol levels. The laboratory based study used the human SH-SY5Y cells (bone marrow cells).

- The study found that dolichol levels were significantly decreased by simvastatin.

This chapter presents evidence that statins can adversely affect health by depleting vital and necessary nutrients such as:

- Vitamin A
- Vitamin E
- Coenzyme Q10
- Zinc
- Copper
- Selenium
- Dolichols

The depletion of these nutrients can have negative health consequences regarding: Energy levels, clogged arteries, the immune system, cancer, cardiovascular disease, asthma, hormone imbalance or deficiency, low sperm count, cell damage or cell death, poor brain function, nervous disorders, depression, and neurodegenerative diseases such as Alzheimer's.

Chapter 18

How statins poison us

The scientific papers in this chapter describe the processes and mechanisms of how statin drugs exert their toxic effects.

You will learn that statins poison every cell in the body by blocking the production of a molecule called mevalonate. You are then shown the myriad of diseases and conditions caused and exacerbated by blocking mevalonate. The chapter is then devoted to scientific evidence of how statins can damage our DNA and how these drugs execute their poisonous and toxic effects that are the cause of a plethora of ill health.

Paper 422:
The Mevalonate Pathway

Food is turned into a compound called *acetyl-CoA*. In the mevalonate pathway this is then eventually converted into another compound called *3-hydroxy-3-methyglutaryl coenzyme A (HGM CoA)*. An enzyme called *HMG-CoA reductase* should then convert the *3-hydroxy-3-methyglutaryl coenzyme A (HGM CoA)* into mevalonate, a precursor of cholesterol.

Statin drugs work by inhibiting the *HMG-CoA reductase* enzyme from doing this task and unfortunately thereby ultimately stops the body producing cholesterol. This is unfortunate as cholesterol is a vital nutrient needed by the body.

As noted above, mevalonate is also the precursor to many other beneficial nutrients and compounds such as dolichols, heme A, prenylated proteins, isopentenyl adenine, ubiquinone and selenoproteins. By stopping the production of mevalonate, statins also have the disastrous effect of stopping the production of these essential and vital compounds.

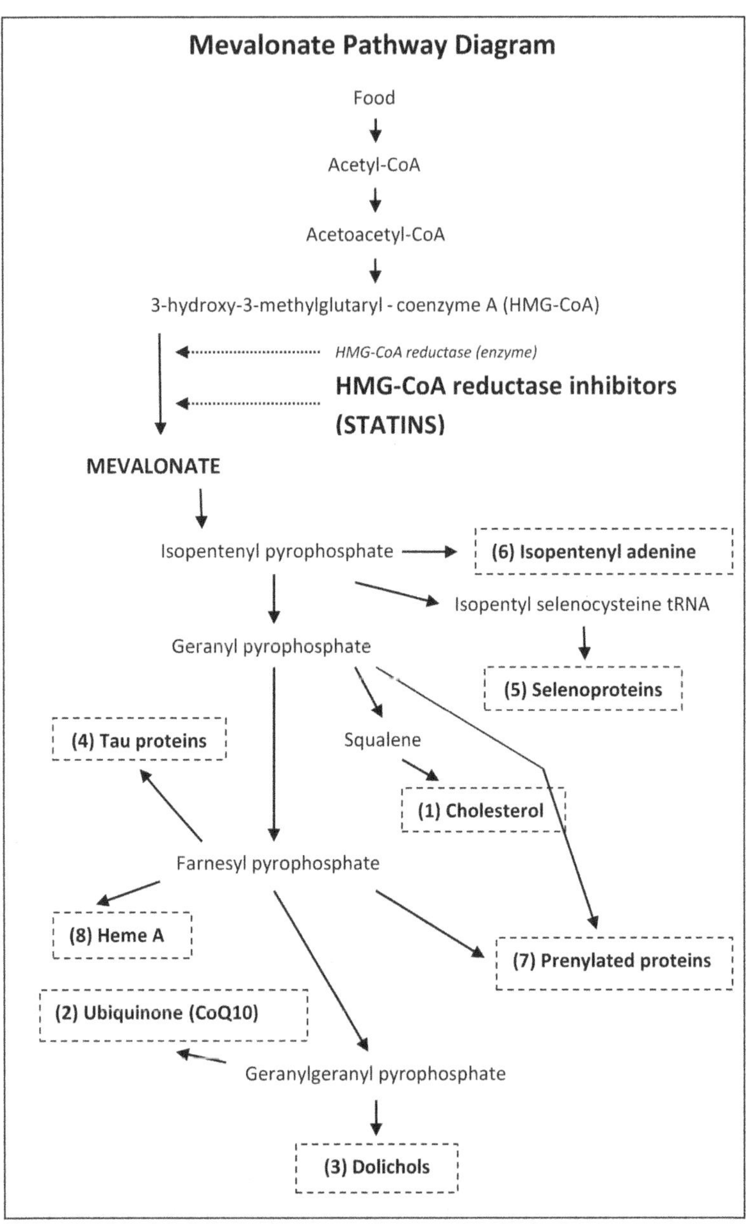
Mevalonate Pathway Diagram
Food
Acetyl-CoA
Acetoacetyl-CoA
3-hydroxy-3-methylglutaryl - coenzyme A (HMG-CoA)
HMG-CoA reductase (enzyme)
HMG-CoA reductase inhibitors
(STATINS)
MEVALONATE
Isopentenyl pyrophosphate
(6) Isopentenyl adenine
Isopentyl selenocysteine tRNA
Geranyl pyrophosphate
(5) Selenoproteins
(4) Tau proteins
Squalene
(1) Cholesterol
Farnesyl pyrophosphate
(8) Heme A
(7) Prenylated proteins
(2) Ubiquinone (CoQ10)
Geranylgeranyl pyrophosphate
(3) Dolichols

A brief examination follows of the consequences statin drugs have on these fundamental and necessary health providing nutrients and compounds.

(1) Cholesterol

Cholesterol is probably the most important substance in the body. Without cholesterol we would die. It does many things to keep us alive. It is the main precursor in the synthesis of many crucial hormones including vitamin D3 (the sunlight hormone); the steroid hormones cortisol, cortisone, and aldosterone in the adrenal glands; and the sex hormones progesterone, estrogen, and testosterone. It is so important that almost every cell in the body can make it. Cholesterol is crucial for the body to function.

Low cholesterol is associated with many health problems including:

- abscess of the anal and rectal region
- abscess of the intestine
- abscess on the brain
- abscess on the spinal cord
- accidents
- adrenal failure
- adrenal hormones deficiency
- aggression
- AIDS
- aldosterone deficiency
- Alzheimer's
- androstenedione deficiency
- antisocial personality disorder
- appendicitis
- arthropathy
- asbestosis
- asthma
- autism
- bacteraemia
- bartholin cyst
- behavioural problems
- bile acid deficiency
- boils
- bronchitis
- cancer
- carbuncle
- cardiac death
- cardiovascular disease
- cell membranes impairment
- cellulitis
- cervicitis
- childbirth problems
- chlamydia
- cholangitis
- chronic obstructive pulmonary disease
- colds
- colon cancer
- conduct disorder
- corticosterone deficiency
- coughs
- Crohn's

- dementia
- depression
- digestive system disorders
- diverticulosis
- early death
- eczema
- emphysema
- empyema
- encephalitis
- endocarditis
- endotoxic shock
- estrogen deficiency
- fatigue
- gangrene
- gastrointestinal diseases
- genito-urinary infections
- gonorrhoea
- gout
- heart attack
- heart disease
- heart failure
- hemodynamics
- hemorrhagic stroke
- hepatitis B
- hepatitis C
- herpes
- homicides
- hormone deficiency
- hyperactivity
- impaired cognition
- impetigo
- infections
- infective myositis
- inflammatory bowel disease
- influenza
- injury
- insomnia
- intermittent claudication
- intestinal infections
- intracerebral hemorrhage
- irritability
- ischemic heart disease
- ischemic stroke
- kidney disease
- laryngitis
- liver disease
- lung disease
- lymphadenitis
- lymphocytes
- mediastinitis
- memory loss
- meningitis
- meningococcal sepsis
- mental disorder
- minor illnesses
- muscle-skeletal infections
- myelin deficiency
- myelitis
- oophoritis
- nerve cell deterioration
- nonischemic systolic heart failure
- nonvascular disease
- osteomyelitis
- pancreatic cancer
- Parkinson's
- pelvic inflammatory disease
- periostitis
- photosensitivity
- pilonidal cyst
- pleurisy
- pneumonia
- pneumuconiosis
- poor health
- poor social interaction

- progesterone
- pulmonary congestion
- pulmonary fibrosis
- pyoderma
- respiratory system disease
- retarded embryonic development
- rhinitis
- rheumatic pneumonia
- rheumatoid arthritis
- ringworm
- rotavirus
- runny nose
- salmonella
- salpingitis
- schizophrenia
- self-injury
- septicaemia
- septic shock
- sinusitis
- skin rash
- slow growth
- Smith-Lemli-Opitz syndrome
- sore throat
- stroke
- sudden cardiac death
- sudden death
- suicide
- synapse impairment
- syphilis
- tantrums
- T-cells impairment
- testosterone deficiency
- thrush
- tonsillitis
- trauma
- trichomoniasis
- trichotillomania
- tuberculosis
- ulcerative colitis
- urinary tract infections
- vaginitis
- vascular disease
- venereal diseases
- violence
- viral hepatitis
- vitamin A deficiency
- vitamin D deficiency
- vitamin E deficiency
- vitamin K deficiency
- weak immune system

(2) Ubiquinone (coenzyme Q10)

Ubiquinone is vital to the production of energy in the body and is also a potent antioxidant.

Depleted levels of ubiquinone are linked to:

- chronic physical and mental fatigue
- muscle pain
- weak immune system
- increased risk of obesity
- neurological disorders (Parkinson's, Huntington's disease and amyotrophic lateral sclerosis)
- heart failure
- pancreatitis

- hepatitis
- peripheral neuropathy
- rhabdomyolysis
- shortness of breath
- fluid retention

(3) **Dolichols**

Dolichols play an important role in cell vitality, immune system health and in helping the body build proteins and other important compounds.

Dolichols exist in the cells of all living creatures. Low dolichol levels can cause such health problems as:

- decrease in energy
- compromised immune system
- hormone imbalance or deficiency
- low sperm count
- cell damage or cell death
- poor brain function
- nervous disorders
- depression
- suicide
- neurodegenerative diseases such as Alzheimer's
- aggressiveness
- hostility

(4) **Tau protein**

Statins cause the formation of abnormal tau protein.
This abnormal tau protein is linked to:

- amyotrophic lateral sclerosis
- Alzheimer's
- frontal lobe dementia
- multiple system atrophy (degenerative neurological disorder)
- Parkinson's
- other neurodegenerative diseases

(5) **Selenoproteins**

Selenoproteins are proteins that have antioxidant activity.
A deficiency in selenoproteins may lead to:

- neurological damage
- developmental delay

- impaired movement co-ordination
- poor memory
- muscle damage

(6) Isopentenyl adenine

Isopentenyl adenine is vital for DNA replication in the cell cycle. DNA is the blueprint of a cell. So without isopentenyl adenine there is no blueprint, and without the blueprint the cell will die before it can replicate.

(7) Prenylated proteins

Prenylated proteins are involved in many functions.
Disruption of prenylated proteins are associated with:

- disruption in cell wall maintenance
- abnormal endocytosis (the process of cells absorbing molecules such as proteins)
- failed cell replication
- subnormal cell growth
- disordered cell signalling
- underdeveloped cytoskeleton (the cells internal skeleton)
- faulty nervous system development
- depleted energy production

(8) Heme A

Heme A is a molecule that plays a part in many processes:
Low levels of heme A may lead to:

- depleted energy production in cells
- DNA damage
- muscle pain
- neuron damage
- cell death
- premature aging

Paper 423:

Essential role for mevalonate in DNA replication

Quesney-Huneeus V et al Essential role for mevalonate synthesis in DNA replication. *Proceedings of the National Academy of Sciences of the United States of America* 1979 Oct;76(10):5056-60

S-phase (synthesis phase) is the part of the cell cycle in which DNA is replicated. Precise and accurate DNA replication is necessary to prevent genetic abnormalities which often lead to cell death or disease.

Dr Valeria Quesney-Huneeus led a team of researchers that included Dr Marvin Siperstein who investigated the relationship between activity of the enzyme 3-hydroxy-3-methylglutaryl (HMG) CoA reductase and DNA synthesis by using cultured cells.

The study found:

- A marked increase in activity of HMG CoA reductase was consistently observed at or just prior to the S-phase burst of DNA synthesis part of the cell cycle.
- When a statin (compactin) was introduced into the culture, the HMG CoA reductase activity was suppressed, and specifically the normal S-phase burst of DNA synthesis was totally prevented.
- The statin-induced inhibition of DNA synthesis could be completely reversed within minutes by the addition of mevalonate, (the product of the HMG CoA reductase reaction).
- By contrast, addition of cholesterol had no effect upon DNA synthesis in statin-treated cells.

This study shows that statins can block DNA replication by inhibiting mevalonate production. However, this toxic effect was not due to statins blocking cholesterol, but to statins blocking another compound derived from mevalonate.

Dr Quesney-Huneeus concluded: "*The major finding of the present study is that mevalonate, or a product of mevalonate, is essential for the initiation of DNA replication, specifically during the S phase of the cell cycle. Moreover, the results indicate that this function of mevalonate in regulating DNA replication is independent of its conversion to cholesterol*".

Paper 424:
Isopentenyladenine is essential for DNA synthesis

Quesney-Huneeus V et al Isopentenyladenine as a mediator of mevalonate-regulated DNA replication. *Proceedings of the National Academy of Sciences of the United States of America* 1980 Oct;77(10):5842-6

The previous study by Dr Valeria Quesney-Huneeus *(see paper 423)* demonstrated that blocking 3-hydroxy-3-methylglutaryl-CoA reductase with statins (compactin) suppresses DNA synthesis specifically during the S-phase of the cell cycle, and the statin-induced inhibition of DNA synthesis could be completely reversed by mevalonate (the product of the HMG CoA reductase reaction).

This study sought to ascertain which compounds derived from mevalonate controls DNA replication by using cultured cells.

The compounds studied were:

- o Isopentenyladenine
- o Zeatin (an analogue of isopentenyladenine)
- o Isopentenyladenosine
- o Dolichol
- o Coenzyme Q10
- o Adenine
- o Adenosine

The study revealed:

- Of the compounds studied, only isopentenyladenine and its analogue, zeatin, could substitute for mevalonate in restoring DNA replication in statin-blocked cells.
- These two derivatives from mevalonate proved to be at least 100 times more active than mevalonate, and both restored DNA replication to normal within 15 min of their being added to the cell culture.
- In addition, isopentenyladenine, like mevalonate, stimulated DNA synthesis specifically during the S-phase of the cell cycle.

This study shows that DNA replication is blocked by statins by inhibiting isopentenyladenine production.

Dr Quesney Huneeus concluded: *"These findings indicate that isopentenyladenine or a closely related derivative may mediate the regulatory role of mevalonate in DNA replication"*.

Paper 425:
Cholesterol and isopentenyl are essential in the cell cycle

Quesney-Huneeus V et al The dual role of mevalonate in the cell cycle. *Journal of Biological Chemistry* 1983 Jan 10;258(1):378-85

Dr Quesney-Huneeus notes that it is well established that cholesterol is required for cell growth. Previous studies *(see papers 423 and 424)* have found mevalonate (specifically effective is its derivative isopentenyl adenine) plays an essential role in S phase DNA replication. It was shown that statins block S-phase DNA replication by inhibiting mevalonate.

The present study was designed to determine the relationship in the cell cycle between the known requirement for cholesterol and the effect of mevalonate and isopentenyladenine on the cell cycle by using cultured cells.

Short description of the Cell cycle:

- G0 phase (Gap 0): A resting phase where the cell has left the cycle and has stopped dividing.
- G1 phase (Gap 1): Cells increase in size in Gap 1 and prepare for DNA replication.
- S phase (synthesis): DNA replication occurs during this phase.
- G2 phase (Gap 2): During the gap between DNA synthesis and mitosis, the cell will continue to grow and prepare to divide.
- M phase (mitosis): Cell growth stops at this stage and cellular energy is focused on the orderly division into two daughter cells.

The study discovered:

- Cholesterol is essential at the early and mid-G1 phases of the cell cycle.
- Isopentenyladenine is required at the late G1-S interphase of the cell cycle.
- Cholesterol is needed at the G0 (resting phase) of the cell cycle.
- Cells treated with statins had retarded progression, or stopped progression through the cell cycle.

This study shows that statins can interfere with the cell cycle by inhibiting cholesterol or isopentenyladenine.

Dr Quesney-Huneeus comments: "*The major finding of the present study is that cholesterol, either endogenously synthesized from mevalonate or supplied exogenously, is specifically required early in G1, to permit the cell to undertake the growth phase that is characteristic of passage from early to late GI in preparation for DNA replication".*

Also: "*It is likely, therefore, as we have previously suggested that isopentenyl adenine or a closely related purine may mediate the effect of mevalonate in initiating DNA replication".*

Paper 426:
Laboratory testing reveals statins cause DNA damage

Gajski G et al Application of cytogenetic endpoints and comet assay on human lymphocytes treated with atorvastatin in vitro. *Journal of Environmental Science and Health* 2008 Jan;43(1):78-85

Using laboratory techniques over a three-day period, the study investigated the potential of atorvastatin to damage DNA in human lymphocytes. (Lymphocytes are white blood cells that are a major part of the immune system.)

- The study found that lymphocyte cells exposed to atorvastatin had significantly increased structural chromosome aberrations and DNA damage compared to lymphocyte cells not exposed to atorvastatin.

Paper 427:
Statin treatment associated with significant muscle mitochondrial DNA depletion

Schick BA et al Decreased skeletal muscle mitochondrial DNA in patients treated with high-dose simvastatin. *Clinical Pharmacology and Therapeutics* 2007 May;81(5):650-3

Mitochondrial DNA contains 37 genes, all of which are essential for normal mitochondrial function. Thirteen of these genes provide instructions for making enzymes involved in oxidative phosphorylation. Oxidative phosphorylation is a process that uses oxygen and simple sugars to create adenosine triphosphate (ATP), the cell's main energy source.

Any depletion of muscle mitochondrial DNA may lead to muscle weakness and/or liver failure, and more rarely, brain abnormalities.

"Floppiness", feeding difficulties and developmental delays are common symptoms.

The aim of this study, conducted by Dr Brian A Schick and colleagues from the University of British Columbia, was to determine whether muscle mitochondrial DNA levels are altered during statin therapy. This clinical trial included 43 patients, aged 31 to 69 years, who had their levels of muscle mitochondrial DNA measured at the start of the study and again after eight weeks. The subjects were placed into three groups:

- o Simvastatin 80 mg per day.
- o Atorvastatin 40 mg per day.
- o Placebo.

The study identified:

- A significant decrease in muscle mitochondrial DNA levels was observed in the simvastatin group and a smaller decrease in levels in the atorvastatin group.
- Half the patients in the simvastatin group had a greater than 50% decrease in muscle mitochondrial DNA levels.
- 13% of the patients in the atorvastatin group had a greater than 50% decrease in muscle mitochondrial DNA levels.

The study shows that statin treatment may be associated with significant muscle mitochondrial DNA depletion.

Dr Schick concluded: "*Given that statin therapy is often life-long, the large decrease (47%) observed raises concern about the potential long-term effect of statins on mitochondrial DNA and skeletal muscle mitochondria*".

Paper 428:
Adverse effects of statins – mechanisms and consequences

Bełtowski J et al Adverse effects of statins – mechanisms and consequences. *Current Drug Safety* 2009 Sep;4(3):209-28

Dr Jerzy Bełtowski, a specialist in internal medicine, describes mechanisms and consequences of the adverse effects of statins.

- Statins inhibit the enzyme, 3-hydroxy-3-methylglutarylcoenzyme A reductase. This reduces the amount of 3-hydroxy-3-methylglutarylcoenzyme A that is converted to mevalonate and therefore reducing cholesterol (mevalonate is a precursor for cholesterol).

- Apart from cholesterol, mevalonate is also the substrate for the synthesis of nonsteroid isoprenoids (isoprenoids are molecules that play a wide variety of roles in physiological processes and as intermediates in the biological synthesis of other important molecules) including farnesylpyrophosphate, geranylgeranylpyrophosphate, coenzyme Q, dolichol, isopentenyladenosine, Heme A etc.
- The adverse effects of statins result from impaired protein prenylation, (prenylation regulates protein-membrane interactions), deficiency of coenzyme Q involved in mitochondrial electron transport (energy production) and antioxidant protection, abnormal protein glycosylation (glycosylation is the enzymatic process that attaches carbohydrates to proteins or other organic molecules) due to dolichol shortage, or deficiency of selenoproteins.
- Myopathy (muscle disease) is the most frequent side effect of statins, and in some cases may have a form of severe rhabdomyolysis. Other adverse effects include liver damage, peripheral neuropathy, impaired heart function and autoimmune diseases.

Paper 429: Molecular basis of statin-associated myopathy

Vaklavas C et al Molecular basis of statin-associated myopathy. *Atherosclerosis* 2009 Jan;202(1):18-28

Dr Christos Vaklavas, an Assistant Professor from the University of Texas Medical School at Houston reviews how statins cause side effects in muscles (myopathy).

- Statins can interfere with protein modification at multiple levels.
- They can affect protein prenylation. (Protein prenylation plays a key role in the localization and function of many proteins. Localization to cellular membranes is required for many proteins to function properly.)
- Statins can adversely affect selenoprotein synthesis. (Selenium is important for a healthy immune system, it has a protective

effect against some forms of cancer, it may enhance male fertility, it can decrease cardiovascular disease mortality, and give protection from asthma.)

- Statins can interfere with the biosynthesis of dolichols. (Dolichols are involved in the process of protein glycosylation. Glycosylation is critical for a wide range of biological processes.)
- Statin-induced myopathy may be also associated with mitochondrial dysfunction.

Paper 430:
Statins alter protein prenylation

Roskoski R Protein prenylation: a pivotal posttranslational process. *Biochemical and Biophysical Research Communications* 2003 Mar 28;303(1):1-7

Professor Robert Roskoski, a Professor of Biochemistry and Molecular Biology at Louisiana State University Health Sciences Centre, explains the effects of statins on protein prenylation.

Statins inhibit the formation of the isoprenoids; geranylgeranyl-pyrophosphate and farnesyl-pyrophosphate. Isoprenoids are a large and diverse class of naturally occurring organic chemicals derived from the mevalonate pathway.

These isoprenoids play a vital role in attaching fatty substances to proteins, a process called protein prenylation. Prenylated proteins are used in a wide array of cellular functions related to cell growth, differentiation, cytoskeletal function and vesicle trafficking.

Below is a list of some prenylated proteins and their functions.

- H-ras: Growth, differentiation
- K-rasA: Growth, differentiation
- K-rasB: Growth, differentiation
- N-ras: Growth, differentiation
- 20; 50 Oligoadenylate synthetase 1: Growth, differentiation, and apoptosis
- RaplA: Regulation of cell adhesion
- RaplB: Activation of the MEK-ERK cascade
- Rac1: Secretion at plasma membrane
- RalA: Regulation of actin cytoskeleton
- Cdc42/G25K: Filopodia formation

- RhoA: Assembly of actin stress fibres and focal adhesion sites
- RhoB: Assembly of actin stress fibres and focal adhesion sites; gene transcription via SRF
- Rab2: Vesicular trafficking
- Rab3a: Vesicular trafficking
- HDJ2: Protein import into mitochondria, co-chaperone of Hsc70
- Inositol-1,4,5-trisphosphate-5-phosphatase II: Inactivates inositol trisphosphate
- Ptp4a1: Protein–tyrosine phosphatase
- S. cerevisiae RAS2: Adenylyl cyclase activation
- Heterotrimeric G-protein (c-subunit): Serpentine receptor linked
- S. cerevisiae a-factor: Mating pheromone
- R. toruloides Rhodotorucine A: Mating pheromone
- Lamin A: Nuclear membrane component
- Lamin B: Nuclear membrane component
- Cenp-F: Centromere (kinetochore) protein for G2— transition
- Phosphorylase kinase, a-subunit: Muscle glycogen metabolism
- Phosphorylase kinase, a-subunit: Liver glycogen metabolism
- Phosphorylase kinase, b-subunit: Muscle glycogen metabolism
- Transducin (c-subunit): Vision
- Retinal cGMP phosphodiesterase a-subunit: Vision
- Retinal cGMP phosphodiesterase b-subunit: Vision
- Rhodopsin kinase: Vision
- RhoE: Regulation of the actin cytoskeleton
- Rap2a: Function unknown
- Rap2b: Function unknown
- Rheb: Function unknown
- PxF: Peroxisome assembly
- Interferon induced guanylate binding protein-1: Binds GMP, GDP, and GTP in macrophages
- Interferon induced guanylate binding protein-2: Binds GMP, GDP, and GTP in macrophages

The total number of prenylated proteins is about 150.

Professor Roskoski notes: *"Although the function of many of the prenylated proteins is known in broad strokes, there is much to learn about the functions of many of these proteins including unimagined nuances of signal transduction"*.

Proper protein prenylation is required for the healthy function of many cells in the body. Taking statins reduces the protein prenylation activities in the body via suppressing the production of the isoprenoids needed to carry out this activity. This is a highly undesirable side effect of statins.

Paper 431: Statins worsen inflammation in peripheral arterial disease patients

DePalma RG et al Statins and biomarkers in claudicants with peripheral arterial disease: cross-sectional study. *Vascular* 2006 Jul-Aug;14(4):193-200

Studies have demonstrated that elevated interleukin-6 levels (small signalling molecules used for cell signalling) and elevated Tumor necrosis factor (TNF-alpha R1) levels (primary role of TNF is in the regulation of immune cells) are a risk for peripheral arterial disease and heart disease and that higher levels increase the risk.

Dr Ralph Depalma, a Professor of Surgery, investigated the effect of statins in patients with peripheral arterial disease. The study included 47 subjects with peripheral arterial disease not taking statins, 53 peripheral arterial disease subjects taking statins and 21 healthy medication-free men.

The study observed:

- The healthy medication-free men had the lowest interleukin-6 and TNF-alpha R1 levels.
- Those with peripheral arterial disease taking statins had 47% increased interleukin-6 levels compared to those not taking statins.
- Those with peripheral arterial disease taking statins had 23% increased TNF-alpha R1 levels compared to those not taking statins.

This study suggests statins worsen inflammation in peripheral arterial disease patients.

Paper 432: Possible mechanisms of how statins cause diabetes

Brault M et al Statin treatment and new-onset diabetes: A review of proposed mechanisms. *Metabolism* 2014 Jun;63(6):735-45

Head researcher Marilyne Brault led a team of investigators from McGill University to review the mechanisms that may be involved between statins and diabetes. Brault notes that new-onset diabetes has been observed in clinical trials and meta-analyses involving statin therapy.

- Statins affect insulin secretion through direct, indirect or combined effects on calcium channels in pancreatic β-cells.
- Statins reduce the expression of glucose transporter 4 (GLUT 4). GLUT 4 is a protein that transports glucose from the bloodstream into cells. Reduced GLUT 4 in response to statins results in hyperglycemia (high blood sugar) and hyperinsulinemia (excess levels of insulin in the blood).
- Statin therapy decreases other important molecules such as coenzyme Q10, farnesyl pyrophosphate, geranylgeranyl pyrophosphate and dolichol; their depletion leads to reduced intracellular signalling.
- Statins interference with intracellular insulin signalling pathways via inhibition of necessary phosphorylation events (phosphorylation influences protein enzymes) and reduction of small GTPase action (GTPases are key proteins in many critical biological processes such as hormonal and sensory signals, and the protein building ribosome's).
- Statins can decrease levels of peroxisome proliferator activated receptor gamma and CCAAT/enhancer-binding protein which regulate glucose levels.
- Statins may also diminish levels of leptin and adiponectin which also play a role in regulating glucose levels.

Paper 433:
Statins can trigger autoimmune diseases and also contribute to the development of some types of cancer

Noël B Autoimmune disease and other potential side-effects of statins. *Lancet* 2004 Jun 12;363(9425):2000

Dr Bernard Noel from the University Hospital of Lausanne, states that severe autoimmune diseases have been reported with statin use. He notes:

- An unexpected number of autoimmune diseases have been reported in patients treated with statins.

- Most of these patients had systemic lupus erythematosus but dermatomyositis, autoimmune hepatitis, and pemphigoides have been reported.
- Unlike usual drug reactions, skin eruptions have been noted many months or even years after starting treatment.
- Side effects generally improve after drug discontinuation, but not necessarily in serological disease, (antibodies in the serum formed in response to an infection, against other foreign proteins or to one's own proteins in instances of autoimmune disease).
- In many reported cases, antinuclear antibodies are still positive many months after interruption of drug treatment. The causal relation between drug intake and autoimmune disease can, therefore, be difficult to establish and many cases are probably not reported.
- Several pathogenic mechanisms have been postulated in statin-induced systemic lupus erythematosus.
  - o Cell death which has an important role in systemic lupus erythematosus might be exacerbated or triggered by statins.
  - o Release of nuclear antigens into the circulation could cause production of pathogenic autoantibodies.
  - o Systemic lupus erythematosus is characterised by a shifting of T helper 1 to T helper 2 immune responses, causing B-cell reactivity and production of pathogenic autoantibodies. Statins and selenoprotein inhibition can aggravate this event.
- Epidemiological study and clinical trial findings suggest that selenoprotein inhibition might heighten the risk of prostate and colon cancer.

Dr Noel concludes: "*Statins could not only trigger autoimmune diseases but also contribute to the development of some types of cancer*".

Paper 434:
Statins increase the risk of many cancers, neurodegenerative disorders and a myriad of infectious diseases

Goldstein MR et al The double-edged sword of statin immunomodulation. *International Journal of Cardiology* 2009 June 12;135(1):128-30

Internist Dr Mark Goldstein reviewed the evidence concerning statins and their effects on disease.

Dr Goldstein review indicated:

- Statins may be harmful in certain segments of the population.
- Statins have been shown to increase the concentration of regulatory T cells (Tregs). There is evidence that this increases the risk of many cancers, particularly in the elderly.
- Furthermore, a statin induced increase in Tregs may be detrimental in neurodegenerative disorders, such as amyotrophic lateral sclerosis; and a myriad of infectious diseases. These include, but are not limited to, human immunodeficiency virus, hepatitis B virus, hepatitis C virus, and varicella zoster virus.

Dr Goldstein concludes: "*These issues need our attention, and call for a heightened state of vigilance among those prescribing statins*".

Paper 435: Incidence, risk factors and mechanisms that lead to statin induced muscle disease

Sewright KA et al Statin myopathy: incidence, risk factors, and pathophysiology. *Current Atherosclerosis Reports* 2007 Nov;9(5):389-96

This paper, authored by Dr Kimberly Sewright, discusses the incidence, risk factors and mechanisms that lead to statin induced myopathy (muscle disease).

- Incidence rates of muscle-related complaints predicted from statin clinical trials may underestimate rate of occurrence of these side effects in clinical practice.
- Among the risk factors for statin associated myopathy are interaction with other drugs, high-dose statin treatment, aging, and diabetes.
- The mechanism of statin-induced myopathy include decreases in mevalonate pathway products (cholesterol, heme A, coenzyme Q10, dolichols, prenylated proteins, selenoproteins), mitochondrial dysfunction, alterations in gene expression, and genetic predisposition.

Paper 436:
Statins may disrupt regulation of calcium levels

Guis S et al In vivo and in vitro characterization of skeletal muscle metabolism in patients with statin-induced adverse effects. *Arthritis and Rheumatism* 2006 Aug 15;55(4):551-7

The aim of the study was to determine what causes could account for the adverse effects of statins in skeletal muscle. 11 patients with increased creatine kinase levels and muscle pains after statin treatment were evaluated in the study.

- The 11 patients reported symptoms of muscle pain, cramps, and exercise intolerance 2–60 months after the onset of treatment
- Investigations indicated that 77% of the patients tested had impaired calcium regulation.

The study findings raise the possibility that statins may induce calcium regulation impairment which could contribute to their toxic effects on muscle.

Paper 437:
How statins cause muscle damage

Hanai J et al The muscle-specific ubiquitin ligase atrogin-1/ MAFbx mediates statin-induced muscle toxicity. *Journal of Clinical Investigation* 2007 Dec;117(12):3940-51

In 2001, scientists from the Harvard Medical School discovered the atrogin-1 gene, which plays a major role in muscle atrophy. (Muscle atrophy is the wasting or loss of muscle tissue.)

In this study, Dr Junichi Hanai led a team of researchers from the Beth Israel Deaconess Medical Centre. Dr Hanai notes that statins can lead to a number of side effects in muscle, including muscle fibre breakdown. This study sought to find the mechanisms of how statins may induce muscle injury. Since atrogin-1 plays a key role in the development of wasting in skeletal muscle, the study investigated if statins might "turn on" this gene.

The study comprised of three separate experiments to test this hypothesis.

- The first experiment examined the expression of the atrogin-1 gene in biopsies of 19 human patients (eight of the patients had muscle pain/damage while using statins). The results showed that atrogin-1 expression was significantly higher among the statin users.

- The second experiment studied statins' effects on cultured muscle cells treated with various concentrations of lovastatin. Compared with control samples, the lovastatin-treated cells became progressively thinner and more damaged. However, the cells lacking the atrogin-1 gene were resistant to statins' deleterious effects.
- Thirdly statins were tested on zebra fish. These tests also found that lovastatin led to muscle damage and as the lovastatin levels increased, so too was the damage. Again, (as in the cultured muscle cells) fish lacking the atrogin-1 gene were resistant to statin-induced damage.

Dr Hanai concluded: *"Collectively, our human, animal, and in vitro findings shed light on the molecular mechanism of statin-induced myopathy (muscle damage) and suggest that atrogin-1 may be a critical mediator of the muscle damage induced by statins"*.

Paper 438: Statins impair mitochondrial function

Sirvent P et al Muscle mitochondrial metabolism and calcium signalling impairment in patients treated with statins. *Toxicology and Applied Pharmacology* 2012 Mar 1;259(2):263-8

Mitochondria are the energy factories of the cells. They are organelles that take in nutrients, break them down, and creates energy for the cell. The process of creating cell energy is known as cellular respiration. Most of the chemical reactions involved in cellular respiration happen in the mitochondria.

Dr Pascal Sirvent an Assistant Professor at Montpellier University evaluated the effect of statins on mitochondrial function.

Patients treated with statins showed impairment of mitochondrial respiration that involved:

- Damage to the complex I protein. (Complex I is a protein that plays a vital role in mitochondrial energy production.)
- Altered frequency and amplitude of calcium sparks. (Calcium sparks are small, intense bursts of calcium that occur in cells

from cardiac muscle, skeletal muscle, and smooth muscle. Calcium sparks regulate calcium in these muscle cells.)

Dr Sirvent concluded: "*The muscle problems observed in statin-treated patients appear thus to be related to impairment of mitochondrial function and muscle calcium homeostasis*".

Paper 439: Statin treatment associated with depleted levels of coenzyme Q10 and cytochrome oxidase

Duncan AJ et al Decreased ubiquinone availability and impaired mitochondrial cytochrome oxidase activity associated with statin treatment. *Toxicology Mechanisms and Methods* 2009 Jan;19(1):44-50

This study, headed by Dr Andrew Duncan, investigated the involvement of statins in impaired cellular energy production. Mitochondria are the cells power plants, and coenzyme Q10 (ubiquinone) and cytochrome oxidase (complex IV) are vital enzymes needed in cellular energy production.

- Two patients experienced muscle problems following treatment with simvastatin (40 mg per day) and cyclosporin (used to treat arthritis and inflammatory disease) (patient 1) and simvastatin (40 mg per day) and itraconazole (used to treat fungal infections) (patient 2).
- Analysis of the two patients skeletal muscle revealed a decreased ubiquinone status (77 and 132; reference range: 140-580 pmol/mg) and decreased complex IV activity (0.006 and 0.007 reference range: 0.014-0.034).
- To assess statin treatment in the absence of possible pharmacological interference from cyclosporin or itraconazole, primary astrocytes (cells from the central nervous system) were cultured with lovastatin.
- Lovastatin treatment resulted in a decrease in ubiquinone (statin treatment 97.9 versus control 202.9 pmol/mg), and a decrease in complex IV activity (statin treatment 0.008 versus control: 0.011).

Dr Duncan concludes: "*These data, coupled with the patient findings, indicate a possible association between statin treatment, decreased ubiquinone status, and loss of complex IV activity*".

Paper 440: Statins may cause muscle damage and impair cellular energy production

Gambelli S et al Mitochondrial alterations in muscle biopsies of patients on statin therapy. *Journal of Submicroscopic Cytology and Pathology* 2004 Jan;36(1):85-9

Oxidative metabolism is part of the process of cellular energy production involving mitochondria.

Dr Simona Gambelli from the University of Siena reports of the results of clinical and biopsy study of nine patients on statin therapy suffering from various muscle problems.

Biopsy findings showed signs of muscle damage and mitochondrial changes such as:

- Subsarcolemmal accumulation of mitochondria: This is where clumps of diseased mitochondria accumulate in the subsarcolemmal region (just under the cell membrane) of skeletal, cardiac, or smooth muscle cells.
- Morphological alterations of mitochondria: Changes in the shape and structure of mitochondria are indicative of damage.
- Presence of Cox-negative fibres: Cox (cytochrome c oxidase or Complex IV) is an important enzyme involved in mitochondria energy production. Cox-negative fibres (Cox deficient fibres) indicate an absence or deficiency of the enzyme.

Dr Gambelli concluded: *"These findings confirm that statins may cause muscle damage and impair oxidative metabolism"*.

Paper 441: Statins cause muscular pain

Sinzinger H et al Isoprostane 8-epi-PGF2α is frequently increased in patients with muscle pain and/or CK-elevation after HMG-Co-enzyme-A-reductase inhibitor therapy. *Journal of Clinical Pharmacy and Therapeutics* Volume 26 Issue 4, Pages 303 – 310

Muscle pains with or without creatine kinase-elevation are among the most frequently observed side-effects in patients on various statins. This study sought to find the changes associated with this side-effect.

This study examined levels of isoprostane 8-epi-PGF2alpha, (high levels are a marker of cellular oxidation injury), (oxidation injury is damage that occurs to the cells and tissues of the brain and body by highly reactive substances known as free radicals), in patients who were taking statin drugs. The patients isoprostane 8-epi-PGF2alpha levels were measured at the start of the study, when muscle problems manifested and different time intervals after withdrawing the respective statin.

The study found:

- The majority of patients with muscular side-effects show elevated 8-epi-PGF2alpha levels.
- Stopping statin therapy resulted in a normalization of the values in all patients.

Professor Helmut Sinzinger from the University of Vienna, who headed the study, concluded: *"These findings indicate a significant involvement of oxidative injury in the muscular side-effects of statins"*.

Paper 442: Statins alter gene expression which may cause muscle pain with exercise

Urso ML et al Changes in ubiquitin proteasome pathway gene expression in skeletal muscle with exercise and statins. *Arteriosclerosis, Thrombosis and Vascular Biology* 2005 Dec;25(12):2560-6

The study leader was Research Scientist Dr Maria Urso, whose research interests include delineating the complex molecular basis of skeletal muscle atrophy at both the gene and protein level in skeletal muscle. In this study, Dr Urso examined gene expression changes in response to exercise and statin treatment. The study included eight healthy men, aged 18 to 30, who were given atorvastatin (80 mg per day) or placebo.

The results from the study indicated:

- The effects of statin and exercise on gene expression showed that 56 genes were differentially expressed with 18% involved in the ubiquitin proteasome pathway and 20% involved in protein folding and catabolism, and apoptosis. (The ubiquitin proteasome pathway is responsible for the recognition and degradation of the majority of proteins in skeletal muscle. Proteins are the biological workhorses that carry out vital functions in every cell. To carry out their task, proteins must fold into a complex three-dimensional structure and a misfolded protein may poison the cells around it. Catabolism is the set of metabolic pathways that breaks down molecules into smaller units to release energy. Apoptosis is the process of programmed cell death.)

- There was a four-fold increase in a ubiquitin proteasome pathway F-box protein called FBXO3. (F-box proteins are involved in protein degradation and repair in skeletal muscle.)

Dr Urso speculates that: *"Statins may alter the response of muscle to exercise stress by altering the action of the ubiquitin proteasome pathway, protein folding, and catabolism, disrupting the balance between protein degradation and repair"* and concludes that the study may *"implicate involvement of the ubiquitin proteasome pathway in skeletal muscle in response to combined exercise and statin treatment, possibly explaining the onset of myalgia (muscle pain) with exertion"*.

Paper 443:
Statins damage skeletal muscle

Draeger A et al Statin therapy induces ultrastructural damage in skeletal muscle in patients without myalgia. *Journal of Pathology* 2006 Sep;210(1):94-102

The head investigator of the study was Dr Annette Draeger, a Professor of Cell Biology.

Dr Draeger notes that muscle pain and weakness are frequent complaints in patients receiving statins. Many patients with muscle pain have creatine kinase levels that are either normal or only marginally elevated, and no obvious structural defects have been reported in patients with muscle pain.

In this study, skeletal muscle biopsies from statin-treated and non-statin-treated patients were examined using both electron microscopy and biochemical approaches to compare patterns of muscle damage.

The study observed:

- The biopsies found clear evidence of skeletal muscle damage in statin-treated patients.

- The damage has a characteristic pattern that includes breakdown of the T-tubular system (continuation of the cell surface membrane) and subsarcolemmal (cell membrane) rupture.
- These characteristic structural abnormalities observed in the statin-treated patients were reproduced by extraction of cholesterol from skeletal muscle fibres and analysed in a test tube.

Dr Draeger concluded: *"These findings support the hypothesis that statin-induced cholesterol lowering per se contributes to myocyte (muscle cell or muscle fibre) damage"*.

Paper 444:
Statins linked with mitochondrial dysfunction

De Pinieux G et al Lipid-lowering drugs and mitochondrial function: effects of HMG-CoA reductase inhibitors on serum ubiquinone and blood lactate/pyruvate ratio. *British Journal of Clinical Pharmacology* 1996 Sep;42(3):333-7

Ubiquinone (coenzyme Q10) is a substance that is found in almost every cell in the body and helps convert food into energy by the mitochondrial respiratory chain. It may also help with heart-related conditions, because it can improve energy production in cells, prevent blood clot formation, and act as an antioxidant.

Low levels of coenzyme Q10 may lead to mitochondrial dysfunction. Mitochondrial dysfunction is a mechanism behind many metabolic, age-related, neurodegenerative and psychiatric diseases or health conditions.

Mitochondrial cytopathies represent a group of multisystem disorders which affect the muscle and nervous systems.

Mitochondrial myopathies are a group of neuromuscular diseases caused by damage to the mitochondria. Nerve cells in the brain and muscles require a great deal of energy, and are particularly damaged when mitochondrial dysfunction occurs.

Elevated lactate/pyruvate ratios are associated with mitochondrial cytopathies and mitochondrial myopathies.

Dr Gonzague De Pinieux and his colleagues evaluated the effect of cholesterol lowering drugs on coenzyme Q10 levels and on mitochondrial function assessed by the blood lactate/pyruvate ratio.

This study included 80 patients, some of whom were treated with statins and 20 healthy control subjects.

The study revealed:

- Coenzyme Q10 levels were lower in statin-treated patients than in untreated patients.
- Lactate/pyruvate ratios were significantly higher in patients treated by statins than in untreated patients or healthy control subjects.

Dr De Pinieux finishes: "*We conclude that statin therapy can be associated with high blood lactate/ pyruvate ratio suggestive of mitochondrial dysfunction. Low serum levels of ubiquinone were also observed*".

Paper 445: Simvastatin effects on skeletal muscle: relation to decreased mitochondrial function and glucose intolerance

Larsen S et al Simvastatin effects on skeletal muscle: relation to decreased mitochondrial function and glucose intolerance. *Journal of the American College of Cardiology* 2013 Jan 8;61(1):44-53

Dr Steen Larsen investigated the possible mechanism of the prevalent side effect of statin induced muscle pain. The study included ten simvastatin-treated patients and nine well-matched control subjects.

The study observed:

- Simvastatin-treated patients had an impaired glucose tolerance and displayed a decreased insulin sensitivity index.
- Simvastatin-treated patients had a reduced coenzyme Q10 content.
- Simvastatin-treated patients had a reduced mitochondrial oxidative phosphorylation capacity. (Oxidative phosphorylation is a vital part of the cellular energy process.)

Dr Larsen concludes: "*These simvastatin-treated patients were glucose intolerant. A decreased coenzyme Q(10) content was accompanied by a decreased maximal mitochondrial oxidative phosphorylation capacity in the simvastatin-treated patients. It is plausible that this finding partly explains the muscle pain and exercise intolerance that many patients experience with their statin treatment*".

Paper 446: List of some drugs that may cause side effects when coadministered with statins

Hamilton-Craig I Statin-associated myopathy. *Medical Journal of Australia* 2001 Nov 5;175(9):486-9

This paper was authored by Professor Ian Hamilton-Craig, an academic cardiologist. Professor Hamilton-Craig notes that myopathy (muscle disease) can be caused by all statins.

In this review he finds:

- The risk of myopathy is increased by: the use of high doses of statins, concurrent use of fibrates, concurrent use of hepatic cytochrome P450 inhibitors, acute viral infections, major trauma, surgery, hypothyroidism and other conditions.
- Cytochrome P450 are enzymes that give protection against potential toxicity from the foods and drugs (including statins) that we ingest by breaking down and eliminating the toxic substance. These enzymes are found primarily within liver cells as well as many other cell types. Cytochrome P450 inhibitors inhibit the effectiveness of cytochrome P450 enzymes and thereby increase the levels of statins in the body which leads to increased toxicity and more side effects.

Cytochrome P450 inhibitors include:

- o Amiodarone (cordarone)
- o Azole antifungals; fluconazole (*diflucan*), itraconazole (*sporanox*), ketoconazole (*nizoral*), posaconazole (*noxafil, posanol*), voriconazole (*vfend*)
- o Calcium channel blockers; (*amlodipine, diltiazem, verapamil*)
- o Cyclosporine (*neoral*)
- o Danazol (*cyclomen*)
- o Dronedarone (*multaq*)
- o Fibric acid derivatives; (*fenofibrate, gemfibrozil*)
- o Glyburide
- o Grapefruit/grapefruit Juice
- o Macrolide antibiotics; clarithromycin (*biaxin*), erythromycin
- o Nefazodone
- o Phenytoin (*dilantin*)
- o Protease Inhibitors; atazanavir (*reyataz*), boceprevir (*victrelis*), darunavir (*prezista*), fosamprenavir (l*exiva*, *telzir*), indinavir

(*crixivan*), lopinavir/ritonavir (*kaletra*), nelfinavir (*viracept*), ritonavir (*norvir*), saquinavir (*invirase*), telaprevir (*incivek*), tipranavir (*aptivus*)
- o Ranolazine (*ranexa*)
- o Telithromycin (*ketek*)
- o Ticagrelor (*brilinta*)

Paper 447:
How statins cause cognitive problems

Kraft R et al A cell-based fascin bioassay identifies compounds with potential anti-metastasis or cognition-enhancing functions. *Disease Models and Mechanisims* 2013 Jan;6(1):217-35

Fascin is a protein that has diverse roles in the developmental and physiological regulation of cellular morphology and function. Studies have revealed that excess fascin promotes cancer, whereas insufficient fascin disrupts brain development.

This study was designed to test the effect of drugs on fascin. Drugs that blocked fascin could serve as anti-cancer agents, whereas drugs that enhanced fascin could improve neurocognitive function and behaviour in people with brain disorders. The study tested 1,040 different drugs on cultured neuron cells. The drugs tested included four types of statins.

The study found:

- 34 drugs that could potentially block fascin.
- 48 drugs that could potentially enhance fascin.
- The study also revealed that four drugs induced neurotoxic *"beads-on-a-string"* swelling effect on the neurons. These four drugs were all statins: A*torvastatin* (lipitor), *lovastatin* (mevacor), *rosuvastatin* (crestor) and *pravastatin* (pravachol).
- The statin-induced swelling the *beads-on-a-string* effect was called so because that's what it looked like under a microscope.
- The beadlike swelling interrupted the flow of information along the nerve cells, so that the cells could not grow branches properly.
- When the statins were removed, the beadlike bulges disappeared and the cells quickly returned to normal growth.

The *beads-on-a-string* effect may explain why many statin users develop cognitive problems. The statin-induced swelling could slow down and impact thinking, judgment and behaviour. It may also explain why cognition improves when people stop taking statins, as the swelling may subside thus allowing uninterrupted flow of information.

Paper 448:
Statins may be implicated in neurodegenerative diseases

Kannan M et al Mevastatin accelerates loss of synaptic proteins and neurite degeneration in aging cortical neurons in a heme-independent manner. *Neurobiology of Aging* 2010 Sep;31(9):1543-53

This study investigated the effects of statins on cultured neurons.
The study discovered:

- Statins impaired synaptic proteins (heightened risk of neurodegenerative diseases).
- Statins reduced N-methyl-d-aspartate receptor currents (N-methyl-d-aspartate receptor currents help in memory function.)
- Statins accelerated neurodegeneration associated with aging.

To conclude: Statins exert a neurotoxic effect in cultured neurons and may be implicated in neurodegenerative diseases such as Parkinson's, Alzheimer's, Amyothrophic Lateral Sclerosis, Multiple Sclerosis and Huntington's.

Paper 449:
Statins implicated in multiple sclerosis

Smolders I et al Simvastatin interferes with process outgrowth and branching of oligodendrocytes. *Journal of Neuroscience Research* 2010 Nov 15;88(15):3361-75

Oligodendrocytes are a type of brain cell. Oligodendrocytes are responsible for producing a fatty protein, called myelin, which insulates axons, the long extensions of nerve cells (neurons). I.E. myelin is the protective sheath coating our nerve fibres. Myelinated axons transmit nerve signals much faster than unmyelinated ones. Each oligodendrocyte can supply myelin for several axons and each axon can be supplied by several oligodendrocytes. Oligodendrocytes wrap the myelin around the axons in thin sheets like rolled up paper.

Oligodendrocytes are the cell type that is predominantly affected in multiple sclerosis.

Any adverse effects on oligodendrocytes and myelin are detrimental and are implicated in multiple sclerosis.

The study, headed by Dr Inge Smolders from Hasselt University, focused on the effects of simvastatin on oligodendrocytes and myelin in cultured cells.

The study revealed:

- Cholesterol is required for the growth of oligodendrocytes.
- Statins inhibited the growth of oligodendrocytes.
- Statins inhibited the growth of myelin.

Dr Smolders finishes: "*We conclude that simvastatin treatment has detrimental effects on oligodendrocyte process outgrowth, the prior step in (re)myelination, thereby mortgaging long-term healing of multiple sclerosis lesions*".

Paper 450:
Statins use as a pathway to multiple sclerosis

Klopfleisch S et al Negative Impact of Statins on Oligodendrocytes and Myelin Formation In Vitro and In Vivo. *Journal of Neuroscience* December 10, 2008, 28(50):13609-13614

This German study, led by Dr Steve Klopfleisch, investigated the relationship between statins and myelin formation in cultured cells and in a trial.

The findings of the investigations were as follows:

- Cholesterol is a major component of myelin.
- Statins are drugs which lower cholesterol levels.
- Lower cholesterol levels disrupt oligodendrocytes from producing myelin.
- Lack of myelin allows lesions to form on the neurons, which disrupts signals between the brain and other parts of the body leading to multiple sclerosis.

Dr Klopfleisch concluded: "*Long-term application (of statins) may negatively influence the intrinsic remyelinating capacity, not only in multiple sclerosis patients, but also in other demyelinating diseases of the central nervous system*".

Paper 451:
Statins can produce abnormalities in myelin

Maier O et al Lovastatin induces the formation of abnormal myelin-like membrane sheets in primary oligodendrocytes. *Glia* 2009 Mar;57(4):402-13

As seen in *papers 449 and 450* oligodendrocytes are a type of brain cell, their principle function is to provide support to axons (nerve cells) and to produce the myelin sheath. Myelin is an insulating layer that forms around nerves, including those in the brain and spinal cord. Cholesterol is a major component of myelin. The purpose of the myelin sheath is to allow impulses to transmit quickly and efficiently along the nerve cells. If myelin is damaged, the impulses slow down. This can cause diseases such as multiple sclerosis.

This study investigated the effect of statins on the formation of myelin in cultured oligodendrocytes.

The study identified:

- Oligodendrocytes treated with lovastatin, did form extensive myelin sheets, however, these sheets were devoid of the major myelin proteins; myelin basic protein and proteolipid protein.
- Experiments revealed that lovastatin blocks the transport of the genetic information of myelin basic protein into oligodendrocytes.
- Proteolipid protein production was only mildly affected by lovastatin. However, lovastatin treatment prevented the movement of proteolipid protein to the cell surface.

The results of the study show that statins can produce abnormalities in myelin, which may have adverse implications in diseases such as multiple sclerosis.

Paper 452:
Statins are neurotoxic to developing brain cells

Pavlov OV et al An in vitro study of the effects of lovastatin on human fetal brain cells. *Neurotoxicology and Teratology* 1995 Jan-Feb;17(1):31-9

The central nervous system (brain and spinal cord) consists of neurons and glial cells. Neurons are nerve cells that are the basic building blocks of the nervous system and glial (astrocyte) cells provide support and protection for neurons.

Cholesterol is vital for the growth and development of neuronal and glial cells. Cholesterol is produced by the glial cells for the use by neurons.

In this study, senior researcher Oleg Pavlov headed a team from the Institute of Experimental Medicine in St. Petersburg. The study used various cultures of embryonic brain cells (neurons and astrocytes) to analyse the direct effects of lovastatin on developing human central nervous system cells.

The study found:

- Lovastatin stopped cholesterol production in astrocytes as well as in glial-neuronal reaggregated cultures.
- The renewal of astrocyte cells was inhibited by lovastatin.
- Exposure of human brain cells to lovastatin resulted in detrimental ultrastructural changes in neuronal and glial cells and led to cell death.

Lovastatin was shown to have adverse effects on the central nervous system and Pavlov concluded: *"Our data suggest that lovastatin is neurotoxic to developing brain cells"*.

Paper 453:
Statins change tau proteins – implications for Alzheimer's

Meske V et al Blockade of HMG-CoA reductase activity causes changes in microtubule-stabilizing protein tau via suppression of geranylgeranylpyrophosphate formation: implications for Alzheimer's disease. *European Journal of Neuroscience* 2003 Jan;17(1):93-102

This study set out to determine the effects of statins on the protein tau. Tau are proteins that stabilize the cytoskeleton (microfilaments and microtubules - the internal scaffolding) in cells and are abundant in neurons. Alzheimer's disease can result when tau proteins become defective (tangled) and no longer stabilize the cellular skeleton properly.

In the laboratory, lovastatin was added to neuron cultures. The study was carried out by Dr Volker Meske and a team of researchers from Charité University Hospital.

The study observed:

- The neuritic network was affected and eventually was completely destroyed.
- This process was marked by alterations in the microfilament and microtubule system.
- The distribution and phosphorylation (phosphorylation is vital for regulating proteins) of protein tau changed.
- There was a transient increase in tau phosphorylation followed by apoptosis (cell death).
- All of the above effects could be linked to the lack of geranylgeranylpyrophosphate. (geranylgeranylpyrophosphate is blocked by statins and is needed in DNA synthesis and cell replication).

Dr Meske concluded: "*Our data demonstrate that lovastatin concentrations able to suppress not only cholesterol but also geranylgeranylpyrophosphate formation may evoke phosphorylation of tau reminiscent of preclinical early stages of Alzheimer's disease and, when prolonged, apoptosis*".

Paper 454: Dr says clinicians should be aware of cognitive impairment and dementia as potential adverse effects associated with statin therapy

King DS et al Cognitive impairment associated with atorvastatin and simvastatin. *Pharmacotherapy* 2003 Dec;23(12):1663-7

Dr Deborah King, an Assistant Professor of Clinical Pharmacy Practice at the University of Mississippi, reports of two women who experienced significant cognitive impairment related to statin therapy. One woman took atorvastatin, and the other first took atorvastatin, then was rechallenged with simvastatin.

Both of the patients showed decreased cognition that was slow in onset, with progressively worsening symptoms related to statin therapy. In both patients, the cognitive impairment completely resolved within one month after statin discontinuation.

Patient 1

- A 67-year-old woman was been treated for high blood pressure, "high" cholesterol and type two diabetes.
- The patient was taking levothyroxine, hormone replacement therapy, glyburide, lisinopril, metoprolol, and atorvastatin. Two months before the patient's visit, her atorvastatin dosage had been increased from 10 mg to 20 mg/day. The patient had been taking 10 mg/day for one year with no reported adverse effects. No other changes to the patient's drug regimen had been made.
- The patient experienced new-onset cognitive impairment, which was reported by the patient and her family. Significant impairment in short-term memory was demonstrated on mental status examination. Her family reported behaviour changes characterized by mood alteration, lack of interest in routine activities, diminished memory, and social impairment.
- Atorvastatin was discontinued, and one month later, the patient and her family noted a dramatic improvement in her mood, memory, motivation, and a return to normal functioning. Repeated mental status examination also demonstrated remarkable improvement in her short-term memory.

Patient 2

- A 68-year-old woman came to a hypertension referral center for initial evaluation. She reported a 20-year personal medical history of high blood pressure. The patient had no known drug allergies, no history of smoking or alcohol consumption, and no psychiatric history or memory impairment. She reported an active lifestyle, with a healthy diet and routine, structured exercise at least five days per week; her long-term drug regimen consisted of lisinopril, estradiol, and atenolol.
- The patient's assessment revealed intact memory with normal judgment and insight. Although her blood pressure was not optimally controlled, physical examination was unremarkable. Hydrochlorothiazide was added to her drug regimen at her initial visit. After laboratory assessment revealed "high" cholesterol, atorvastatin 10 mg per day was begun.

- Approximately nine months after the initial visit, the patient's daughter reported noticeable memory impairment, cognitive decline, and behaviour changes. According to the daughter, the patient was forgetting scheduled routine social events and appointments. She also neglected her longstanding exercise program and had complaints of weakness in her extremities and a lack of energy. The daughter felt that the progressive cognitive decline and symptoms were associated with the start of atorvastatin therapy.
- The patient discontinued atorvastatin on her own, which resulted in both physical and cognitive improvement in one week, as reported by the patient and her daughter.
- The patient was rechallenged with atorvastatin one month after her symptoms resolved, and the cognitive impairment and other symptoms returned three weeks later.
- Atorvastatin was again discontinued; no other changes were made in concurrent drugs. After one month, the patient reported memory improvement and resolution of weakness and tiredness. Mental status examination demonstrated a return to baseline. She had also resumed her routine exercise and social activities.
- She then started Simvastatin 20 mg per day.
- Approximately seven weeks later, the patient and her daughter called to report a return of the memory impairment and cognitive decline. The patient also had complaints of lower extremity weakness and aches.
- Simvastatin was discontinued and, once again, her symptoms resolved in three weeks.

Cholesterol is essential in the formation of myelin. (Myelin is a substance rich in fats and proteins that forms layers around the nerve fibres and acts as insulation. The nerve can be likened to an electrical cable; the axon, or nerve fibre that transmits the nerve impulse, is like the copper wire; and the myelin sheath is like the insulation around the wire. Myelin is present in both the central nervous system and the peripheral nervous system.)

Statin-induced dementia may be caused by statins decreasing the amount of central nervous system cholesterol below the critical value necessary for the formation of myelin. Inadequate myelin production results in demyelination of nerve fibres in the central nervous system, resulting in memory loss.

Once the offending statin is removed from the patient's system, myelin stores are replenished and mental status returns to normal. In the two patients, who received simvastatin, mental status returned to normal within one month of discontinuing the statin.

In addition to demyelination of nerves in the central nervous system, nerves in the peripheral nervous system may be affected. Patients may experience tingling sensations of the extremities and loss of the sense of touch secondary to peripheral nervous system demyelination. The second patient experienced some peripheral adverse effects.

Dr. King concludes: "*Clinicians should be aware of cognitive impairment and dementia as potential adverse effects associated with statin therapy*".

Paper 455:
How statins cause male infertility

Niederberger C Atorvastatin and male infertility: is there a link? *Journal of Andrology* 2005 Jan-Feb;26(1):12

The author of the paper, Dr Craig Niederberger, is Head of the Department of Urology in the College of Medicine at the University of Illinois

Dr Niederberger notes that some doctors have noticed many men on Lipitor (atorvastatin) have low sperm motility. Sperm motility describes the ability of sperm to "swim" properly towards an egg to enable a successful pregnancy.

Coenzyme Q10 (ubiquinone) is a vitamin-like substance produced by the body.

Dr Niedberger relays how sperm motility may be affected by statins by the following mechanism:

- Statins inhibit the production of Coenzyme Q10. Even a brief exposure to atorvastatin causes a marked decrease in blood Coenzyme Q10 concentrations.
- Coenzyme Q10 is vital for energy production and is also an important antioxidant. Both these properties are vital for sperm motility.
- Coenzyme Q10 is present in high concentrations in semen and high levels of coenzyme Q10 correlate with increased sperm motility.

- A study reported CoQ10 supplementation in infertile men with asthenozoospermia (the medical term for reduced sperm motility) resulted in a significant increase in sperm motility.

Paper 456: Simvastatin has deleterious effects on human first trimester placental cells

Kenis I et al Simvastatin has deleterious effects on human first trimester placental explants. *Human Reproduction* 2005 Oct;20(10):2866-72

A group led by Dr Irina Kenis, explored the effects of statins on the placenta. The study compared cultured human first trimester placental cells exposed to small doses of simvastatin with cells not exposed to simvastatin.

The study revealed:

- Compared with unexposed cells, simvastatin sharply inhibited the migration of extravillous trophoblast cells. (The migration of extravillous trophoblast cells into the uterus is a vital stage in the establishment of pregnancy.)
- Compared with unexposed cells, simvastatin inhibited the formation of trophoblast cells.
- Compared with unexposed cells, simvastatin led to more cell death in the trophoblast cells.
- Progesterone levels were significantly reduced in the simvastatin-treated cells in comparison with unexposed cells. (Progesterone keeps the placenta functioning properly and the uterine lining healthy and thick.)
- Human chorionic gonadotropin levels were reduced in the simvastatin-treated cells in comparison with unexposed cells. (Human chorionic gonadotropin is a hormone produced during pregnancy and should almost double every 48 hours in the beginning of a pregnancy. Human chorionic gonadotropin levels that do not rise appropriately may indicate a problem with the pregnancy.)

Dr Kenis concludes: *"Simvastatin adversely affects human first trimester trophoblast. These effects may contribute to failure of the implantation process and be deleterious to the growth potential of the placenta"*.

Paper 457:
How statins adversely affect the immune system

Sun D et al Lovastatin inhibits bone marrow-derived dendritic cell maturation and upregulates proinflammatory cytokine production. *Cellular Immunology* 2003 May;223(1):52-62

In a laboratory setting, Dr Dongxu Sun from the University of Texas Health Science Centre at San Antonio, investigated the effects of lovastatin on the maturation and functional changes of bone marrow-derived dendritic cells. (Dendritic cells act as messengers between the innate and the adaptive immune systems.)

The study discovered:

- Lovastatin inhibited the maturation of dendritic cells in a dose-dependent manner.
- Lovastatin up-regulated dendritic cells pro-inflammatory cytokine production. (A proinflammatory cytokine is a cytokine (a small protein involved in cell signalling) which promotes systemic inflammation. Due to their proinflammatory action, they tend to make a disease worse by producing fever, inflammation, tissue destruction, and, in some cases, even shock and death.)
- When mevalonate was added, these adverse effects were prevented. (Mevalonate is inhibited by statins.)

Dr Sun concludes: *"These results indicate that lovastatin may inhibit bone marrow-derived dendritic cells maturation and up-regulate cytokine production through a mevalonate dependent pathway, and may cause adverse effects on either innate or adaptive immunity"*.

Paper 458:
What happens to your immune system when you take statins?

Benati D et al Opposite effects of simvastatin on the bactericidal and inflammatory response of macrophages to opsonized S. aureus. *Journal of Leukocyte Biology* 2010 Mar;87(3):433-42

Phagocytes are white blood cells that protect the body by ingesting harmful toxins, bacteria and dead and dying cells. Cytokines (Tumor necrosis factor alpha (TNFa) and cyclooxygenase 2 (COX-2), are molecules that trigger and sustain inflammation.

Staphylococcus aureus is a bacterium that is frequently found in the human respiratory tract and on the skin. It is a common cause of skin infections (e.g. boils), respiratory disease (e.g. sinusitis), and food poisoning.

Dr Daniela Benati and colleagues from the University of Siena, examined the effects of simvastatin on the immune system. The study used human phagocytes that were pre-treated with carrier or simvastatin, alone or in association with mevalonate, and subsequently incubated with *Staphylococcus aureus*.

The study found:

- Phagocyte activity was blocked by simvastatin. This effect by simvastatin was reversed by mevalonate.
- TNFa and COX-2 activity was enhanced by simvastatin compared with carrier-treated controls. This effect by simvastatin was reversed by mevalonate.
- Mevalonate is inhibited by statins.

The results of the study show that statins impair the ability of phagocytes to kill dangerous pathogens, but enhance the production of cytokines that cause excessive inflammation.

Dr Benati concludes: *"By enhancing TNFa and COX-2 production while impairing the mechanisms responsible for bacterial killing in macrophages exposed to opsonized bacteria, simvastatin may contribute to establish a state of undesirable, "gratuitous" inflammation in chronically treated patients"*.

The papers in this chapter have given detailed evidence of how statin drugs can promote and worsen an almost endless list of diseases and conditions that damage our body.

- The mechanisms of how stains cause DNA damage and interrupt the cell cycle are described.
- An explanation of why energy is sapped when taking statins is given.
- Descriptions of the processes involved are explained of how muscle pain and muscle damage are almost inevitable when on statin therapy.

- Evidence is shown that statins may worsen heart function.
- The reasons behind the surge in diabetes in statin users are portrayed.
- A depiction is presented of the premise of how statins initiate autoimmune diseases.
- Theories of how statins may exacerbate cancer risk are put forward.
- Information is presented as to why statins cause a decline in cognition which may lead to neurodegenerative disease such as Parkinson's, Alzheimer's, dementia, amyothrophic lateral sclerosis, multiple sclerosis and Huntington's.
- Male fertility may be adversely affected by statins as are the risk of problem pregnancies and birth defects.
- Statins decrease the function of the immune system.
- Details are given that describe how statins damage proteins, enzymes, minerals, antioxidants, cellular structure, brain cells, pancreatic β-cells, energy production, mitochondria, immune system regulation, glucose regulators, calcium regulation, hormonal signalling molecules, sensory signalling molecules, and how they damage DNA and alter gene expression.

Statin and cholesterol expert Dr Malcolm Kendrick sums up the impact of statin use: "*I believe statins have substantial side effects which can significantly affect quality of life*".

Chapter 19

Who decides what are "healthy" cholesterol levels?

After reading the preceding chapters about the harms of lowering your cholesterol levels with statins (or any cholesterol lowering drug), you may be wondering why we are being virtually compelled to hammer our cholesterol levels to lower and lower numbers.

In November 1985, The National Heart, Lung, and Blood Institute (NHLBI) inaugurated the National Cholesterol Education Program (NCEP) to increase awareness among health professionals and the public that elevated blood cholesterol is a cause of coronary heart disease, and that reducing elevated blood cholesterol levels will contribute to the reduction of coronary heart disease.

The NHLBI is a division of the National Institutes of Health (NIH) who are an agency for the United States Department of Health and Human Services (HHS), also known as the Health Department, which is a cabinet-level department of the U.S. federal government who have the remit of protecting the health of all Americans and providing essential human services.

In a nutshell, the National Cholesterol Education Program was formed to persuade the medical profession and the general public that lower cholesterol levels are good for your health.

However, the medical profession were far from united that cholesterol levels needed to be lowered. Eminent cardiologist Dr Eliot Corday was concerned at the clamour to a wholesale cutting of cholesterol levels.

Dr Corday began the research that led to the development of cardiac catheterization. Another of his discoveries was that *electrocardiogram* (ECG) readings changed dramatically in patients with coronary heart disease. He also played a central role in developing continuous ECG recordings in ambulatory patients.

Lastly, he began the radioisotope studies that became the forerunner of modern nuclear cardiology. His contributions to four new fields – catheterization, stress testing, ambulatory ECG monitoring, and nuclear cardiology – made him among the best known cardiologists of his time. He was also the consulting cardiologist for many of the USA's Presidents. Dr Corday has been described as a giant of cardiology.

Dr Corday had this to say about the National Cholesterol Education Program in February 1989: "*In the last year the medical profession has become alarmed about the continuing statements on radio and television and in the daily newspapers and national magazines encouraging the public to be aware of their cholesterol levels. The large anticholesterol advertising campaign initiated by the National Cholesterol Education Program (NCEP) of the National Heart, Lung, and Blood Institute (NHLBI) encourages the public to 'know your blood cholesterol and bring it down'. Even at a cholesterol level of around 200 mg/dl, the NCEP recommends anticholesterol dietary interventions*".

He notes that a survey of practicing physicians revealed 80% believed that cessation of smoking and controlling high blood pressure was a means to prevent heart disease, but only 30% considered cholesterol levels played a major role.

Dr Corday analysed two massive clinical trials that had been postulated to support a cholesterol lowering regime, The Multiple Risk Factor Interventional Trial (MRFIT) and The Lipid Research Clinic Coronary Primary Prevention Trial (LRC-CPPT).

Regarding the findings of MRFIT Dr Corday concluded: "*The results of MRFIT can hardly be used to support a nationwide blood cholesterol reducing program*" and of (LRC-CPPT) he finished: "*There was no difference in total mortality between the two groups*". (One group had been taking a cholesterol lowering drug, cholestyramine, the other group was taking placebo.)

He also examined a more recent trial, The Helsinki Heart Study, which tested the effects of another cholesterol lowering drug, gemfibrozil. Again Dr Corday noted that there was no difference in mortality rates between those taking the drug and those taking placebo.

After this analysis of the three trials Dr Corday stated: "*To extrapolate the results of these studies to propose dietary interventions in the entire population is misleading at best and intellectually dishonest at worst*".

Despite Dr Corday's comments and despite the concerns of a large section of the medical community, the cholesterol lowering juggernaut had begun.

How was the National Cholesterol Education Program born?

Daniel Steinberg was a proponent of the theory that high cholesterol causes heart disease. This claim in part was based on animal experiments. However, the animals used most frequently in these experiments were vegetarian rabbits and mice, simply because omnivorous or carnivorous animals show small or no vascular effects when their cholesterol is raised by diet. Also no animal study has ever produced a heart attack solely by raising an animal's cholesterol.

Steinberg was the Chairman of the Council on Arteriosclerosis, American Heart Association. On November 12, 1969 he stated: "*It is now good medical practice to treat-and I use the word advisedly-people who have definite hyperlipoproteinemia (elevated cholesterol)*".

Steinberg was co-chair of the aforementioned Lipid Research Clinics Coronary Primary Prevention Trial (LRC-CPPT). The trial included 3,806 men with alleged high cholesterol. The men received either the bile acid sequestrant cholestyramine (a cholesterol lowering drug) or placebo.

The results, which were released in January 1984 revealed:

- 96.43% of men taking cholestyramine were alive at the end of the trial.
- 96.26% of men taking placebo were alive at the end of the trial.

Despite the fact the study revealed men had virtually the same death rates no matter what their cholesterol levels or LDL cholesterol levels were, Steinberg stated: "*The positive result of the CPPT trial prompted the NIH to convene a panel of experts to advise whether the evidence was now strong enough to justify policy recommendations regarding control of cholesterol. The panel, which I [Daniel Steinberg] chaired, reached unanimous agreement on an interim set of guidelines and recommended that the NIH initiate a national program (National Cholesterol Education Program) to educate patients and practitioners on the importance of controlling blood cholesterol levels*".

In 1984, Steinberg was the scientific advisor at the pharmaceutical giant, Merck.

In May 1984, Merck got Lovastatin approved for human testing by the Food and Drug Administration (FDA). The FDA are an agency responsible for the control and safety of food and drugs.

In 1985, Steinberg chaired a panel that put Scott Grundy, another proponent of cholesterol lowering, in charge of the NCEP.

To deliver their message to the public the NCEP constituted the adult treatment panel (ATP). The ATP was a panel that contained representatives from medical and professional health associations, voluntary health organisations and government agencies.

The aim of the panel was to develop guidelines for detection, evaluation, and treatment of high blood cholesterol in adults. The ATP guidelines are the most widely used guidelines regarding cholesterol levels. These guidelines are periodically updated. So far five sets of guidelines have been published.

The timeline is as follows:

- ATP-I published in 1988.
- ATP-II published in 1993.
- ATP-III published in 2001.
- ATP-III update published in 2004.
- The fifth set of guidelines published in 2013, were named the 2013 ACC/AHA Guidelines (American College of Cardiology/ American Heart Association).

To help understand the nature of these NCEP guidelines the following will be described:

- An examination of their recommendations.
- The studies the panels used as evidence
- The personnel in the panels.
- The impact of each new guideline.

Paper 459:
Adult Treatment Panel-I (ATP-I) 1988

Before the 1988 ATP guidelines Dr Eliot Corday observed that a cholesterol level of 250 mg/dL (6.5 mmol/L) was considered the upper limit of normal.

Recommendations

ATP-1 recommended the following:

ATP-I Total cholesterol levels classification and recommendation

Cholesterol Level	**Classification**
Less than 200 mg/dl (5.1 mmo/L)	Desirable
200 – 239 mg/dL (5.1 – 6.2 mmol/L)	Borderline High
Over 240 mg/dL (6.2 mmol/L)	High
	Recommendation
Less than 200 mg/dl (5.1 mmo/L)	Check every 5 years
200 – 239 mg/dL (5.1 – 6.2 mmol/L) without CHD or 2 risk factors	Low fat diet and annual check
200 – 239 mg/dL (5.1 – 6.2 mmol/L) with CHD or 2 risk factors	Low fat diet and/or cholesterol lowering drugs depending on LDL levels
Over 240 mg/dL (6.2 mmol/L)	Low fat diet and/or cholesterol lowering drugs depending on LDL levels

ATP-I LDL cholesterol levels classification and recommendations

LDL Cholesterol Level	**Classification**
Less than 130 mg/dL (3.4 mmol/L)	Desirable
130 – 159 mg/dL (3.4 – 4.1 mmol/L)	Borderline High
Over 160 (4.1 mmol/L)	High
	Recommendation
Over 160 mg/dL (4.1 mmol/L) and without CHD or 2 risk factors	Low fat diet to bring LDL below 160 mg/dL (4.1 mmol/L)

LDL Cholesterol Level	Classification
Over 130 mg/dL (3.4 mmol/L) and with CHD or 2 risk factors	Low fat diet to bring LDL below 130 mg/dL (3.4 mmol/L)
Over 190 mg/dL (4.9 mmol/L) and without CHD or 2 risk factors	Low fat diet and cholesterol lowering drugs to bring LDL below 160 mg/dL (4.1 mmol/L)
Over 160 mg/dL (4.1 mmol/L) and with CHD or 2 risk factors	Low fat diet and cholesterol lowering drugs to bring LDL below 130 mg/dL (3.4 mmol/L)

Risk factors constituted:

- o Male sex
- o Family history of premature CHD
- o Cigarette smoking
- o High blood pressure
- o Low levels of high density lipoprotein (HDL) cholesterol
- o Diabetes
- o Stroke
- o Peripheral vascular disease
- o Severe obesity

Studies

From the references in the ATP-I document, it can be seen that data from eight trials were considered for the panel to put forward the above cutting of desirable cholesterol levels.

The eight trials were:

- MRFIT. (Follow up.) The Multiple Risk Factor Interventional Trial (low cholesterol v high cholesterol).
- LRC-CPPT. The Lipid Research Clinic Coronary Primary Prevention Trial (cholestyramine v placebo).
- CDP Niacin. Coronary Drug Project (niacin v placebo).
- CDP Clofibrate. Coronary Drug Project (clofibrate v placebo).
- Oslo diet heart study (cessation of smoking and low fat diet v normal living).

- 7 countries trial (Japanese cholesterol levels 165 mg/dL (4.26 mmol/L) v USA cholesterol levels 240 mg/dL 6.19 mmol/L.)
- WHO Clofibrate. (Plus one year follow up.) The World Health Organisation Clofibrate Trial (clofibrate v high cholesterol).
- Helsinki Heart Study. (Follow up.) (Gemfibrozil v placebo.)

The following table reports the percentage of people still alive at the end of the trials.

Percentage of people still alive at the end of the trials

Trial Name	Number in Trial	% of people alive at the end of the trial in treatment group	% of people alive at the end of the trial in control group
MRFIT	361,662	97.60	97.90
LRC-CPPT	3,806	96.43	96.26
CDP Niacin	8,341	48.00	41.80
CDP Clofibrate	8,341	42.20	41.80
Oslo diet heart study	1,232	97.35	96.18
7 countries trial	3,338	17.90	16.40
WHO Clofibrate	10,627	96.96	97.60
Helsinki Heart Study	4,081	95.06	95.92

When the total number of people in each trial is taken into consideration, the data reveals that 0.14% more people were alive who were taking placebo or with higher cholesterol levels at the end of the trials than the people taking cholesterol lowering drugs or with lower cholesterol levels. To sum up: All the low fat diets and cholesterol lowering drugs (with their side effects) made no difference to death rates.

The personnel of the ATP-I panel

Below is a table of the panel members and their relationships with pharmaceutical companies that sell cholesterol lowering drugs (mainly statins). These relationships may have developed before, during or after the publication of ATP-I.

ATP-I panel member name and relationships with pharmaceutical companies that sell cholesterol lowering drugs

ATP-I panel member name	Relationships with pharmaceutical companies that sell cholesterol lowering drugs
Dewitt Goodman	Research funding from Merck
Stephen Hulley	None
Luther Clark	Honoraria for educational presentations from Abbott, AstraZeneca, Bristol-Myers Squibb, Merck, and Pfizer; Received grant/research support from Abbott, AstraZeneca, Bristol-Myers Squibb, Merck, and Pfizer.
C E Davis	None
Valentin Fuster	Payments from Merck and Pfizer for speaking
John Larosa	Payments from Pfizer and honoraria for speaking or consulting from Bristol Myers Squibb, Merck & Co, Novartis and Bayer
Albert Oberman	Payments from Pfizer for travel expenses and meals
Ernst Schaefer	Consultant at Amarin; AstraZeneca; DuPont; Merck & Co., Inc.; Roche Pharmaceuticals; Unilever Payments from Merck for speaking. Holds stock with Boston Heart Lab.
Daniel Steinberg	Scientific advisor for Merck
W Virgil Brown	Consulting fees from Abbott Laboratories, Amgen, Anthera, Genzyme, Pfizer Inc., LipoScience, and Merck & Co and has received honoraria related to speaking from Abbott Laboratories, LipoScience, and Merck & Co.

ATP-I panel member name	Relationships with pharmaceutical companies that sell cholesterol lowering drugs
Scott Grundy	Has given lectures to health professionals on cholesterol management in which cholesterol-lowering drugs are discussed and for which he received honoraria that were funded by the following companies: Merck, Pfizer, Sankyo, Schering Plough, Kos, Abbot, Bristol-Myers Squibb and AstraZeneca. Also, Grundy has consultant agreements to serve on scientific advisory boards of Pfizer, Sanofi, and AstraZeneca.
Diane Becker	Unrestricted grants from Atherotech, Novartis Pharmaceuticals Corporation, and Pfizer Inc.
Edwin Bierman	Grant from The Upjohn Company, owned by Pfizer
Jacqueline Sooter-Bochenek	None
Rebecca Mullis	Nonc
Neil Stone	Financial relationship with Abbott, AstraZeneca, Merck, Pfizer, Sanofi-Aventis, and Schering-Plough, and has served as a consultant to Abbott, AstraZeneca, Merck, Pfizer, Reliant, Schering-Plough
Donald Hunninghake	Research Grants from AstraZeneca, Bristol Myers Squibb, KOS, Merck, Merck Schering Plough, Novartis, Pfizer, Schering Plough; Speaking Honorarium: AstraZeneca, KOS, Merck, Pfizer
Jacqueline Dunbar	None
Henry Ginsberg	Research grants from AstraZeneca; Isis Pharmaceuticals/Genzyme, Merck, Reliant, Roche, Sanofi and Takeda. He has also received speakers' Bureau/Honoraria payments from Abbott, AstraZeneca, Bristol-Myers Squibb, Merck, Merck/Schering-Plough, Novartis, Pfizer, Roche, Sanofi and Takeda.

ATP-I panel member name	Relationships with pharmaceutical companies that sell cholesterol lowering drugs
Roger Illingworth	Grants and research support from AstraZeneca Pharmaceuticals LP. He has participated in the Speakers Bureau for Kos Pharmaceuticals Inc., Merck & Co Inc., Pfizer Inc., Schering-Plough Corporation and has acted as a consultant for AstraZeneca Pharmaceuticals LP, and Sankyo Pharma.
Harold Sadin	None
Gustav Schonfeld	Participated in studies that were supported by grants from Merck Research Laboratories
James Cleeman	Has served for 25 years as founding Coordinator of the National Cholesterol Education Program at the NHLBI and spearheaded the US effort to lower cholesterol levels.
Hollis Bryan Brewer	Received honoraria from AstraZeneca, Pfizer, Lipid Sciences, Merck, Merck/Schering-Plough, Fournier, Tularik, Esperion, and Novartis; he has served as a consultant for AstraZeneca, Pfizer, Lipid Sciences, Merck, Merck/Schering-Plough, Fournier, Tularik, Sankyo, and Novartis.
Nancy Ernst	NHLBI employee
William Friedewald	Involved in trials where the following companies provided study medications, equipment, or supplies; Abbott Laboratories, Amylin Pharmaceutical, AstraZeneca Pharmaceuticals, Bayer HealthCare, GlaxoSmithKline Pharmaceuticals, King Pharmaceuticals, Merck, Novartis Pharmaceuticals, Omron Healthcare, Sanofi-Aventis, and Takeda Pharmaceuticals.
Jeffery Hoeg	NHLBI employee
Basil Rifkind	NHLBI employee
David Gordon	NHLBI employee

Out of the 29 members of the panel, 18 members have had or have financial relationships with pharmaceutical companies who market cholesterol lowering drugs, five members worked at the NHLBI (who set up the ATP panel) and six had no obvious ties.

Impact of the recommendations

Figures show that about 261,000 people were taking cholesterol lowering medication in the USA in 1983. With the impact of the ATP-I guidelines that figure rose to 1,309,000.

Summary of ATP-I

The members of ATP-I recommended that desirable cholesterol levels be reduced by 20% with evidence that showed people with lower cholesterol levels or who use cholesterol lowering drugs do not live longer than people with higher cholesterol levels. Over 75% of the panel members have at some time developed financial relationships with pharmaceutical companies who market cholesterol lowering drugs, or were employed by the organisation that set up the panel. The panel's recommendations resulted in a five-fold increase in the use of cholesterol lowering drugs.

Paper 460: Adult treatment Panel-II (ATP-II) 1993

Recommendations

ATP-II recommended the following:

ATP-II Total cholesterol levels classification and recommendation

Cholesterol Level	Classification
Less than 200 mg/dl (5.1 mmo/L)	Desirable
200 – 239 mg/dL (5.1 – 6.2 mmol/L)	Borderline High
Over 240 mg/dL (6.2 mmol/L)	High
	Recommendation
Less than 200 mg/dl (5.1 mmo/L) with HDL above 35 mg/dL (0.9 mmol/L) without CHD	Check every 5 years. Provided education on low fat diet, exercise and risk factor reduction.

Cholesterol Level	Classification
Less than 200 mg/dl (5.1 mmo/L) with HDL below 35 mg/dL (0.9 mmol/L) without CHD	Reinforced education on low fat diet, exercise and risk factor reduction. Re-evaluated in 1-2 years – low fat diet or no action depending on LDL levels.
200 – 239 mg/dL (5.1 – 6.2 mmol/L) without CHD or 2 risk factors and HDL above 35 mg/dL (0.9 mmol/L)	Reinforced education on low fat diet, exercise and risk factor reduction. Re-evaluated in 1-2 years – low fat diet and/or drugs depending on LDL levels.
200 – 239 mg/dL (5.1 – 6.2 mmol/L) without CHD but with 2 or more risk factors and/or HDL below 35 mg/dL (0.9 mmol/L)	Low fat diet and/or cholesterol lowering drugs depending on LDL levels
Over 240 mg/dL (6.2 mmol/L)	Low fat diet and/or cholesterol lowering drugs depending on LDL levels

ATP-II LDL cholesterol levels classification and recommendations

LDL Cholesterol Level	Classification
Less than 130 mg/dL (3.4 mmol/L)	Desirable
130 – 159 mg/dL (3.4 – 4.1 mmol/L)	Borderline High
Over 160 (4.1 mmol/L)	High
	Recommendation
Less than 130 mg/dl (3.4 mmo/L) without CHD	Check cholesterol and HDL within 5 years. Provided education on low fat diet, exercise and risk factor reduction.

LDL Cholesterol Level	Classification
130 – 159 mg/dL (3.4 – 4.1 mmol/L) without CHD and with fewer than 2 risk factors	Provided information on Step 1 (low fat) diet. Re-evaluated annually. Reinforced education on low fat diet, exercise and risk factor reduction.
130 – 159 mg/dL (3.4 – 4.1 mmol/L) without CHD but with 2 or more risk factors	Low fat diet to bring LDL below 130 mg/dL (3.4 mmol/L)
160 – 189 mg/dL (4.1 – 4.8 mmol/L) without CHD and fewer than 2 risk factors	Low fat diet to bring LDL below 160 mg/dL (4.1 mmol/L)
Over 190 mg/dL (4.9 mmol/L) without CHD and fewer than 2 risk factors	Low fat diet and cholesterol lowering drugs to bring LDL below 160 mg/dL (4.1 mmol/L)
Over 160 mg/dL (4.1 mmol/L) without CHD but with 2 or more risk factors	Low fat diet and cholesterol lowering drugs to bring LDL below 130 mg/dL (3.4 mmol/L)
Less than 100 mg/dL (2.6 mmol/L) With CHD	Low fat diet and receive individual instruction on diet and exercise.
More than 100 mg/dL (2.6 mmol/L) With CHD	Low fat diet and cholesterol lowering drugs to bring LDL below 100 mg/dL (2.6 mmol/L)

Risk factors constituted:

- Age: Males over 45, females over 55 or premature menopause without estrogen replacement therapy
- Family history of premature CHD (definite heart attack or sudden death before 55 in father or other male first-degree relative, or before 65 in mother or other female first-degree relative).
- Current cigarette smoking
- High blood pressure (over 140/90 or on blood pressure medication)
- Low HDL (less than 35 mg/dL (0.9 mmol/L)

- Diabetes
- o High HDL (over 60 mg/dL (1.5 mmol/L) was considered protective.

The changes in ATP-II compared to ATP-I are:

- Low HDL may result in a low fat diet prescription even if total cholesterol is below 200 mg/dl (5.1 mmo/L). HDL was not considered in ATP-I.
- All patients with CHD have a LDL target of less than 100 mg/dL (2.6 mmol/L). All CHD patients could possibly receive cholesterol lowering drugs if a low fat dietary intervention did not reduce LDL levels. In ATP-I the target LDL was 130 mg/dL (3.4 mmol/L) and cholesterol lowering drugs were only to be prescribed if LDL was more than 160 mg/dL (4.1 mmol/L).

Studies

Page four of the ATP-II report says: "*The demonstration that cholesterol lowering prevents CHD is the cornerstone of both the public health and clinical approach to controlling high blood cholesterol. Beyond the beneficial effect of cholesterol lowering on CHD rates, however, lies the question of whether reduction of blood cholesterol levels extends the life span*".

A meta-analysis of 19 randomised clinical intervention trials of cholesterol reduction is quoted to back up the "cornerstone" of ATP-II.

That "cornerstone" is titled: "*An analysis of randomized trials evaluating the effect of cholesterol reduction on total mortality and coronary heart disease incidence*". The paper was authored by Ingar Holme from Ullevaal Hospital in Oslo and was published in *Circulation* 1990 December issue 82(6) pages 1916-1924.

The 19 trials are:

- MRFIT. The Multiple Risk Factor Interventional Trial (extra medical care re; blood pressure, smoking, dietary advice for lowering cholesterol v usual care).
- Oslo diet heart study (cessation of smoking and low fat diet v normal living).
- WHO factory. World Health Organisation Factory Trial (cessation of smoking, lowering of blood pressure and lowering of cholesterol v normal living).

- Acheson clofibrate trial. (Clofibrate v none.)
- Carlson clofibrate and nicotinic acid trial. (Clofibrate and nicotinic acid v none.)
- Research committee of the Scottish Society of Physicians trial. (Clofibrate v placebo.)
- CDP. Coronary Drug Project Trial. (Clofibrate and niacin v placebo.)
- Newcastle upon Tyne physicians trial. (Clofibrate v placebo.)
- Dorr colestipol hydrochloride trial. (Colestipol hydrochloride v placebo.)
- Dayton unsaturated fat trial. (Diet with higher levels of unsaturated fat v normal diet.)
- Leren cholesterol lowering diet trial. (Cholesterol lowering diet v normal diet.)
- MRC soya-bean. Medical Research Council soya-bean oil Trial (soya-bean diet v normal diet.)
- MRC low fat. Medical Research Council low fat diet trial. (Low fat diet v normal diet.)
- Rose corn oil trial. (Low fat diet v normal diet.)
- Woodhill low fat low cholesterol trial. (Low fat low cholesterol diet v normal diet.)
- LRC-CPPT. The Lipid Research Clinic Coronary Primary Prevention Trial (cholestyramine v placebo.)
- WHO Clofibrate. The World Health Organisation Clofibrate Trial (clofibrate v high cholesterol.)
- Helsinki Heart Study. (Gemfibrozil v placebo.)
- Minnesota Coronary Survey. (Low saturated fat diet v normal diet.)

Percentage of people still alive at the end of the trials

Trial Name	Number in Trial	% of people alive at the end of the trial in treatment group	% of people alive at the end of the trial in control group
MRFIT	12,866	95.87	95.96
Oslo diet heart study	1,232	97.35	96.18
WHO factory	49,784	95.94	96.32
Acheson	95	51.06	58.33
Carlson	558	91.39	90.68
Scottish physicians	537	90.90	90.47
CDP	5,011	75.06	74.57
Newcastle physicians	497	88.93	81.02
Dorr	2,278	96.77	95.74
Dayton	846	58.96	58.05
Leren	412	78.65	75.24
MRC soya-bean	393	85.92	83.50
MRC low fat	252	83.73	81.39
Rose	80	88.88	96.15
Woodhill	468	83.11	88.18
LRC-CPPT	3,806	96.43	96.26
WHO Clofibrate	10,627	97.59	98.35
Helsinki Heart Study	4,081	97.80	97.93
Minnesota Coronary Survey	9,775	94.55	94.72

When the total number of people in each trial is taken into consideration, the data reveals that 0.18% more people were alive who were taking placebo or with higher cholesterol levels or on their normal diet at the end of the trials than the people taking cholesterol lowering drugs or with lower cholesterol levels or on low fat diets. To sum up: All the low fat diets and cholesterol lowering drugs (with their side effects) made no difference to death rates.

The personnel of the ATP-II panel

Below is a table of the panel members and their relationships with pharmaceutical companies that sell cholesterol lowering drugs (mainly statins). These relationships may have developed before, during or after the publication of ATP-II.

ATP-II panel member name and relationships with pharmaceutical companies that sell cholesterol lowering drugs

ATP-II panel member name	Relationships with pharmaceutical companies that sell cholesterol lowering drugs
Scott Grundy	Has given lectures to health professionals on cholesterol management in which cholesterol-lowering drugs are discussed and for which he received honoraria that were funded by the following companies: Merck, Pfizer, Sankyo, Schering Plough, Kos, Abbot, Bristol-Myers Squibb and AstraZeneca. Also, Grundy has consultant agreements to serve on scientific advisory boards of Pfizer, Sanofi, and AstraZeneca.
David Bilheimer	Employment history includes, NHBLI, Merck, Novartis and Mannkind
Alan Chait	Served as a consultant to Merck (USA), Pfizer, Novo Nordisk, Novartis, AstraZeneca, and Takeda
Luther Clark	Honoraria for educational presentations from Abbott, AstraZeneca, Bristol-Myers Squibb, Merck, and Pfizer; Received grant/research support from Abbott, AstraZeneca, Bristol-Myers Squibb, Merck, and Pfizer

ATP-II panel member name	Relationships with pharmaceutical companies that sell cholesterol lowering drugs
Margo Denke	Honoraria and travel expense reimbursement from Merck. She has also participated on the speakers bureau for Merck, Merck/Schering-Plough, and Schering-Plough
Richard Havel	Supported by an educational grant from Merck Sharp & Dohme
William Hazzard	Research support from Merck Institute for Aging and Health and received Pfizer Scholars Grants
Stephen Hulley	None
Donald Hunninghake	Research Grants from AstraZeneca, Bristol Myers Squibb, KOS, Merck, Merck Schering Plough, Novartis, Pfizer, Schering Plough; Speaking Honorarium: AstraZeneca, KOS, Merck, Pfizer
Robert Kreisberg	Research grant from Merck & Company and supported by an unrestricted educational grant from Pfizer, Inc.
Penny KrisEtherton	Research grant from GlaxoSmithKline
James McKenney	Speaker honorarium: AstraZeneca LP, Kos Pharmaceuticals, Merck & Co. and Pfizer, Inc. Research Grants: AstraZeneca LP, GlaxoSmithKline, Kos Pharmaceuticals, Merck & Co., Pfizer, Inc., Schering-Plough, and Takeda. Consultant Services: AstraZeneca LP, Kos Pharmaceuticals, Merck & Co., Pfizer, Inc., and Sankyo Pharma Inc.
Michael Newman	None
Ernst Schaefer	Consultant at Amarin; AstraZeneca; DuPont; Merck & Co., Inc.; Roche Pharmaceuticals; Unilever Payments from Merck for speaking. Holds stock with Boston Heart Lab.

ATP-II panel member name	Relationships with pharmaceutical companies that sell cholesterol lowering drugs
Burton Sobel	Consultant Merck. Research funding from GlaxoSmithKline, Bristol-Myers Squibb Medical Imaging, Merck, Abbott Laboratories, and Pfizer. Research financial support from Abbott Laboratories, Bayer Diagnostics, J.R. Carlso Laboratories, Eli Lilly, Merck Sante and Novartis Pharmaceuticals.
Carolyn Somelofski	None
Milton Weinstein	Research supported by an unrestricted grant from Merck and Co. Paid consultant at OptumInsight, which has received funding from Pfizer for research studies.
Hollis Bryan Brewer	Received honoraria from AstraZeneca, Pfizer, Lipid Sciences, Merck, Merck/Schering-Plough, Fournier, Tularik, Esperion, and Novartis; he has served as a consultant for AstraZeneca, Pfizer, Lipid Sciences, Merck, Merck/Schering-Plough, Fournier, Tularik, Sankyo, and Novartis.
James Cleeman	Has served for 25 years as founding Coordinator of the National Cholesterol Education Program at the NHLBI and spearheaded the US effort to lower cholesterol levels
Karen Donato	Developed a scientific statement which received unrestricted educational grants from AstraZeneca, Bristol-Myers Squibb, Sanofi-Aventis, and Metabolic Syndrome Institute (Solvay Pharmaceuticals and Abbott Laboratories)
Nancy Ernst	NHLBI employee
Jeffery Hoeg	NHLBI employee
Basil Rifkind	NHLBI employee
Jacques Rossouw	NHLBI employee

ATP-II panel member name	Relationships with pharmaceutical companies that sell cholesterol lowering drugs
Christopher Sempos	NHLBI employee
Joanne M. Gallivan	NHLBI employee
Maureen Harris	None
Laurie Quint-Adler	None

Out of the 28 members of the panel, 17 members have had or have financial relationships with pharmaceutical companies who market cholesterol lowering drugs, six members worked at the NHLBI (who set up the ATP panel) and five had no obvious ties.

Impact of the recommendations

One of the panel members, Christopher Sempos, estimated that the recommendation would result in 12.7 million Americans taking cholesterol-lowering drugs. This estimate reflects approximately 4 million adults with established coronary heart disease and 8.7 million without established coronary heart disease. In 1988 around 1,309,000 people were taking cholesterol lowering medication.

Summary of ATP-II

The members of ATP-II recommended that further restrictions of cholesterol levels were appropriate with evidence that showed people with lower cholesterol levels or who use cholesterol lowering drugs do not live longer than people with higher cholesterol levels. Over 80% of the panel members have at some time developed financial relationships with pharmaceutical companies who market cholesterol lowering drugs, or were employed by the organisation that set up the panel. The panel's recommendations resulted in a near ten-fold increase in the use of cholesterol lowering drugs compared to ATP-I.

The next five studies played a major part in Adult Treatment Panel-III recommendations.

Paper 461: Doctor says that an individual patient, despite many years of investment in taking statins, gets virtually nil health benefit

Spence D The treatment paradox. *British Medical Journal* Jan 12, 2008; 336(7635): 100

Dr Des Spence, a General Practitioner from Scotland analysed the results of the West of Scotland Coronary Prevention Study (WOSCOPS). WOSCOPS was a double-blind, randomised, placebo controlled study that was designed to determine the effects of pravastatin in men with "high cholesterol" and no history of heart attack. The study included 6,595 men, 45 to 64 years of age, with average cholesterol levels of 7.0 mmol/l (272 mgdL) to receive pravastatin (40 mg each evening) or placebo. The average follow-up period was 4.9 years.

Interestingly approximately 81,000 men (no women) from the West of Scotland were screened for the study before the 6,595 were handpicked. This may have been because the investigators reasoned these men were at the highest risk of heart disease. However, this begs the question *"Are the results of the study applicable to the general population?"*

He observes:

- It wasn't by chance that the west of Scotland was chosen. The participants were men aged between 45 and 64 in the most socially deprived area in western Europe.
- More than three quarters (78%) were current or former smokers, and their average cholesterol concentration was 7 mmol/l (270mg/dL). If lowering of cholesterol concentration was going to work anywhere it was going to work here.
- The study ran for five years and those taking statins had an absolute reduction of a derisory 0.7% in cardiovascular mortality.
- This corresponds to a number needed to treat of 143 men over five years to prevent one cardiovascular death.
- This figure can be annualised to give 715 to prevent one cardiovascular death. So, putting it crudely, some 714 patients a year gain no benefit from treatment, even in the highest risk population in the world.

Dr Spence concludes: *"This is the 'treatment paradox': that an individual patient, despite many years of investment in taking statins, gets virtually nil health benefit. Patients might rightly scratch their heads and complain about mis-selling if the numbers were presented in this way".*

Paper 462: More patients die when taking statins in the AFCAPS/TexCAPS study

Downs JR et al Primary prevention of acute coronary events with lovastatin in men and women with average cholesterol levels: results of AFCAPS/TexCAPS. Air Force/Texas Coronary Atherosclerosis Prevention Study. *Journal of the American Medical Association* 1998 May 27;279(20):1615-22

This study investigated the effect of statin treatment on men and women without cardiovascular disease, with average total cholesterol and average low-density lipoprotein cholesterol (LDL) levels and below-average high-density lipoprotein cholesterol (HDL) levels. The study included 5,608 men and 997 women who were given either lovastatin (20-40 mg daily) or placebo and followed for an average of 5.2 years.

- The study found that more patients died who were given statins compared to patients given placebo.

Paper 463: Adverse effects caused by statins

Grossman CM Cholesterol reduction, heart disease, and mortality. *Annals of Internal Medicine* 1997 Apr 15;126(8):661

This paper, by Dr Charles M Grossman, analyses the (4S) Scandinavian Simvastatin Survival Study. The study investigated the effects of statins on patients with existing coronary heart disease. The study was a randomised in a double-blind trial and included 4,444 patients with angina pectoris or previous heart attack. The study lasted for 5.4 years and the patients received either simvastatin or placebo.

Dr Grossman noted at the start of the study, compared with the simvastatin group, the placebo group contained:

- o 58 more patients with a major Q wave infarction. (A Q wave is represented in an electrocardiogram (ECG). Patients with

major Q waves have significantly higher death rates than patients with moderate or minor Q waves).
- o 32 more patients with a one to five year history of angina.
- o 21 more patients with both angina and a heart attack.

Regarding the study he found:

- More men died from heart disease in the placebo group. (Dr Grossman commented that the extra heart disease deaths in men in the placebo group: *"may have resulted from differences in the two groups and that the attempt at randomisation may have failed").*
- Despite the placebo group starting with more patients with a worse grade of heart disease, more women died of heart disease in the simvastatin group.

Regarding adverse effects by the end of the trial, the findings revealed:

- Patients in the simvastatin group had a 17% increased risk of edema compared with patients in the placebo group.
- Patients in the simvastatin group had a 2% increased risk of abdominal pain compared with patients in the placebo group.
- Patients in the simvastatin group had a 12% increased risk of atrial fibrillation compared with patients in the placebo group. (Atrial fibrillation is a heart condition that causes an irregular and often abnormally fast heart rate.)
- Patients in the simvastatin group had a 37% increased risk of constipation compared with patients in the placebo group.
- Patients in the simvastatin group had a 26% increased risk of gastritis compared with patients in the placebo group.
- Patients in the simvastatin group had a 17% increased risk of diabetes compared with patients in the placebo group.
- Patients in the simvastatin group had a 16% increased risk of muscle pain compared with patients in the placebo group.
- Patients in the simvastatin group had a 19% increased risk of headaches compared with patients in the placebo group.
- Patients in the simvastatin group had a 5% increased risk of insomnia compared with patients in the placebo group.
- Patients in the simvastatin group had a 7% increased risk of vertigo compared with patients in the placebo group.

- Patients in the simvastatin group had a 5% increased risk of bronchitis compared with patients in the placebo group.
- Patients in the simvastatin group had a 28% increased risk of sinusitis compared with patients in the placebo group.
- Patients in the simvastatin group had a 50% increased risk of eczema compared with patients in the placebo group.
- Patients in the simvastatin group had a 3% increased risk of urinary tract infections compared with patients in the placebo group.

Paper 464:
Statins may cause a huge rise in breast cancer risk

Sacks FM et al The effect of pravastatin on coronary events after myocardial infarction in patients with average cholesterol levels. Cholesterol and Recurrent Events Trial investigators. *New England Journal of Medicine* 1996 Oct 3;335(14):1001-9

This study, named the Cholesterol and Recurrent Events Trial (CARE) investigated the effects of statins in patients with coronary disease, who have average (below 240 mg/dL or 6.2 mmol/L) cholesterol levels. The study was a double-blind, placebo controlled trial lasting five years and included 4,159 patients who received either 40 mg of pravastatin per day or placebo.

The study found:

- Those taking statins had a 19% reduced risk of death from coronary heart disease compared to placebo.
- Those taking statins had a 45% increased risk of death due to cardiovascular but noncoronary causes compared to placebo.
- Those taking statins had a 100% increased risk of violent death compared to placebo.
- Those taking statins had a 9% increased risk of death from cancer compared to placebo.
- Those taking statins had a 7% increased risk of any cancer compared to placebo.
- Women taking statins had a 1100% increased risk of breast cancer compared to placebo.

Dr Uffe Ravnskov, an expert in cholesterol, statins and heart disease, commented in his book 'The Cholesterol Myths': *"Considering the large number of participants, this result doesn't seem particularly impressive... In fact, the reduction in coronary heart disease deaths was offset by the fact that in the treatment (statin) group a few more had died from other causes".*

Paper 465: Three workers from Bristol-Myers Squibb (the manufacturers of pravastatin) are co-workers in study (funded by Bristol-Myers Squibb) to examine the efficacy of pravastatin

Tonkin A et al Prevention of cardiovascular events and death with pravastatin in patients with coronary heart disease and a broad range of initial cholesterol levels. The Long-Term Intervention with Pravastatin in Ischaemic Disease (LIPID) Study Group. *New England Journal of Medicine* 1998 Nov 5;339(19):1349-57

This study, (The Long-Term Intervention with Pravastatin in Ischaemic Disease or LIPID), investigated the effects of statins on death rates from coronary heart disease and overall death rates in patients with existing coronary heart disease and a broad range of cholesterol levels. The study was a double-blind, randomised, placebo controlled trial, included 9,014 patients who were 31 to 75 years of age and who were followed for an average of 6.1 years. The patients received either pravastatin (40 mg daily) or placebo.

- Patients were excluded from the trial if they had had a clinically significant medical or surgical event within three months of the study, and if they had suffered heart failure, kidney or liver disease.
- 11,106 patients were originally chosen for the trial. Before the study started the patients entered an eight-week 'run-in' phase to see if they could tolerate the pravastatin treatment. Nearly 20% of the patients dropped out in this run-in phase.
- By the end of the study 19% of the patients assigned to treatment with pravastatin had permanently stopped taking the drug.
- The study was funded by Bristol-Myers Squibb who produce pravastatin.
- Three of the co-workers in the study (M. Gandy, J. Joughin, J. Seabrook) came from Bristol-Myers Squibb.

Payments have also been received by some members of the research team from pharmaceutical companies (including Bristol-Myers Squibb) in the cholesterol lowering industry, they include:

- The chair of the study, Dr Andrew Tonkin, has received research grants from Bristol-Myers Squibb, AstraZeneca, Merck Sharpe & Dohme, and has been a member of Advisory boards for AstraZeneca, Merck Sharpe & Dohme and Pfizer.
- David Colquhoun has received research support from Bristol-Myers Squibb, AstraZeneca, Pfizer, Merck Sharpe Dohme, Fornier Pharma, Solvay, Schering-Plough, Abbott, Sanofi, and Boehringer Ingelheim. He has been on the speakers' bureau of, received honoraria from, and served as a consultant for AstraZeneca, Pfizer, Merck Sharpe Dohme, Abbott, Servier, and Fornier Pharma.
- Harvey White has received consulting fees and lecture fees from The Medicines Company and Sanofi-Aventis and received grant support from The Medicines Company, Sanofi-Aventis, Proctor & Gamble, Schering Plough, and Eli Lilly Co.
- Peter Thompson has received honoraria from Pfizer for educational lectures related to treatment of dyslipidemia. He has also given educational lectures for Astra Zeneca, Bristol Myers Squibb. He has received research grants from Bristol Myers Squibb, Merck, Pfizer, and has served on advisory boards for Astra Zeneca, Bristol Myers Squibb and Sanofi Aventis.
- The results of the study revealed that 172 patients needed to be given statins every year to prevent one major coronary event. Put another way, for every 172 patients given pravastatin every year, 171 received no cardiovascular benefit from the drug.
- Patients taking pravastatin had a higher risk of side effects than patients on placebo.

Adverse event data from this study and six other pravastatin double-blind, placebo-controlled trials were pooled. The other studies were; West of Scotland Coronary Prevention Study (WOSCOPS); Cholesterol and Recurrent Events study (CARE); Pravastatin Limitation of Atherosclerosis in the Coronary Arteries study (PLAC I); Pravastatin, Lipids and Atherosclerosis in the Carotids study (PLAC II); Regression Growth Evaluation Statin Study (REGRESS);

and Kuopio Atherosclerosis Prevention Study (KAPS). These trials involved a total of 10,764 patients treated with pravastatin 40 mg and 10,719 patients treated with placebo.

The pooled results of the studies revealed:

- Patients in the pravastatin group had a 1.5% increased risk of rash (including dermatitis) compared with patients in the placebo group.
- Patients in the pravastatin group had a 11% increased risk of edema compared with patients in the placebo group.
- Patients in the pravastatin group had a 7.7% increased risk of fatigue compared with patients in the placebo group.
- Patients in the pravastatin group had a 2.2% increased risk of chest pain compared with patients in the placebo group.
- Patients in the pravastatin group had a 10% increased risk of fever compared with patients in the placebo group.
- Patients in the pravastatin group had a 15% increased risk of weight gain compared with patients in the placebo group.
- Patients in the pravastatin group had a 2% increased risk of musculoskeletal pain compared with patients in the placebo group.
- Patients in the pravastatin group had a 11% increased risk of muscle cramp compared with patients in the placebo group.
- Patients in the pravastatin group had a 6.2% increased risk of musculoskeletal traumatism compared with patients in the placebo group.
- Patients in the pravastatin group had a 11% increased risk of dizziness compared with patients in the placebo group.
- Patients in the pravastatin group had a 25% increased risk of sleep disturbance compared with patients in the placebo group.
- Patients in the pravastatin group had a 2.1% increased risk of anxiety compared with patients in the placebo group.
- Patients in the pravastatin group had a 6.6% increased risk of 'pins and needles' compared with patients in the placebo group.
- Patients in the pravastatin group had a 3.8% increased risk of urinary tract infections compared with patients in the placebo group.

- Patients in the pravastatin group had a 5% increased risk of upper respiratory tract infections compared with patients in the placebo group.
- Patients in the pravastatin group had a 11% increased risk of a cough compared with patients in the placebo group.
- Patients in the pravastatin group had a 2.2% increased risk of influenza compared with patients in the placebo group.
- Patients in the pravastatin group had a 8.5% increased risk of pulmonary (lung) infection compared with patients in the placebo group.
- Patients in the pravastatin group had a 4.4% increased risk of sinus abnormality compared with patients in the placebo group.
- Patients in the pravastatin group had a 9.6% increased risk of bronchitis compared with patients in the placebo group.
- Patients in the pravastatin group had a 3% increased risk of visual disturbance (includes blurred vision and double vision) compared with patients in the placebo group.
- Patients in the pravastatin group had a 10% increased risk of a viral infection compared with patients in the placebo group.

In addition to the events listed above, events of probable, possible, or uncertain relationship to pravastatin-treated patients included the following: Scalp hair abnormality (including alopecia), urticarial (hives), sexual dysfunction, libido change, flushing, allergy, muscle weakness, vertigo, insomnia, memory impairment, neuropathy (including peripheral neuropathy), taste disturbance.

The following events have also been reported with pravastatin: Myopathy, rhabdomyolysis, immune-mediated necrotizing myopathy, dysfunction of certain cranial nerves, peripheral nerve palsy, cognitive impairment (e.g. memory loss, forgetfulness, amnesia, memory impairment, confusion), anaphylaxis, angioedema, lupus erythematosus-like syndrome, polymyalgia rheumatica, dermatomyositis, vasculitis, purpura, hemolytic anaemia, arthritis, arthralgia, asthenia, photosensitivity, chills, malaise, toxic epidermal necrolysis, erythema multiforme (including Stevens-Johnson syndrome), abdominal pain, constipation, pancreatitis, hepatitis (including chronic active hepatitis), cholestatic jaundice, fatty change in liver, cirrhosis, fulminant hepatic necrosis, hepatoma, fatal and non-fatal hepatic failure, a variety of skin changes (e.g. nodules, discoloration, dryness of mucous membranes, changes to hair/nails), urinary abnormality (including dysuria, frequency, nocturia), shortness of breath, enlargement of breast tissue in males, anaemia, thrombocytopenia, and leukopenia.

- To conclude: The study was not representative of a real world setting. Some patients were excluded because of specified criteria, nearly a fifth of those chosen for the study dropped out in the 'run-in' phase, by the end of the study another fifth of the patients had permanently stopped taking the drug, the study was funded by the manufacturer of the drug (Bristol Myers Squibb), employees of Bristol Myers Squibb were members of the research team and many of the other researchers had extensive links with other pharmaceutical companies in the cholesterol lowering industry. Every year 99.41% of patients received no cardiovascular benefit from the drug and many suffered from adverse side effects.

Paper 466:
Adult treatment Panel-III (ATP-III) 2001

Recommendations

ATP-III recommended the following:

ATP-III Total cholesterol levels classification

Total Cholesterol Level	Classification
Less than 200 mg/dl (5.1 mmo/L)	Desirable
200 – 239 mg/dL (5.1 – 6.2 mmol/L)	Borderline High
Over 240 mg/dL (6.2 mmol/L)	High
HDL Level	
Less than 40 mg/dL (1.03 mmol/)	Low
More than 60 mg/dL (1.55 mmol/L)	High (Desirable)

ATP-III LDL cholesterol levels classification and recommendations

LDL Cholesterol Level	Classification
Less than 100 mg/dL (2.6 mmol/L)	Optimal
Less than 130 mg/dL (3.4 mmol/L)	Above optimal
130 – 159 mg/dL (3.4 – 4.1 mmol/L)	Borderline High
160 – 189 mg/dL (4.1 – 4.9 mmol/L)	High
Over 190 mg/dL (4.9 mmol/L)	Very High
	Recommendation
Less than 130 mg/dL (3.4 mmol/L) without CHD or Risk Equivalents and fewer than 2 risk factors	Public Health Messages on Healthy Life Habits. Re-evaluation: 5 Years.
130 – 159 mg/dL (3.4 – 4.1 mmol/L) without CHD or Risk Equivalents and fewer than 2 risk factors	Public Health Messages on Healthy Life Habits. Re-evaluation: 1 Year
160 – 189 mg/dl (4.1 – 4.9 mmo/L) without CHD or Risk Equivalents and fewer than 2 risk factors	TLC and optional cholesterol lowering drug to bring LDL below 160 mg/dL (4.1 mmol/L)
Over 190 mg/dL (4.9 mmol/L) without CHD or Risk Equivalents and fewer than 2 risk factors	TLC and cholesterol lowering drug to bring LDL below 160 mg/dL (4.1 mmol/L)
Less than 130 mg/dL (3.4 mmol/L) without CHD or Risk Equivalents and with 2 or more risk factors and less than 10% Framingham risk	Control Other Risk Factors. Public Health Message on Healthy Life Habits. Re-evaluation in 1 Year.

LDL Cholesterol Level	Classification
130 – 159 mg/dL (3.4 – 4.1 mmol/L) without CHD or Risk Equivalents and with 2 or more risk factors and less than 10% Framingham risk	TLC and optional cholesterol lowering drug to bring LDL below 130 mg/dL (3.4 mmol/L)
Over 160 mg/dL (4.1 mmol/L) without CHD or Risk Equivalents and with 2 or more risk factors and less than 10% Framingham risk	TLC and cholesterol lowering drug to bring LDL below 130 mg/dL (3.4 mmol/L)
Less than 130 mg/dL (3.4 mmol/L) without CHD or Risk Equivalents and with 2 or more risk factors and 10-20% Framingham risk	Control Other Risk Factors. Public Health Message on Healthy Life Habits. Re-evaluation in 1 Year.
More than 130 mg/dL (3.4 mmol/L) without CHD or Risk Equivalents and with 2 or more risk factors and 10-20% Framingham risk	TLC and cholesterol lowering drug to bring LDL below 130 mg/dL (3.4 mmol/L)
Less than 100mg/dL (2.6 mmol/L) with CHD or Risk Equivalents or more than 20% Framingham risk	TLC and control other risk factors
100 – 129 mg/dL (2.6 – 3.4 mmol/L) with CHD or Risk Equivalents or more than 20% Framingham risk	TLC and optional cholesterol lowering drug to bring LDL below 100 mg/dL (2.6mmol/L)
More than 130 mg/dL (3.4 mmol/L) with CHD or Risk Equivalents or more than 20% Framingham risk	TLC and cholesterol lowering drug to bring LDL below 100 mg/dL (2.6mmol/L) and other Therapeutic Options.

ATP-III Triglyceride levels classification

Triglyceride Level	Classification
Less than 150 mg/dl (1.68 mmo/L)	Normal
150 – 199 mg/dL (1.68 – 2.24 mmol/L)	Borderline High
200 – 499 mg/dL (2.26 – 5.64 mmol/L)	High
Over 500 mg/dL (5.65 mmol/L)	Very High

Risk factors constituted:

- Age: Males over 45, females over 55
- Family history of premature CHD (definite heart attack or sudden death before 55 in father or other male first-degree relative, or before 65 in mother or other female first-degree relative.
- Current cigarette smoking
- High blood pressure (over 140/90 or on blood pressure medication)
- Low HDL (less than 40 mg/dL (1.03 mmol/L)
    - o High HDL (over 60 mg/dL (1.5 mmol/L) was considered protective.

Public Health Message – maintain a desirable body weight, consume a healthy diet, exercise regularly, avoid smoking, and drink alcohol in moderation.

Therapeutic options include intensifying LDL-lowering dietary or drug therapies, emphasizing weight reduction and increased physical activity, adding drugs to lower triglycerides or raise HDL cholesterol (nicotinic acid or fibrates), and intensifying control of other risk factors.

TLC. Therapeutic Lifestyle Changes:

- TLC diet:
- Low saturated fat (less than 7% of calories, low cholesterol (less than 200 mg per day) diet.
- Increase in fibre and plant stanols/sterols.
- Weight management.
- Increased exercise.

CHD and CHD Equivalents:

- CHD disease
- Carotid artery disease
- Peripheral arterial disease
- Abdominal aortic aneurysm
- Diabetes

Framingham risk: Calculator used to estimate the ten-year cardiovascular risk of an individual.

ATP-III also recommended the following:

- People with multiple metabolic risk factors (metabolic syndrome) may be candidates for intensified therapeutic lifestyle changes. The aim of this is to lower LDL. Intensified therapeutic lifestyle changes include:
    - o Intensified weight management
    - o Increased physical activity
    - o Treatment for high blood pressure
    - o Prevention of blood clots
    - o Treat low HDL and elevated triglycerides
- Treatment of elevated triglycerides: The aim of this is to lower LDL. If triglycerides are still more than 200 mg/dL (2.26 mmol/L) after LDL goal is reached, then a secondary target is set for Non HDL cholesterol.
- Treatment of Non-HDL (Total cholesterol minus HDL). Targets are 30 mg/dL (0.77 mmol/L) more than LDL targets.

The changes in ATP-III compared to ATP-II are:

- Diabetes now classed the same as CHD
- Framingham ten-year heart disease calculator used
- Metabolic syndrome patients identified for treatment
- LDL of 100 mg/dL (2.6 mmol/L) now classed as optimal
- People with high triglycerides identified for treatment
- Encourages the use of dietary fibre and plant stanol/sterols to lower LDL

Studies

The recommendations from ATP-III were largely based on data from five major clinical statin trials.

The five trials were:

- WOSCOPS. West of Scotland Coronary Prevention Study (pravastatin v placebo).
- AFCAPS/TEXCAPS. Air Force/Texas Coronary Atherosclerosis Prevention Study (lovastatin v placebo).
- 4S. Scandinavian Simvastatin Survival Study (simvastatin v placebo).
- CARE. Cholesterol and Recurrent Events Trial (pravastatin v placebo).
- LIPID. Long-Term Intervention with Pravastatin in Ischaemic Disease Trial (pravastatin v placebo).

Percentage of people still alive at the end of the trials

Trial Name	Number in Trial	% of people alive at the end of the trial in treatment group	% of people alive at the end of the trial in control group
WOSCOPS	6,595	96.78	95.90
AFCAPS/ TEXCAPS	6,605	97.57	97.66
4S	4,444	89.96	85.80
CARE	4,159	91.35	90.56
LIPID	9,014	88.96	85.93

When the total number of people in each trial is taken into consideration, the data reveals that 1.76% more people were alive who were taking statins at the end of the trials than the people taking placebo. To sum up: Trials with statin drugs, with their carefully chosen participants, (and with all their side effects), made virtually no difference to death rates.

The personnel of the ATP-III panel

Below is a table of the panel members and their relationships with pharmaceutical companies that sell cholesterol lowering drugs (mainly statins). These relationships may have developed before, during or after the publication of ATP-III.

ATP-III panel member name and relationships with pharmaceutical companies that sell cholesterol lowering drugs

Scott Grundy	Has given lectures to health professionals on cholesterol management in which cholesterol-lowering drugs are discussed and for which he received honoraria that were funded by the following companies: Merck, Pfizer, Sankyo, Schering Plough, Kos, Abbot, Bristol-Myers Squibb and AstraZeneca. Also, Grundy has consultant agreements to serve on scientific advisory boards of Pfizer, Sanofi, and AstraZeneca
Diane Becker	Unrestricted grants from Atherotech, Novartis Pharmaceuticals Corporation, and Pfizer Inc.
Luther Clark	Honoraria for educational presentations from Abbott, AstraZeneca, Bristol-Myers Squibb, Merck, and Pfizer; received grant/research support from Abbott, AstraZeneca, Bristol-Myers Squibb, Merck, and Pfizer
Richard Cooper	None
Margo Denke	Honoraria and travel expense reimbursement from Merck. She has also participated on the speakers bureau for Merck, Merck/Schering-Plough, and Schering-Plough.
Wm. James Howard	Research Grants/Contracts: Pfizer, AstraZeneca Honoraria: Pfizer, AstraZeneca, Merck, Schering-Plough, Abbott, Sankyo Consultantship: Merck, Schering-Plough Speakers Bureau: Pfizer, AstraZeneca, Merck, Schering-Plough, Abbott, Sankyo
Donald Hunninghake	Research Grants from AstraZeneca, Bristol Myers Squibb, KOS, Merck, Merck Schering Plough, Novartis, Pfizer, Schering Plough; Speaking Honorarium: AstraZeneca, KOS, Merck, Pfizer

Roger Illingworth	Grants and research support from AstraZeneca Pharmaceuticals LP. He has participated in the Speakers Bureau for Kos Pharmaceuticals Inc., Merck & Co, Inc., Pfizer, Inc., Schering-Plough Corporation and has acted as a consultant for AstraZeneca Pharmaceuticals LP, and Sankyo Pharma.
Russell Luepker	Chairs NHLBI advisory boards
Patrick McBride	Grants and/or research support from Pfizer, Merck, Parke-Davis, and AstraZeneca; has served as a consultant for Kos Pharmaceuticals, Abbott, and Merck; and has received honoraria from Abbott, Bristol-Myers Squibb, Novartis, Merck, Kos Pharmaceuticals, Parke-Davis, Pfizer, and DuPont
James McKenney	Speaker honorarium: AstraZeneca LP, Kos Pharmaceuticals, Merck & Co. and Pfizer, Inc. Research Grants: AstraZeneca LP, GlaxoSmithKline, Kos Pharmaceuticals, Merck & Co., Pfizer, Inc., Schering-Plough, and Takeda. Consultant Services: AstraZeneca LP, Kos Pharmaceuticals, Merck & Co., Pfizer, Inc., and Sankyo Pharma, Inc.
Richard Pasternak	Served as a consultant for and received honoraria from Merck, Pfizer, and Kos Pharmaceuticals, and has received grants from Merck and Pfizer.
Neil Stone	Financial relationship with Abbott, AstraZeneca, Merck, Pfizer, Sanofi-Aventis, and Schering-Plough, and has served as a consultant to Abbott, AstraZeneca, Merck, Pfizer, Reliant, Schering-Plough
Linda Van Horn	Research grant Roche Bioscience
Hollis Bryan Brewer	Received honoraria from AstraZeneca, Pfizer, Lipid Sciences, Merck, Merck/Schering-Plough, Fournier, Tularik, Esperion, and Novartis; he has served as a consultant for AstraZeneca, Pfizer, Lipid Sciences, Merck, Merck/Schering-Plough, Fournier, Tularik, Sankyo, and Novartis.

James Cleeman	Has served for 25 years as founding Coordinator of the National Cholesterol Education Program at the NHLBI and spearheaded the US effort to lower cholesterol levels
Nancy Ernst	NHLBI employee
David Gordon	NHLBI employee
Daniel Levy	Participated in CME activity supported by an independent educational grant from Merck & Co., Inc.
Basil Rifkind	NHLBI employee
Jacques Rossouw	NHLBI employee
Peter Savage	NHLBI employee
Steven Haffner	GlaxoSmithKline, Novartis, Pfizer; speakers bureau membership – AstraZeneca, GlaxoSmithKline, Merck, Novartis, Pfizer; consultancy – AstraZeneca, GlaxoSmithKline, Merck, Novartis, Pfizer; honorarium recipient – AstraZeneca, GlaxoSmithKline, Merck, Novartis, Pfizer.
David Orloff	Serves as a consultant to Amylin, AstraZeneca Pharmaceuticals LP, Bristol-Myers Squibb, Glaxo-SmithKline, ISIS, Merck & Co., Inc., Novo Nordisk, Pfizer Inc, Roche, Takeda Pharmaceuticals, Vivus, and Wyeth; and owns stock in Abbott Laboratories Inc., Amgen, Genentech, Genzyme, Johnson & Johnson, Eli Lilly, Merck & Co., Inc., Pfizer Inc, and Wyeth
Michael Proschan	Involved in research where medications supplied by Pfizer Inc, AstraZeneca, and Bristol-Myers Squibb and financial support provided by Pfizer.
J. Sanford Schwartz	Has served as a consultant for and/or conducted research funded by Bristol-Myers Squibb, AstraZeneca, Merck, Johnson & Johnson-Merck, and Pfizer.

Christopher Sempos	NHLBI employee
Susan Shero	NHLBI employee
Elaine Z. Murray	Staff member
Susan A. Keller	Staff member

Out of the 30 members of the panel, 18 members have had or have financial relationships with pharmaceutical companies who market cholesterol lowering drugs, eight members were employees at the NHLBI (who set up the ATP panel) and four had no obvious ties.

Impact of the recommendations

Dr Donald Fedder, a researcher from the University of Maryland, estimated the ATP-III guidelines would result in 36.2 Americans eligible to take cholesterol lowering medication. In 1993 around 12.7 million were on drugs to lower cholesterol.

Summary of ATP-III

The members of ATP-III recommended that wider use of cholesterol lowering drugs (statins) be initiated to further push down cholesterol levels. This advice was given using evidence from trials in which the participants had been carefully selected. Despite this, the results of the trials revealed virtually no difference in death rates. Over 85% of the panel members have at some time developed financial relationships with pharmaceutical companies who market cholesterol lowering drugs, or were employed by the organisation that set up the panel. The panel's recommendations resulted in a near three-fold increase in the use of cholesterol lowering drugs compared to ATP-II.

The next five studies played a major part in Adult Treatment Panel-III Update recommendations.

Paper 467:
Doctor puts results of statin study into perspective

Ravnskov U Statins as the new aspirin. Conclusions from the heart protection study were premature. *British Medical Journal* 2002 Mar 30;324(7340):789

This study, (The Heart Protection Study), investigated the effects of statins in patients who had heart disease or were at a high risk of heart disease. The study lasted five years and included 20,536 UK adults (aged 40-80 years) with coronary disease, other occlusive arterial disease, or diabetes who were randomly allocated to receive 40 mg simvastatin daily or placebo.

- 32,145 patients were originally chosen for the trial. Before the study started the patients entered a six-week 'run-in' phase to see if they could tolerate the simvastatin treatment. Over 36% of the patients dropped out in this 'run-in' phase.
- The results of the study revealed that 163 patients needed to be given statins every year to prevent one major coronary event. Put another way, for every 163 patients given simvastatin every year, 162 received no cardiovascular benefit from the drug.

Dr Uffe Ravnskov analysed the figures from the trial and noted the study showed that after five years of taking a statin a patient would have a 87.1% chance of been alive, whereas without taking statins the patient would have a 85.4% chance of been alive.

He commented: "*The way the results were presented exaggerates the benefit for the individual patient. The most interesting figure is survival because most myocardial infarctions heal with minimal cardiac dysfunction, if any. Tell a patient that his chance not to die in five years without statin treatment is 85.4% and that simvastatin treatment can increase this to 87.1 %. With these figures in hand I doubt that anyone should accept a treatment whose long-term effects are unknown*".

Dr Ravnskov outlined a few of the risks: "*For example, it was claimed that the study presented uniquely reliable evidence that simvastatin is not carcinogenic. But the study went on for about five years only, just like other statin trials. It is not possible to say anything about the risk of cancer because it takes decades to disclose chemical carcinogenesis in human beings. Heavy smoking, for example, does not induce lung cancer in five years. Low cholesterol concentrations have been related to depression, cognitive impairment, and suppression of the immune system*".

Paper 468: Statins offer no benefit to the elderly

Shepherd J et al Pravastatin in elderly individuals at risk of vascular disease (PROSPER): a randomised controlled trial. *Lancet* 2002 Nov 23;360(9346):1623-30

The aim of the trial was to ascertain the effects of pravastatin treatment in elderly men and women aged 70-82. The study involved 2,804 men and 3,000 women (total 5,804) with a history of, or risk factors for, vascular disease. They were assigned into groups of either a statin (pravastatin) or placebo and the study lasted for just over three years.

- 23,770 individuals were originally assessed for inclusion in the trial. 16,714 were rejected by the researchers for a number of reasons which included;
    - A history of stroke, transient ischemic attack and amputation because of vascular disease.
    - Any surgery requiring an overnight hospital stay.
    - Poor cognitive function.
    - History of cancer.
    - Heart failure, pacemaker, atrial fibrillation or other arrhythmia or Wolfe-Parkinson syndrome.
    - Organ transplant.
    - Alcohol or drug abuse.
    - Inability to tolerate medication.
    - Abnormal laboratory findings.
- Before the study started the 7,056 chosen patients entered a four-week 'run-in' phase to see if they could tolerate the pravastatin treatment. Nearly 18% of the patients dropped out in this 'run-in' phase.
- The study was supported by an investigator initiated grant from Bristol-Myers Squibb (the manufacturer of pravastatin).
- Many of the authors of the study had financial ties with Bristol-Myers Squibb and other pharmaceutical companies involved in the cholesterol lowering industry. The following statement was included in the study paper:
    - Conflict of interest statement: The authors declare the following arrangements with the sponsoring company or other companies, or both, making competing products.

> Consultancy agreements: J Shepherd, M B Murphy, I Ford, B M Buckley, S M Cobbe, J W Jukema, C J Packard. Research support, honoraria, travel grants: J Shepherd, G J Blauw, M B Murphy, E L E M Bollen, B M Buckley, S M Cobbe, I Ford, A Gaw, M Hyland, J W Jukema, P W Macfarlane, A E Meinders, J Norrie, C J Packard, D J Stott, R G J Westendorp.

The results of the study revealed:

- Heart disease was higher in the placebo group.
- Stroke and cancer risk was higher in the pravastatin group.
- Total death rates were virtually identical in both groups.

To conclude: The study was not representative of a real world setting. Over 75% of possible patients for inclusion in the study were not included for various reasons. The study was paid for by Bristol-Myers Squibb (the manufacturer of pravastatin). Many of the study authors have received payments from Bristol-Myers Squibb and other statin manufacturers.

Despite the skewed study design in favour of pravastatin, the lead author of the study, Dr James Shepherd, had to admit: "*There was no observed difference in all-cause mortality*".

Paper 469:
Statin treatment may increase the risk of death from cancer

ALLHAT Officers and Coordinators for the ALLHAT Collaborative Research Group. Major outcomes in moderately hypercholesterolemic, hypertensive patients randomized to pravastatin vs. usual care: The Antihypertensive and Lipid-Lowering Treatment to Prevent Heart Attack Trial (ALLHAT-LLT). *Journal of the American Medical Association* 2002 Dec 18;288(23):2998-3007

This study, which lasted for six years, was designed to determine whether pravastatin compared with patients usual medical care, reduces death rates in patients aged 55 or older who have high cholesterol and blood pressure and other heart disease risk factors. 10,355 participants were enrolled in the study and were assigned into two groups where they received either 40 mg of pravastatin a day or their usual medical care.

The researchers found at the end of the six-year study:

- Total death rates were virtually identical in both groups.
- Heart disease death rates were virtually identical in both groups.
- Those who took statins had an increased risk of death from cancer and suicide/homicide/accidental death compared to those who did not take statins.
- 23% of those in the pravastatin group had stopped taking it.

The results of this study show that statin treatment is not tolerated by a large percentage of patients and also suggest that it may increase the risk of death from cancer.

Paper 470:
Doctor questions the benefits of atorvastatin

Devroey D et al ASCOT-LLA: questions about the benefits of atorvastatin. *Lancet* 2003 Jun 7;361(9373):1985-6

This paper, headed by Dr Dirk Devroey from the University of Brussels, analysed the Anglo-Scandinavian Cardiac Outcomes Trial—Lipid Lowering Arm (ASCOT-LLA) conducted by Peter Sever and colleagues. The ASCOT-LLA study investigated the effects of atorvastatin for the prevention of coronary heart disease in high risk patients with high blood pressure but without previous heart disease and with cholesterol levels less than 6.5 mmol/L (251 mg/dL). The study included 10,305 patients who were randomly assigned to receive atorvastatin 10 mg per day or placebo. The study was due to last for five years but was terminated after 3.3 years.

Dr Devroey found:

- The benefit of atorvastatin was not significant in patients with diabetes, left-ventricular hypertrophy, and previous vascular disease.
- Women in the placebo group had less incidence of major coronary events than women in the atorvastatin group.
- The results among women accord with the findings of the Antihypertensive and Lipid-Lowering Treatment to Prevent Heart Attack Trial (ALLHAT-LLT), in which pravastatin did not reduce all-cause mortality, myocardial infarction, or fatal coronary heart disease.

- The finding that atorvastatin had no effect on total mortality accords with the results of previous primary prevention studies.
- Why was ASCOT-LLA stopped prematurely after 3.3 years when no significant reduction in mortality could be shown? During the first three years of the study, there was no decreasing trend in mortality.
- In addition, there was even a non-significant trend towards a disadvantage with atorvastatin for fatal and non-fatal heart failure, peripheral arterial disease, and development of diabetes mellitus or renal impairment.

Dr Devroey commented *"We dispute the conclusions of Peter Sever and colleagues about the beneficial effects of atorvastatin as presented in the Anglo-Scandinavian Cardiac Outcomes Trial—Lipid Lowering Arm (ASCOT-LLA)"*.

Devroey concluded: *"Atorvastatin offers no additional benefit above antihypertensive treatment for the reduction of fatal and non-fatal cardiovascular events in women, patients with diabetes, and those with left-ventricular hypertrophy or previous vascular disease-and all this without affecting mortality"*.

As noted above, the authors of the ASCOT-LLA trial, Peter Sever and colleagues, reported beneficial findings for atorvastatin.

Interestingly there were 14 authors of the ASCOT-LLA trial and all of them served as consultants to and received travel expenses, payment for speaking at meetings, or funding for research from pharmaceutical companies marketing lipid-lowering drugs, including Merck Sharp and Dohme, Bristol-Myers Squibb, Astra-Zeneca, Sanofi, Schering, Servier, Pharmacia, Bayer, Novartis, Aventis Pfizer. The 14 authors; (Peter S Sever, Björn Dahlöf, Neil R Poulter, Hans Wedel, Gareth Beevers, Mark Caulfield, Rory Collins, Sverre E Kjeldsen, Arni Kristinsson, Gordon T McInnes, Jesper Mehlsen, Markku Nieminen, Eoin O'Brien and Jan Östergren) also received financial support from Pfizer (who manufacture atorvastatin) to cover administrative and staffing costs of ASCOT, and travel, accommodation expenses or both incurred by attending relevant meetings.

Would Peter Sever and colleagues report beneficial findings for statins if they weren't so intimately involved with the pharmaceutical companies that market statin drugs?

Paper 471: Patients in statin studies are carefully selected and monitored

Murphy SA et al Effect of intensive lipid-lowering therapy on mortality after acute coronary syndrome (a patient-level analysis of the Aggrastat to Zocor and Pravastatin or Atorvastatin Evaluation and Infection Therapy-Thrombolysis in Myocardial Infarction 22 trials). *American Journal of Cardiology* 2007 Oct 1;100(7):1047-51

This study discusses two randomised, double-blind trials, which compared the effects of moderate cholesterol lowering with standard-dose statin therapy with intensive cholesterol lowering with high-dose statin therapy in patients who had suffered an acute coronary syndrome.

The two trials were the Pravastatin or Atorvastatin Evaluation and Infection Therapy-Thrombolysis In Myocardial Infarction 22 (PROVE-IT-TIMI 22) trial and the Aggrastat to Zocor (A to Z) trial.

The PROVE-IT-TIMI 22 trial compared 40 mg of pravastatin daily (moderate statin therapy) with 80 mg of atorvastatin daily (intensive statin therapy).

In the A to Z trial patients received either placebo for four months followed by 20 mg per day of simvastatin thereafter (moderate statin therapy) or 40 mg per day of simvastatin for one month followed by 80 mg per day thereafter (intensive statin therapy).

This study was a pooled analysis of the two trials. The combined studies included 8,658 post-acute coronary syndrome patients who were followed for up to three years.

Adverse effects in the PROVE-IT-TIMI 22 trial:

- The rates of discontinuation of treatment because of an adverse event were very high in the trial. 30.4% in the intensive statin therapy atorvastatin group and 33% in the moderate statin therapy pravastatin group had discontinued at two years.
- The intensive statin therapy atorvastatin group had a 22% increased risk of having to discontinue taking the statin because of myalgias or muscle aches or elevations in creatine

kinase levels compared to the moderate statin therapy pravastatin group.

- The intensive statin therapy atorvastatin group had a 200% increased risk of elevations in alanine aminotransferase levels that were more than three times the upper limit of normal compared to the moderate statin therapy pravastatin group.
- The intensive statin therapy atorvastatin group had significantly more liver-related side effects compared to the moderate statin therapy pravastatin group.

Adverse effects in the A to Z trial:

- The rates of discontinuation of treatment because of an adverse event were also very high in this trial. 34% in the intensive statin therapy atorvastatin group and 32% in the moderate statin therapy pravastatin group discontinued prematurely.
- The intensive statin therapy atorvastatin group had a 19% increased risk of having to discontinue taking the statin because of muscle related adverse events compared to the moderate statin therapy pravastatin group.
- The intensive statin therapy atorvastatin group had a 130% increased risk of elevations in alanine aminotransferase and aspartate aminotransferase levels that were more than three times the upper limit of normal compared to the moderate statin therapy pravastatin group.
- The intensive statin therapy atorvastatin group had a 787% increased risk of muscle disease compared to the moderate statin therapy pravastatin group.
- Three patients developed rhabdomyolysis in the intensive statin therapy atorvastatin group.

Dr Christopher Cannon, who was lead investigator in the PROVE-IT-TIMI 22 trial commented: *"It is important to note that our safety and efficacy results were obtained in a carefully selected and monitored study population... Patients in clinical practice generally have more coexisting conditions than did our patients, and they may not tolerate a high-dose statin regimen... Thus, clinicians must take these factors into account when applying the results of our trial in clinical practice".*

Paper 472: Adult treatment Panel-III Update (ATP-III Update) 2004

Recommendations

ATP-III Update recommended the following:

ATP-III Update did not classify cholesterol or LDL levels. So the presumption may be that the classification was the same as ATP-III. ATP-III Update also recommended no change for people without CHD or Risk Equivalents and fewer than 2 risk factors.

ATP-III Update LDL cholesterol levels recommendations

LDL Cholesterol Level	Recommendation
Less than 130 mg/dL (3.4 mmol/L) without CHD or Risk Equivalents and with 2 or more risk factors and 10-20% Framingham risk	TLC and control other risk factors. Public Health Message on Healthy Life Habits. Re-evaluation in 1 Year. Optional cholesterol lowering drug to bring LDL below 100mg/dL (2.6 mmol/L). At least 30-40% reduction in LDL levels should be achieved.
More than 130 mg/dL (3.4 mmol/L) without CHD or Risk Equivalents and with 2 or more risk factors and 10-20% Framingham risk	TLC and cholesterol lowering drug to bring LDL below 130 mg/dL (3.4 mmol/L). Optional target of less than 100mg/dL (2.6 mmol/L) with cholesterol lowering drug. At least 30-40% reduction in LDL levels should be achieved.
Less than 100mg/dL (2.6 mmol/L) with CHD or Risk Equivalents or more than 20% Framingham risk	TLC and control other risk factors. Optional target of less than 70mg/dL (1.8 mmol/L) with cholesterol lowering drug. At least 30-40% reduction in LDL levels should be achieved.

LDL Cholesterol Level	Recommendation
100 – 129 mg/dL (2.6 – 3.4 mmol/L) with CHD or Risk Equivalents or more than 20% Framingham risk	TLC and optional cholesterol lowering drug to bring LDL below 100 mg/dL (2.6mmol/L). Optional target of less than 70mg/dL (1.8 mmol/L) with cholesterol lowering drug. At least 30-40% reduction in LDL levels should be achieved.
More than 130 mg/dL (3.4 mmol/L) with CHD or Risk Equivalents or more than 20% Framingham risk	TLC and cholesterol lowering drug to bring LDL below 100 mg/dL (2.6mmol/L) and other Therapeutic Options. Optional target of less than 70mg/dL (1.8 mmol/L) with cholesterol lowering drug. At least 30-40% reduction in LDL levels should be achieved.

Risk factors constituted:

- Age: Males over 45, females over 55
- Family history of premature CHD (definite heart attack or sudden death before 55 in father or other male first-degree relative, or before 65 in mother or other female first-degree relative.
- Current cigarette smoking
- High blood pressure (over 140/90 or on blood pressure medication)
- Low HDL (less than 40 mg/dL (1.03 mmol/L)

CHD includes:

- History of heart attack
- Unstable angina
- Stable angina
- Coronary artery procedures (angioplasty or bypass surgery)
- Evidence of clinically significant blockage of the coronary arteries.

CHD risk equivalents include:

- Peripheral arterial disease
- Abdominal aortic aneurysm

- Carotid artery disease
- Diabetes
- Two or more risk factors with ten-year Framingham risk for CHD more than 20%.

The changes in ATP-III Update compared to ATP-III are:

- In persons with CHD or Risk Equivalents, or more than 20% Framingham risk (high risk), an LDL goal of less than 70 mg/dL is an option.
- For persons without CHD or Risk Equivalents but with two or more risk factors and 10-20% Framingham risk (moderately high risk), an LDL goal of 100mg/dL (2.6 mmol/L) is an option.
- LDL levels should be reduced by at least 30-40%.
- All persons at high risk or moderately high risk who have lifestyle-related risk factors (e.g. obesity, physical inactivity, elevated triglycerides, low HDL, or metabolic syndrome) are candidates for TLC to modify these risk factors regardless of LDL level.

Studies

The recommendations from ATP-III Update were based on data from the following major clinical statin trials.

The trials were:

- HPS. Heart Protection Study (simvastatin v placebo).
- PROSPER. PROspective Study of Pravastatin in the Elderly at Risk (pravastatin v placebo).
- ALLHAT-LLT. Antihypertensive and Lipid-Lowering Treatment to Prevent Heart Attack Trial (pravastatin v usual care).
- ASCOT-LLA. Anglo-Scandinavian Cardiac Outcomes Trial—Lipid Lowering Arm (atorvastatin v placebo).
- PROVE-IT and A to Z. The Pravastatin or Atorvastatin Evaluation and Infection Therapy trial and Aggrastat to Zocor trial (Intensive statin therapy v moderate statin therapy).

Percentage of people still alive at the end of the trials

Trial Name	Number in Trial	% of people alive at the end of the trial in treatment group	% of people alive at the end of the trial in control group
HPS	20,536	87.10	85.40
PROSPER	5,804	89.69	89.49
ALLHAT-LLT	10,355	85.10	84.70
ASCOT	10,305	96.42	95.87
PROVE-IT & A to Z	8,658	96.37	95.31

When the total number of people in each trial is taken into consideration, the data reveals that 1.75% more people were alive who were taking statins at the end of the trials than the people taking placebo. To sum up: Trials with statin drugs, with their carefully chosen participants, (and with all their side effects), made virtually no difference to death rates.

The personnel of the ATP-III Update panel

Below is a table of the panel members and their relationships with pharmaceutical companies that sell cholesterol lowering drugs (mainly statins). These relationships may have developed before, during or after the publication of ATP-III Update.

ATP-III Update panel member name and relationships with pharmaceutical companies that sell cholesterol lowering drugs

Scott Grundy	Has given lectures to health professionals on cholesterol management in which cholesterol-lowering drugs are discussed and for which he received honoraria that were funded by the following companies: Merck, Pfizer, Sankyo, Schering Plough, Kos, Abbot, Bristol-Myers Squibb and AstraZeneca. Also, Grundy has consultant agreements to serve on scientific advisory boards of Pfizer, Sanofi, and AstraZeneca

James Cleeman	Has served for 25 years as founding Coordinator of the National Cholesterol Education Program at the NHLBI and spearheaded the US effort to lower cholesterol levels
Noel Bairey Merz	Received lecture honoraria from Pfizer, Merck, and Kos; she has served as a consultant for Pfizer, Bayer, and EHC (Merck); she has received unrestricted institutional grants for Continuing Medical Education from Pfizer, Procter & Gamble, Novartis, Wyeth, AstraZeneca, and Bristol-Myers Squibb Medical Imaging; she has received a research grant from Merck; she has stock in Boston Scientific, IVAX, Eli Lilly, Medtronic, Johnson & Johnson, SCIPIE Insurance, ATS Medical, and Biosite.
Hollis Bryan Brewer	Received honoraria from AstraZeneca, Pfizer, Lipid Sciences, Merck, Merck/Schering-Plough, Fournier, Tularik, Esperion, and Novartis; he has served as a consultant for AstraZeneca, Pfizer, Lipid Sciences, Merck, Merck/Schering-Plough, Fournier, Tularik, Sankyo, and Novartis.
Luther Clark	Honoraria for educational presentations from Abbott, AstraZeneca, Bristol-Myers Squibb, Merck, and Pfizer; received grant/research support from Abbott, AstraZeneca, Bristol-Myers Squibb, Merck, and Pfizer
Donald Hunninghake	Research Grants from AstraZeneca, Bristol Myers Squibb, KOS, Merck, Merck Schering Plough, Novartis, Pfizer, Schering Plough; Speaking Honorarium: AstraZeneca, KOS, Merck, Pfizer
Richard Pasternak	Served as a consultant for and received honoraria from Merck, Pfizer, and Kos Pharmaceuticals, and has received grants from Merck and Pfizer.

Sidney Smith	Received institutional research support from Merck; he has stock in Medtronic and Johnson & Johnson. Consultant for or on the speakers' bureaus of Bayer Corp., Eli Lilly and Co., GlaxoSmithKline Pharmaceuticals, Pfizer Labs, and Sanofi-Aventis; and has served as a member of the Data Safety Monitoring Board of AstraZeneca Pharmaceuticals.
Neil Stone	Financial relationship with Abbott, AstraZeneca, Merck, Pfizer, Sanofi-Aventis, and Schering-Plough, and has served as a consultant to Abbott, AstraZeneca, Merck, Pfizer, Reliant, Schering-Plough

Out of the nine members of the panel, eight members have had or have financial relationships with pharmaceutical companies who market cholesterol lowering drugs and one member was an employee at the NHLBI (who set up the ATP panel).

Impact of the recommendations

Regarding the ATP-III update recommendations, Dr John Abramson from Harvard Medical school commented: "*Based on these new thresholds, millions more Americans now fall within the eligibility criteria for statin therapy*".

Summary of ATP-III Update

The members of ATP-III Update recommended that wider use of statins be initiated to further push down cholesterol levels. This advice was given using evidence from trials in which the participants had been carefully selected. Despite this, the results of the trials revealed virtually no difference in death rates. All of the panel members have at some time developed financial relationships with pharmaceutical companies who market cholesterol lowering drugs, or were employed by the organisation that set up the panel. The ATP-III Update panel's recommendations resulted in millions more people taking statin drugs compared to ATP-III.

Paper 473:
Petition to the National Institutes of Health seeking an independent review panel to re-evaluate the National Cholesterol Education Program Guidelines

On September 23, 2004 a petition voicing concerns regarding the ATP-III Update was sent to the following people:

- Dr Elias Zerhouni, Director, National Institutes of Health
- Dr Barbara Alving, Acting Director, National Heart, Lung and Blood Institute
- Dr James Cleeman, Director, National Cholesterol Education Program

The petition was signed by 35 prestigious scientists, most of whom have affiliations with major universities.

The signees were:

- o Dr John Abramson, MD Clinical Instructor, Primary Care, Harvard Medical School
- o Professor R. James Barnard, PhD Professor Dept of Physiological Science, UCLA
- o Dr Henry C. Barry, MD, MS Department of Family Practice, Michigan State University
- o Dr Stephen Bezruchka MD, MPH Senior Lecturer, International Health Program, Department of Health Services
- o Assistant Professor Christopher Gardner, PhD Assistant Professor of Medicine, Stanford University
- o Dr Lee Green, MD, MPH Department of Family Medicine, University of Michigan
- o Barry Groves, PhD Independent researcher, Oxford, UK
- o Dr Jerome R Hoffman, MA, MD Prof. of Medicine / Emergency Medicine, UCLA School of Medicine
- o Michael Jacobson, PhD Executive Director
- o Marion Nestle, PhD Paulette Goddard Prof. of Nutrition, Food Studies, & Public Health, New York University
- o Beverly Rockhill, PhD Department of Epidemiology, University of North Carolina
- o Dr Paul J. Rosch, MD, FACP President American Institute of Stress, Clinical Prof. of Medicine & Psychiatry, New York Medical College School of Public Health & Comm. Med., University of Washington
- o Dr Howard Brody, MD, PhD University Distinguished Prof., Michigan State University
- o Dr David L. Brown, MD Prof. of Medicine & Epidemiology, Albert Einstein College of Medicine, Director Interventional Cardiology Beth Israel Medical Centre

- Professor T. Colin Campbell, PhD Jacob Gould Schurman Prof. Emeritus, Nutritional Biochemistry, Cornell University
- Dr Joshua Chodosh, MD, MSHS VA Greater L.A. Health System, Dept. of Research & Development
- Dr Mark H. Ebell MD, MS Deputy Editor American Family Physician, Associate Professor Michigan State University, Athens Primary Care, Athens, GA
- Edward L. Fieg, DO Chief Emergency Services, 74th Medical Group, SGOPE Wright-Patterson USAF Medical Centre
- Dr Linda French, MD Associate Professor, Associate Chair for Clinical Services, Department of Family Practice, College of Human Medicine, Michigan State University, Ctr. for Science in the Public Interest
- Professor Joel M. Kauffman, PhD Professor of Chemistry Emeritus, Dept. of Chemistry & Biochemistry, Univ. of the Sciences in Philadelphia
- Dr Malcolm Kendrick, MbChB, MRCGP Primary Care Physician Bollington Health Centre Cheshire, UK
- Dr Mitzi Krockover, MD Senior Partner Sokolov, Sokolov, Burgess (former director, Iris-Cantor UCLA Women's Health Centre)
- Dr Philip R Lee, MD Consulting Professor Program in Human Biology, Stanford University, Prof. of Social Medicine (Emeritus), School of Medicine, UCSF
- Dr Joel Lexchin MD Associate Professor School of Health Policy and Mgmt., York University
- Dr Susan Love, MD, MBA Dr Susan Love Research Foundation
- Dr Jeffrey Mann, MD Emergency Physician
- Dr Kilmer McCully, MD Chief Pathology & Laboratory Medicine, VA Medical Centre Boston
- Dr Tanja Rundek, MD, PhD Assistant Prof. of Neurology, Department of Neurology, Columbia University, Div. of Stroke and Critical Care
- Dr Kendra Schwartz, MD, MSPH Director of Practice-based Research, Dept. of Family Medicine, Wayne State University
- Dr Morley C. Sutter, MD, PhD Emeritus Professor Univ. of British Columbia
- Dr Susan Troyan, MD Beth Israel Deaconess Med. Ctr., Harvard Medical School

- o Dr Barbara Starfield, MD, MPH Univ. Distinguished Professor, Johns Hopkins University & Medical Institutions
- o Dr Michael Wilkes, MD, PhD,Vice Dean for Education, Professor of Medicine School of Medicine, Univ. of California, Davis
- o Dr James M. Wright, MD, PhD Professor Dept. of Pharmacology & Therapeutics and Medicine, Univ. of British Columbia
- o Associate Professor Margo N. Woods, DSc Associate Prof. of Medicine, Dept. of Family Medicine and Community Health, Tufts University School of Medicine

The main points of the petition were:

- The initial report published in Circulation failed to disclose that eight of its nine authors have financial relationships with drug companies. Such conflicts certainly could affect authors' judgment and undermine public confidence in the report.
- The evidence does not show that statins should be used by women who are at moderately high risk of CVD.
  - o The 2001 guidelines cited six references as evidence that statins reduce the risk of heart disease in moderately high risk women under the age of 65. Not one of the six studies, however, provides significant evidence to support this claim.
  - o Among the five new studies, only ASCOT specifically addresses the benefit of statin therapy in women with multiple risk factors and no history of heart disease. In this study, the women treated with atorvastatin developed 10% more heart disease than the women in the control group.
  - o Therefore, there is still no significant evidence from the "gold standard" of medical research, large randomized clinical trials, showing that women who do not already have heart disease benefit from taking a statin drug.
- The evidence does not show that statins should be used by older persons who are at risk of CVD.
  - o For people above the age of 65 without heart disease, the 2001 guidelines cited nine references to support the claim that stain therapy effectively reduces their risk

of developing heart disease. Again, not one of the nine studies provided significant evidence that statins protect senior citizens without heart disease.

- o Among the latest five studies, only PROSPER looked specifically at this issue. It included more than 3,000 people between the ages of 70 and 82 at elevated risk of, but without, heart disease. The latest NCEP report states that the results of the PROSPER study "support the efficacy of statin therapy in older, high-risk persons without established CVD." In fact, the evidence shows just the opposite. Those treated with a statin did not experience significantly fewer heart attacks and strokes. But they did develop 25% more new cancers than the people in the control group.

- The evidence in the five latest clinical trials for using statins in patients with diabetes is mixed.
  - o Three studies found that statins did not provide significant benefit to people with diabetes.
  - o The new recommendations cite that the HPS's finding that statins reduce the risk of heart disease. However, taking the HPS findings at face value, only one death was prevented each year that 250 diabetic patients were treated with a statin.
- The ALLHAT study did not show a benefit from more than tripling the number of people taking statins.
  - o In ALLHAT, patients at increased risk of heart disease were randomized to receive statin therapy or to be treated by their regular doctor. The results show that tripling the number of people taking statins provides no additional benefit—not to those older or younger, male or female, with or without diabetes, with or without heart disease, and among those without heart disease, not to those with LDL-cholesterol higher or lower than 130 mg/dL (3.4 mmol/L).
  - o The ALLHAT study suggests that treating an additional 25-30 million Americans with statins as suggested by the 2001 and latest NCEP recommendations will provide little, if any, benefit.

- While the latest NCEP report, like the 2001 guidelines before it, notes that lifestyle modification should be a first line of therapy to prevent heart disease, the sad fact is that these recommendations are being largely ignored, partly because the "experts", many of whom have conflicts of interest through their relationships with statin manufacturers, focus ever more attention on lowering cholesterol with expensive drugs. The vast majority of heart disease can be prevented by adopting healthy habits.

The National Cholesterol Education Program group rejected the petition.

Paper 474:
ACC/AHA 2013 panel

The 2013 ACC/AHA panel were originally called the Adult Treatment Panel-IV (ATP-IV) appointed by the NHLBI. ATP-IV had 16 members. All 16 members of the ATP IV Panel transitioned to the ACC/AHA Panel. (ACC – American College of Cardiology and AHA – American Heart Association.)

Recommendations
ACC/AHA 2013 recommended the following:

ACC/AHA 2013 Health status and recommendations

Health status	Recommendation
With no ASCVD, no diabetes, age 40-75, and LDL 70-189 mg/dL (1.8 – 4.9 mmol/L) and less than 5% Pooled Cohort Equations Calculator 10 year ASCVD risk	No statins unless: LDL more than 160 mg/dL or other evidence of genetic high cholesterol. Family history of premature ASCVD. High levels of C-reactive protein. High Coronary Artery Calcium score. Ankle-brachial index less than 0.9. Elevated lifetime risk of ASCVD.

Health status	Recommendation
With no ASCVD, age less than 40 or more than 75 and LDL less than 190 mg/dL (4.9 mmol/L)	No statins unless: LDL more than 160 mg/dL or other evidence of genetic high cholesterol. Family history of premature ASCVD. High levels of C-reactive protein. High Coronary Artery Calcium score. Ankle-brachial index less than 0.9. Elevated lifetime risk of ASCVD.
With no ASCVD, no diabetes, age 40-75, LDL less than 190 mg/dL (4.9 mmol/L) and 5-7.5% Pooled Cohort Equations Calculator 10 year ASCVD risk	Moderate intensity statins
With no ASCVD, no diabetes, age 40-75, LDL less than 190 mg/dL (4.9 mmol/L) and more than 7.5% Pooled Cohort Equations Calculator 10 year ASCVD risk	Moderate or high intensity statins
With diabetes, with no ASCVD, age less than 40 or more than 75 and LDL less than 190 mg/dL (4.9 mmol/L)	Statin therapy should be individualized based on considerations of ASCVD risk reduction benefits, the potential for adverse effects and drug-drug interactions, and patient preferences
With no ASCVD, but with diabetes, age 40-75, and less than 7.5% Pooled Cohort Equations Calculator 10 year ASCVD risk	Moderate intensity statins
With no ASCVD, but with diabetes, age 40-75, and more than 7.5% Pooled Cohort Equations Calculator 10 year ASCVD risk	High intensity statins

Health status	Recommendation
With no ASCVD, age 40-75, but with LDL more than 190 mg/dL (4.9 mmol/L)	High intensity statins
With ASCVD, age over 21, (except women planning a family)	Moderate or high intensity statins

Notes:

- The Pooled Cohort Equations CV ten-year calculator has replaced the Framingham Risk ten-year CVD calculation.
- Atherosclerotic cardiovascular disease (ASCVD) includes coronary heart disease (CHD), stroke, and peripheral arterial disease.
- Family history of premature ASCVD with onset less than 55 years of age in a first degree male relative or less than 65 years of age in a first degree female relative.
- C-reactive protein (CRP) is produced by the liver. High levels of CRP indicate inflammation throughout the body.
- Coronary Artery Calcium score. A higher Coronary Artery Calcium score indicates a higher risk of a cardiac event.
- The Ankle-brachial index result can help diagnose peripheral arterial disease. A lower score may help diagnose peripheral arterial disease.
- Elevated lifetime risk of ASCVD. No details of an elevated lifetime risk of ASCVD were given in the document. The guidance was for doctors to take it into consideration.
- Moderate intensity statins – Daily dose lowers LDL by approximately 30% to 50%.
- High intensity statins – Daily dose lowers LDL by approximately more than 50%.

The main changes in ACC/AHA 2013 included:

- Use of fixed doses of statins rather than LDL targets for the treatment of ASCVD.
- Virtual universal use of statin drugs. Non statin drugs were generally not recommended.
- Use of the Pooled Cohort Equations CV ten-year risk calculator.

Studies

The statin recommendations were based almost exclusively on randomised controlled trials involving statin drugs.

The trials were:

- TNT: Treating to New Targets trial (high dose atorvastatin v moderate dose atorvastatin).
- IDEAL: Incremental Decrease in Endpoints Through Aggressive Lipid lowering trial (high dose atorvastatin v moderate dose simvastatin).
- PROVE-IT and A to Z. The Pravastatin or Atorvastatin Evaluation and Infection Therapy trial and Aggrastat to Zocor trial (Intensive statin therapy v moderate statin therapy).
- ACCORD. Action to Control Cardiovascular Risk in Diabetes trial (simvastatin plus fenofibrate or simvastatin plus placebo).
- SEARCH. Study of the Effectiveness of Additional Reductions in Cholesterol and Homocysteine trial (high dose simvastatin v moderate dose simvastatin).
- SPARCL. Stroke Prevention by Aggressive Reduction in Cholesterol Levels trial (atorvastatin v placebo).
- HATS. HDL-Atherosclerosis Treatment Study (simvastatin plus niacin v placebo)
- MIRACL. Myocardial Ischemia Reduction with Acute Cholesterol Lowering trial (atorvastatin v placebo).
- CORONA. Controlled Rosuvastatin Multinational Trial in Heart Failure trial (rosuvastatin v placebo).
- WOSCOPS. West of Scotland Coronary Prevention Study (pravastatin v placebo).
- 4S. Scandinavian Simvastatin Survival Study (simvastatin v placebo).
- CARE. Cholesterol and Recurrent Events Trial (pravastatin v placebo).
- AFCAPS/TEXCAPS. Air Force/Texas Coronary Atherosclerosis Prevention Study (lovastatin v placebo).
- LIPID. Long-Term Intervention with Pravastatin in Ischaemic Disease Trial (pravastatin v placebo).
- GISSI-P. Gruppo Italiano per lo Studio della Streptochinasi nell'Infarto Miocardico-Prevenzione trial (low cholesterol v high cholesterol).

- LIPS. Lescol Intervention Prevention Study (fluvastatin v placebo).
- HPS. Heart Protection Study (simvastatin v placebo).
- PROSPER. PROspective study of pravastatin in the elderly at risk (pravastatin v placebo).
- ALLHAT-LLT. Antihypertensive and Lipid-Lowering Treatment to Prevent Heart Attack Trial (pravastatin v usual care).
- ASCOT-LLA. Anglo-Scandinavian Cardiac Outcomes Trial—Lipid Lowering Arm (atorvastatin v placebo).
- ALERT. Assessment of LEscol in Renal Transplantation study (fluvastatin v placebo).
- CARDS. Collaborative Atorvastatin Diabetes Study (atorvastatin v placebo).
- ALLIANCE. Aggressive Lipid-Lowering Initiation Abates New Cardiac Events (atorvastatin v usual care).
- ASPEN. Atorvastatin Study for Prevention of Coronary Heart Disease Endpoints in Non-Insulin-Dependent Diabetes Mellitus (atorvastatin v placebo).
- MEGA. Management of Elevated Cholesterol in the Primary Prevention Group of Adult Japanese (pravastatin plus diet v diet).
- JUPITER. Justification for the Use of Statins in Primary Prevention: An Intervention Trial Evaluating Rosuvastatin trial (rosuvastatin v placebo).
- GISSI-HF. Gruppo Italiano per lo Studio della Streptochinasi nell'Infarto Miocardico-Heart Failure trial (rosuvastatin v placebo).
- AURORA. A Study to Evaluate the Use of Rosuvastatin in Subjects on Regular Hemodialysis: An Assessment of Survival and Cardiovascular Events study (rosuvastatin v placebo).
- 4D. Deutsche Diabetes Dialyse Studie (atorvastatin v placebo).
- GREACE. The GREek Atorvastatin and Coronary-heart-disease Evaluation study (atorvastatin v usual care).
- MUSASHI-AMI. MUlticenter Study for Aggressive Lipid Lowering Strategy by HMG-CoA Reductase Inhibitors in Patients with AMI (statins v no statins).
- SEAS. Simvastatin and Ezetimibe in Aortic Stenosis study (simvastatin and ezetimibe v placebo).
- SHARP. Study of Heart and Renal Protection (simvastatin and ezetimibe v placebo).

Percentage of people still alive at the end of the trials

Trial Name	Number in Trial	% of people alive at the end of the trial in treatment group	% of people alive at the end of the trial in control group
TNT	10,001	94.31	94.36
IDEAL	8,888	91.75	91.59
PROVE-IT & A to Z	8,658	96.37	95.31
ACCORD	5,518	92.65	91.97
SEARCH	12,064	84.01	83.92
SPARCL	4,731	90.86	91.08
HATS	80	97.61	97.36
MIRACL	3,086	95.83	95.60
CORONA	5,011	71.04	69.60
WOSCOPS	6,595	96.78	95.90
4S	4,444	89.96	85.80
CARE	4,159	91.35	90.56
AFCAPS/ TEXCAPS	6,605	97.57	97.66
LIPID	9,014	88.96	85.93
GISSI-P	4,253	86.32	92.21
LIPS	1,677	92.29	89.91
HPS	20,536	87.10	85.40
PROSPER	5,804	89.69	89.49
ALLHAT-LLT	10,355	85.10	84.70
ASCOT	10,305	96.42	95.87
ALERT	2,012	86.38	86.88

Trial Name	Number in Trial	% of people alive at the end of the trial in treatment group	% of people alive at the end of the trial in control group
CARDS	2,838	95.70	94.20
ALLIANCE	2,442	90.05	89.63
ASPEN	2,410	94.20	94.30
MEGA	7,832	98.57	98.00
JUPITER	17,802	97.77	97.22
GISSI-HF	4,574	71.24	71.86
AURORA	2,773	54.21	52.31
4D	1,255	52.01	49.68
GREACE	1,600	97.12	95.00
MUSASHI-AMI	486	99.17	99.59
SEAS	1,873	88.87	89.23
SHARP	9,270	94.98	95.07

When the total number of people in each trial is taken into consideration, the data reveals that 0.61% more people were alive who were taking statins at the end of the trials than the people taking placebo. To sum up: Trials with statin drugs, with their carefully chosen participants, (and with all their side effects), made no difference to death rates.

The personnel of ACC/AHA 2013 panel

Below is a table of the panel members and their relationships with pharmaceutical companies that sell cholesterol lowering drugs (mainly statins). These relationships may have developed before, during or after the publication of ACC/AHA 2013.

ACC/AHA 2013 panel member name and relationships with pharmaceutical companies that sell cholesterol lowering drugs

Neil Stone	Financial relationship with Abbott, AstraZeneca, Merck, Pfizer, Sanofi-Aventis, and Schering-Plough, and has served as a consultant to Abbott, AstraZeneca, Merck, Pfizer, Reliant, Schering-Plough
Jennifer Robinson	Research grants from Aegerion, Amarin, Amgen, AstraZeneca, Esperion, Genentech/Hoffman, LaRoche, GlaxoSmithKline, Merck, Sanofi-Aventis/Regeneron
Alice Lichtenstein	Research grant from Merck, Sharp & Dohme
Noel Bairey Merz	Received lecture honoraria from Pfizer, Merck, and Kos; she has served as a consultant for Pfizer, Bayer, and EHC (Merck); she has received unrestricted institutional grants for Continuing Medical Education from Pfizer, Procter & Gamble, Novartis, Wyeth, AstraZeneca, and Bristol-Myers Squibb Medical Imaging; she has received a research grant from Merck; she has stock in Boston Scientific, IVAX, Eli Lilly, Medtronic, Johnson & Johnson, SCIPIE Insurance, ATS Medical, and Biosite.
Conrad Blum	None
Robert Eckel	Consultant for Merck, Pfizer, Abbott, Amylin, Eli Lilly, Esperion, Foodminds, Johnson & Johnson, Novo Nordisk, Vivus. Research grants from GlaxoSmithKline and Sanofi-aventis/ Regeneron
Anne Goldberg	Consultant for Abbott, Roche, ISIS/Genzyme, Sanofi-Aventis, Unilever, Merck. Research grants from Abbott, Aegerion, Amarin, Amgen, Genentech/Roche, GlaxoSmithKline, ISIS/ Genzyme, Merck, Novartis, Reliant, Sanofi-Aventis/Regeneron, Sanofi-Aventis
David Gordon	NHLBI employee

Daniel Levy	Participated in CME activity supported by an independent educational grant from Merck & Co., Inc.
Donald Lloyd-Jones	AstraZeneca, Schering-Plough
Patrick McBride	Grants and/or research support from Pfizer, Merck, Parke-Davis, and AstraZeneca; has served as a consultant for Kos Pharmaceuticals, Abbott, and Merck; and has received honoraria from Abbott, Bristol-Myers Squibb, Novartis, Merck, Kos Pharmaceuticals, Parke-Davis, Pfizer, and DuPont
J. Sanford Schwartz	Has served as a consultant for and/or conducted research funded by Bristol-Myers Squibb, AstraZeneca, Merck, Johnson & Johnson-Merck, and Pfizer.
Susan Shero	NHLBI employee
Sidney Smith	Received institutional research support from Merck; he has stock in Medtronic and Johnson & Johnson. Consultant for or on the speakers' bureaus of Bayer Corp., Eli Lilly and Co., GlaxoSmithKline Pharmaceuticals, Pfizer Labs, and Sanofi-Aventis; and has served as a member of the Data Safety Monitoring Board of AstraZeneca Pharmaceuticals.
Karol Watson	Consultant for Abbott, AstraZeneca, Genzyme, GlaxoSmithKline, Kos, Medtronic, Merck, Novartis, Pfizer
Peter Wilson	Consultant for Merck, XZK. Research grants from Merck and Liposcience

Out of the 16 members of the panel, 13 members have had or have financial relationships with pharmaceutical companies who market cholesterol lowering drugs, two members were employees at the NHLBI (who set up the ATP panel) and one had no obvious ties.

Impact of the recommendations

Professor Michael J. Pencina from the Duke Clinical Research Institute analysed the recommendations from ACC/AHA 2013 and concluded: "*As compared with the ATP-III guidelines, the new guidelines would increase the number of U.S. adults receiving or eligible for statin therapy from 43.2 million (37.5%) to 56.0 million (48.6%). Most of this increase in numbers (10.4 million of 12.8 million) would occur among adults without cardiovascular disease. Among adults between the ages of 60 and 75 years without cardiovascular disease who are not receiving statin therapy, the percentage who would be eligible for such therapy would increase from 30.4% to 87.4% among men and from 21.2% to 53.6% among women. This effect would be driven largely by an increased number of adults who would be classified solely on the basis of their 10-year risk of a cardiovascular event*".

Summary of ACC/AHA 2013

The members of ACC/AHA 2013 recommended a large increase in statin use. This advice was given using evidence from statin trials in which the participants had been carefully selected. Despite this, the results of the trials revealed no difference in death rates. Over 90% of the panel members have at some time developed financial relationships with pharmaceutical companies who market cholesterol lowering drugs, or were employed by the organisation that set up the panel. The ACC/AHA 2013 panel's recommendations resulted in a 29% increase in people taking statin drugs compared to ATP-III Update.

Paper 475:
The new Cardiovascular 10 year risk calculator systematically overestimated heart disease risks by 75–150%

Ridker PM et al Statins: new American guidelines for prevention of cardiovascular disease. *Lancet* 2013 Nov 30;382(9907):1762-5

Professor Paul Ridker from Brigham and Women's Hospital investigated the predictions of heart disease risk in the new Pooled Cohort Equations Cardiovascular ten-year risk calculator.

He evaluated the risk calculator by the following method:

- He used the results from three large completed studies that involved thousands of people and continued for at least a decade.

- o He compared how many heart attacks or strokes had actually occurred in 10 years and how many the risk calculator predicted.
- Professor Ridker found that the new Pooled Cohort Equations Cardiovascular ten-year risk calculator systematically overestimated heart disease risks by 75–150%, roughly doubling the actual risk.

Professor Ridker concluded: *"It is possible that as many as 40–50% of the 33 million middle-aged Americans targeted by the new ACC/AHA guidelines for statin therapy do not actually have risk thresholds that exceed the 7·5% threshold suggested for treatment"*.

This chapter has described how the cholesterol lowering guidelines were initiated and how they have evolved:

- The government funded National Cholesterol Education Program was set up to persuade the medical profession and the public that lower cholesterol levels are better.
- Many eminent members of the medical profession have opposed the 'lower is better' mantra throughout the last few decades.
- The man who headed the National Cholesterol Education Program, Daniel Steinberg, was a scientific advisor for the manufacturer (Merck) of lovastatin.
- In 1988 Steinberg appointed a panel to recommend guidelines for lowering cholesterol levels. Over 75% of the panel had vested interests in the recommendation of a reduction of cholesterol levels. The 1988 panel's recommendations resulted in a five-fold increase in the use of cholesterol lowering drugs. This recommendation was issued despite the scientific evidence showing that lower cholesterol levels did not save lives.
- Five sets of guidelines have been issued over the years since 1988. Every new set of guidelines has substantially increased the number of people recommended for cholesterol lowering drugs.
- The latest set of guidelines in 2013 recommended the use of only statin drugs.
- Before the first set of guidelines were issued, about 261,000 people in the USA were receiving cholesterol lowering drugs.

After the last set of guidelines were given in 2013, 56 million Americans are now eligible to receive statin drugs – a 214-fold increase.

- In all of the five sets of guidelines, the vast majority of the panel members have developed financial interests in cholesterol lowering (especially statin) manufacturers.
- In all of the five sets of guidelines, the panel members have recommended increases in cholesterol lowering medication despite the fact that the evidence they used showed that cholesterol lowering medication does not reduce death rates.
- Most of the evidence was from trials funded by statin manufacturers. Researchers have found that trials funded by the manufacturer are substantially more likely to paint a positive picture of the manufacturer's drug.
    - Patients are selected in a way that will make a positive result more likely.
    - The data is analysed as the trial progresses. If the trial seems to be producing negative data it is stopped prematurely and the results are not published, or if it is producing positive data it may be stopped early so that longer-term effects are not examined.
    - Most trials have a 'run-in' period where anyone who shows signs of suffering from statin side-effects is excluded from the trial.
    - The results of these statin manufacturer funded trials are published in a manner that gives maximum exposure to the supposed benefits of the drug and glosses over the toxic effects of the statins.
- The calculator formula that doctor's use for risk of cardiovascular disease systematically overestimates heart disease risks by 75–150%.

Professor Timothy Noakes from the University of Cape Town in South Africa has researched the scientific literature regarding cholesterol, heart disease and statins. This is what he concluded: "*Focusing on an elevated blood cholesterol concentration as the exclusive cause of coronary heart disease is unquestionably the worst medical error of our time. After reviewing all the scientific evidence, I draw just one conclusion: never prescribe a statin drug for a loved one*".

Chapter 20

Comment by eminent doctors and professors

Professor Noakes is not the only member of the medical profession who believes that statin drugs should not be taken. Many doctors and professors have deep reservations regarding the burgeoning use of statins. For instance, Prof Simon Capewell, an expert in clinical epidemiology at Liverpool University said: *"The recent statin recommendations are deeply worrying, effectively condemning all middle-aged adults to lifelong medications of questionable value"*.

This chapter portrays the views of other eminent doctors and scientists who warn of the toxic dangers of statin drugs.

Paper 476:
The adverse health effects of low cholesterol
Song JX et al Primary and secondary hypocholesterolemia.
Beijing Da Xue Xue Bao (Journal of Peking University)
2010 Oct 18;42(5):612-5

In this review of the literature, Dr Jun-Xian Song from the Peking University People's Hospital, examines the influence of low cholesterol levels (hypocholesterolemia) on health.

His review recorded:

- Low cholesterol levels are common in the population.
- Physicians pay little attention to the diseases, causes and consequences of low cholesterol in clinical practice.
- Low cholesterol levels can result in some adverse events, such as increased death rates, intracerebral hemorrhage, cancer, infection, adrenal failure, suicide and mental disorder.
- Despite the adverse health consequences of low cholesterol, physicians are increasingly prescribing cholesterol lowering treatments such as statin drugs.

With all the adverse health effects of low cholesterol Dr Song concludes: *"It's high time that physicians attached more importance to hypocholesterolemia."*

Paper 477:
Doctor says that low cholesterol levels can lead to permanent cognitive damage, infertility and vitamin deficiencies

Ali S et al Hypocholesterolemia secondary to atorvastatin therapy. *Journal of Ayub Medical College Abbottabad* 2010 Jul-Sep;22(3):225-7

Dr Shafqut Ali notes that cholesterol is essential for all animal life in the world. It is required to build and maintain cell membranes and regulates membrane fluidity. The myelin sheath is rich in cholesterol. Cholesterol is the basic raw molecule for steroid hormones including cortisol, aldesterone in adrenal glands as well as sex hormones, progesterone, estrogens and testosterone in ovaries of females and testes of males respectively. Some research indicates that cholesterol may act as an antioxidant.

Dr Ali describes the case of a man who developed hypocholesterolemia (low cholesterol) while taking statin drugs.

- A 40-year-old male who had suffered a heart attack underwent stenting and was prescribed atorvastatin.
- His cholesterol was 4.3 mmol/l (166 mg/dL) before starting atorvastatin.
- He was advised to restrain from fats and fatty food.
- He remained symptoms free for four weeks and used to walk two to four kilometres comfortably, but after four weeks he started developing symptoms of nightmares, phobias, abnormal thinking, loneliness, insomnia, forgetfulness, un-usefulness for family and community, along with sexual weakness.
- By the end of eight weeks of statins he developed easy fatigability, inability to walk more than one kilometre, restlessness, muscles cramps, impotency, aggressiveness, and finally significant ataxia (loss of co-ordination, balance and speech) along with slowness in writing.
- He considered that these are features of the disease itself and was worried about his cardiac status. He came back to his cardiologist in the sixth week of treatment for review of his cardiac status.

- His cholesterol levels had dropped to 1.7 mmol/l (65 mg/dL).
- The patient's cardiac physician stopped the Atorvastatin, lifted the dietary restrictions and advised him to eat one or two eggs daily.
- With stoppage of Atorvastatin and lifting of the dietary restrictions, recovery started within two weeks and he became symptoms free within five weeks.
- He has since remained symptom free and can walk three kilometres daily comfortably.

Dr Ali concludes that if a: *"Patient remains long period in hypocholesterolemic (low cholesterol) state, it can lead to permanent psychomotor, cognitive, motorsystem damage, hypoadrenalism, infertility in both males and females along with permanent affects of fat soluble vitamins deficiencies"*.

Paper 478:
Direct-to-consumer advertising promotes risky statin use

Niederdeppe J et al Direct-to-consumer television advertising exposure, diagnosis with high cholesterol, and statin use. *Journal of General Internal Medicine* 2013 Jul;28(7):886-93

Direct-to-consumer advertising usually refers to the marketing of pharmaceutical products but can apply in other areas as well. This form of advertising is directed toward patients, rather than healthcare professionals. Forms of direct-to-consumer advertising include TV, print, radio and other mass and social media.

The first author of the paper, Jeff Niederdeppe is an Associate Professor in the Department of Communication at Cornell University. His research examines the mechanisms and effects of mass media campaigns, strategic health messages, and news coverage in shaping health behaviour, health disparities, and social policy. He has published over 70 peer-reviewed articles in communication, public health, health policy and medicine journals.

The objective of this study was to determine the relationship between estimated exposure to direct-to-consumer advertising for statin drugs and two clinical variables: diagnosis with high cholesterol and statin use.

The study unearthed:

- Exposure to statin ads increased the odds of being diagnosed with high cholesterol by 16% to 20 % in both men and women.

- Exposure to statin ads increased statin use by 16% to 22 % in both men and women.
- These associations were driven almost exclusively by men and women at low risk for future cardiac events.

Professor Niederdeppe concluded: "*This study provides new evidence that direct-to-consumer advertising may promote over-diagnosis of high cholesterol and over-treatment for populations where risks of statin use may outweigh potential benefits*".

Paper 479: UK doctors virtually compelled to prescribe statins against their better judgement

Jenkins AJ Might money spent on statins be better spent? *British Medical Journal* 2003 October 18; 327(7420): 933

Dr Arnold Jenkins a General Practioner in the UK comments:

As a general practitioner I wonder how many million pounds sterling the NHS could save by curtailing the prescribing of statins. They are a major cost in my practice, as I am sure they are to many practitioners.

Even in general practice I recognised the Scandinavian simvastatin survival study as a seminal paper on the benefits of statins, and as we used to be taught to evaluate evidence (as opposed to stick to protocols) I read it. I was surprised to learn that more women died in the treated group than in the control group. On discussion with cardiology colleagues I was assured that as the numbers were small it was a statistical anomaly, resolvable by larger studies.

Imagine my delight when I heard of the large heart protection study showing clear benefits in the use of statins for women. On reading this study I was therefore disappointed to find the total mortality data for women missing. I now understand that the total mortality benefit for women did not reach significance and therefore was not published (Louise Bowman, personal communication, 2002).

I do not understand why the censors of this paper do not realise two things.

Firstly, any meta analyses based on this study are likely to be skewed.

Secondly, in such long-term studies total mortality, not improvement in the condition, should be the gold standard for evaluation (euthanasia, for example, provides 100% cure of headache but should be ruled out on the mortality data).

I have yet to find a paper showing a significant reduction in mortality in women for groups treated with statins. It therefore seems that any benefit, if found, will be minimal. Yet we are almost compelled by protocols such as the national service framework for coronary heart disease and local prescribing incentives to prescribe for this subgroup. Also the supporting documentation to the new general medical services contract indicates that such statin prescribing may become a quality indicator.

I wonder whether the money could be better spent or if we should abandon the little evidence based medicine we currently have?

In the UK General Practitioners receive payments from the general medical services contract, via the quality and outcomes framework, for prescribing statins or getting patients total cholesterol levels below 5 mmol/L (193 mg/dL). Virtually the only practical way to get peoples cholesterol levels under 5 mmol/L is to prescribe them statins.

The General Practitioners are awarded points for hitting various targets regarding patients' statin usage and cholesterol levels. In 2013-2014, each point is worth £156.92 in England.

Regarding statins and cholesterol levels, points are awarded as follows:

- Patients with coronary heart disease who have total cholesterol levels of 5 mmol/l or less: 17 points.
- Patients who have had a heart attack and are treated with statins: 10 points.
- Patients with stroke or transient ischaemic attack (mini stroke) who have a record of total cholesterol: 2 points.
- Patients with stroke shown to be non-haemorrhagic, or a history of transient ischaemic attack whose total cholesterol is 5 mmol/l or less. 5 points.
- Patients with peripheral arterial disease in whom total cholesterol is 5 mmol/l or less: 3 points.
- Patients with diabetes whose total cholesterol is 5 mmol/l or less: 6 points.
- Patients with a new diagnosis of high blood pressure aged 30 -75 who are prescribed statins: 10 points.

- Patients aged 40 or over with schizophrenia, bipolar affective disorder and other psychoses who have a record of total cholesterol/HDL cholesterol ratio: 5 points.

The payments for the quality and outcomes framework incentives could be worth up to £141,000 for a general practitioner's practice.

The following article by Dr Catherine Shanahan describes how doctors in the US actually get paid more for writing more statin prescriptions:

You may have read that doctors receive payment or bonuses for prescribing statins, the cholesterol-lowering drugs. I'm a family physician in Kauai, so I'm in a good position to fill in some details about how doctors actually get paid more for writing more statin prescriptions. The mechanism is a little cumbersome to describe clearly, but I'll take a stab at it.

We have a series of "quality measures" that are tracked by the insurance company. One quality measure is the number of mammograms we do on our patients between ages 40 and 69, another is that we send our diabetic patients to the eye doctor once a year for retinal exams. For our patients who carry a diagnosis of "coronary artery disease", we have to write them a prescription for a cholesterol-lowering drug. If any one doctor doesn't follow any one of these imperatives, he loses points toward a cash bonus, and the entire group is similarly penalized. As you can imagine, there is lots of peer pressure to prescribe!

Actually, we don't get our bonus unless the patient goes and buys the drug or gets the test or sees the eye doctor and so on, so it's not enough just to write the prescription, we have to talk up the drug enough to get them to go out and buy it. Currently, there are only a few means by which a person can be labelled as a patient with coronary artery disease. Having a heart attack is one, and having abnormal results on heart tests (like angiograms) is another. Diabetes is now considered a "coronary artery disease equivalent" and so, in the near future, doctors may be required to get all our patients who have type one or type two diabetes to take their statins, or lose more money.

These Health Maintenance Organizations (HMOs) are insurance companies like Blue Cross, which offer their clients (employers and patients) HMO programs. The HMO plan we have is offered by HMSA (Hawaii Medical Service Association). For whatever reason, HMSA wants to offer an HMO program for people, and doctors who participate as providers must comply with the rules of the program and accept payments according to the rules. There are clear benefits to pharmaceutical companies in this structure but no obvious reason why HMSA would want to encourage people to buy expensive drugs that HMSA must pay for. One might speculate that there are some quid-pro-quo relationships between the insurance companies and the pharmaceutical companies, but I have no idea what they are. However, the ties are structured, I feel, as do many other scientists, that these kinds of business relationships lead to behaviours that pose real threats to patient care, and to human health in general. Because industrial connections like this fund most research, they distort the scientific process and are far more insidious, invisible, and totalitarianistic than expensive dinners and trips to Hawaii, which are what the media would have us believe is the sum total of the problem.

By the way, the bonus is actually not a bonus at all. This is where it gets Orwellian. We give up a certain percentage of the payment for accepting HMO patients, and we get it all back, in theory, if we meet all of our quality measures. We never do because of computer glitches which continually fail to track our prescribing, testing, and referring patterns accurately. Nobody can explain why we've agreed to accept HMO insurance plans, but we seem to feel we have no choice. And we will have less choice before long; Medicare is planning to begin similar programs. Each of these programs takes more money away from the doctors and gives it to middle managers, ensures that drug companies get more money, and that expensive tests of limited value are done more often.

Catherine Shanahan MD
Kalaheo, Hawaii

Paper 480:
Doctor's low awareness of statin side effects

Golomb BA et al Statin Adverse Effects: A Review of the Literature and Evidence for a Mitochondrial Mechanism. *American Journal of Cardiovascular Drugs* 2008;8(6):373-418

The lead researcher in this study, Dr Beatrice Golomb, is an Associate Professor of Medicine at the University California San Diego School of Medicine. Dr Golomb reviewed the scientific literature regarding the adverse effects caused by statin drugs.

Dr Golomb found:

- Muscle adverse events were the most reported problem both in the literature and by patients.
- In meta-analyses of randomized controlled trials, muscle adverse events are more frequent with statins than with placebo.
- A number of manifestations of muscle adverse events have been reported, with rhabdomyolysis the most feared.
- Adverse events are dose dependent, and risk is amplified by drug interactions that functionally increase statin potency.
- An array of additional risk factors for statin AEs are those that amplify (or reflect) mitochondrial or metabolic vulnerability, such as metabolic syndrome factors, thyroid disease, and genetic mutations linked to mitochondrial dysfunction.
- Converging evidence supports a mitochondrial foundation for muscle adverse events associated with statins, and both theoretical and empirical considerations suggest that mitochondrial dysfunction may also underlie many nonmuscle statin adverse events.
- Evidence from randomized controlled trials and studies of other designs indicates existence of additional statin-associated adverse events, such as cognitive loss, neuropathy, pancreatic and hepatic dysfunction, and sexual dysfunction.
- Physician awareness of statin adverse events is reportedly low even for the adverse events most widely reported by patients.

Dr Golomb concludes: "*Adverse events of statins are neither vanishingly rare nor of trivial impact. For statins, as for all medications, vigilance for potential adverse events is imperative. Recognition of potential statin adverse events is needed*".

Paper 481:
Do doctors report statin side-effects?

Golomb BA et al Physician Response to Patient Reports of Adverse Drug Effects. *Drug Safety* 2007; 30 (8): 669-675

This study, conducted by Dr Beatrice Golomb, was a patient-targeted survey and sought to assess patients' experience of how physicians responded when patients presented with possible statin adverse drug reactions. The study included 650 adult patients taking statins with self-reported adverse drug reactions. The paper focused on patients' experience of the doctor-patient interaction and the physicians' response when patients report statin adverse drug reactions.

The study revealed:

- 87% of patients spoke to their physician about the possible connection between statin use and their symptom.
- Patients reported that they and not the doctor most commonly initiated the discussion regarding the possible connection of drug to symptom (98% vs. 2% cognition survey, 96% vs. 4% neuropathy survey, 86% vs. 14% muscle survey).
- Physicians were 147% more likely to dismiss than affirm the possibility of a connection between statins and cognition symptoms.
- Physicians were 88% more likely to dismiss than affirm the possibility of a connection between statins and neuropathy symptoms.
- Physicians were 62% more likely to dismiss than affirm the possibility of a connection between statins and muscle symptoms.
- Rejection of a possible connection was reported to occur even for symptoms with strong literature support for a drug connection, and even in patients for whom the symptom met presumptive literature-based criteria for probable or definite drug-adverse effect causality.
- Here are some physicians responses to patients concern about the possible connection between statin use and their symptoms grouped into seven categories: (i) "Attributed to age", (ii) "dismissed importance of symptoms", (iii) "dismissed existence of symptom", (iv) "dismissed relation to statins", (v) "dismissed relation to statins, muscle-specific", (vi) "dismissed relation to statins, cognition-specific", (vii) "disbelief that statins cause adverse drug reactions in general".
    - o *Attributed to age*: "Just normal aging process". "Can expect some problems at your age". "Well, you're no youngster". "You're just getting old".
    - o *Dismissed importance of symptoms*: "Doctor said would have to live with side effects and did not seem to care". "Ignorned complaints about side effects". "Doctor

shrugged and said some people just live with it, then laughed". "Did not seem to be concerned with side effects". "Didn't take seriously". "Made me feel I was alone in my inability to take statins because of 'minor discomfort'".

- o *Dismissed existence of symptom*: "Acted as if it was in imagination". "Doctor suggested it was imagination". "Don't think doctor believed me". "Told me I just didn't like taking pills". "Nothing wrong with me". "It's all in my head". "She 'pooh-poohed' me and said keep taking Lipitor".
- o *Dismissed relation to statins*: "Almost impossible". "Cannot be statins". "Not possible". "Denied possibility". "Can't be". "Said this has nothing to do with the Pravachol". Said that's not a side effect of this drug". "They (doctors) were very skeptical even though I presented Pfizer's own report on side effects". "Statins could not be cause of symptoms". "Neither doctor (internist, neurologist) believed me – my pharmacist suggested Lipitor as a cause". "My chiropractor suggested it may be the Lipitor – my MD didn't think so".
- o *Dismissed relation to statins, muscle-specific*: "Didn't think Lipitor caused muscle weakness because there was no pain". "Wouldn't consider Lipitor the cause of body aches". "Doctor didn't think cramps were caused by statins". "Doctor felt that there was no connection between pain and the statin drugs".
- o *Dismissed relation to statins, cognition-specific*: "Statins do not cause memory loss and may, in fact, help it". "No research linking statins to memory problems". "Doctor said statins would improve (not worsen) memory". "Memory and peripheral neuropathy are not acknowledged side effects of statins". "I was the first to tell him (doctor) about this significant side effect (memory problems, coordinating thoughts/complex tasks) and since then he has had other patients with similar problems".
- o *Disbelief that statins cause adverse drug reactions in general*: "Doctor said there were no side effects". "Doctor had heard of no difficulties". "Said Lipitor has minimum to no adverse drug reactions". "Can't be the statins, thinks it is a miracle drug". "Said that only 1% of patients have side effects".

The data shows that doctors may fail to even contemplate a possible statin adverse reaction which contributes towards low reporting rates of statin adverse reactions.

Dr Golomb concluded: "*Since low reporting rates are considered to contribute to delays in identification of adverse drug reactions, findings from this study suggest that additional putative cases may be identified by targeting patients as reporters, potentially speeding recognition of adverse drug reactions*".

Paper 482:
Professor says there is an urgent need to establish the true incidence of the side effects of statins

Majeed A et al Urgent need to establish the true incidence of the side effects of statins. *British Medical Journal* 2014 Jun 11;348:g3650

Professor Azeem Majeed discusses the urgent need to establish the true incidence of the side effects of statins.

- One key area of the debate about widening the use of statins is the discordance between rates of side effects of statins in clinical trials and in clinical practice.
- In clinical trials, the incidence of side effects from statins is low and similar in the intervention and placebo groups.
- By contrast, observational studies using primary care databases report a much higher rate of potentially serious side effects (such as myopathy and renal failure) in people taking statins.
- Even these rates derived from clinical records may underestimate the true incidence of side effects in people taking statins, because not all patients with side effects inform their doctor and not all doctors enter a relevant diagnostic code in the patient's electronic medical record.
- Many GPs will be familiar with patients who report side effects after starting statins. These side effects are often severe enough for patients to stop taking the drug. Of course, these side effects could be coincidental or psychosomatic and nothing to do with the drug. It is also possible that previous clinical trials (most of which were carried out many years ago) under-recorded the side effects of statins.

Paper 483:
Systematic review finds statins have many adverse effects

Bang CN et al Statin treatment, new-onset diabetes, and other adverse effects: a systematic review. *Current Cardiology Reports* 2014 Mar;16(3):461

Dr Casper Bang from the Cardiology Department of Weill Cornell Medical College, New York, conducted a systematic review of the adverse effects of statins.

His review found:

- The majority of the literature suggests an increased risk of new-onset diabetes in patients treated with statins in a number of different settings and that the risk appears greatest among the more potent statins.
- Furthermore, a dose-response curve has been shown between statin treatment and the development of diabetes.
- Other side effects have been reported such as increased risk of myotoxicity (muscle toxicity), increased liver enzymes, cataracts, mood disorders, dementias, haemorrhagic stroke and peripheral neuropathy, which should maybe be added to the increased risk of new-onset diabetes, when considering the risk- benefit ratio of statin treatment.

Paper 484:
7 million Americans may suffer from statin induced muscle pain

Fernandez G et al Statin myopathy: a common dilemma not reflected in clinical trials. *Cleveland Clinic Journal of Medicine* 2011 Jun;78(6):393-403

In this paper, Dr Genaro Fernandez and his associates from the University of Utah, asked the question: *"Why is statin-induced myopathy (muscle pain) so uncommon in clinical trials"?*

The authors find that in the United States, where an estimated 33 million adults use statins, musculoskeletal pain can be expected to occur in 7 million people, likely induced by statin therapy in 25% of cases.

However, in clinical trials, muscle pain is only reported in 1% to 5% of patients taking the statin drugs.

So why is statin-induced myopathy (muscle pain) so uncommon in clinical trials?

- One reason may be that patients in clinical trials are carefully screened. To minimize toxicity, the clinical trials of statins excluded patients with renal insufficiency, hepatic insufficiency, a history of muscular complaints, and poorly controlled diabetes, as well as patients taking drugs with possible interactions. Large efficacy trials exclude around 30% of the participants in active pre-trial phases.
- Another reason is that these trials were designed to assess the efficacy of statins and were not sensitive to adverse effects like muscle pain. When they looked at myopathy, they focused on rhabdomyolysis—the most severe form—rather than on myalgia, fatigue, or other minor muscle complaints. Additionally, most trials enrolled too few patients and did not have long enough follow-up to reveal infrequent toxicities.
- Despite the strict criteria, a significant number of trial patients discontinued statin therapy during the study period in the Treat to New Targets (TNT) trial. 5% of patients in both the high- and low-dose atorvastatin (Lipitor) groups experienced muscle toxicity, even though 35% of eligible patients had been excluded during the active pre-trial phase.

Paper 485:
Professor concludes that results from statin trials may be considerably flawed

Laporte JR Meta-analysis of side effects of statins shows need for trial transparency. *British Medical Journal* 2014;348:g2940

This article, authored by Professor Joan-Ramon Laporte from the Autonomous University of Barcelona noted the exclusions in statin clinical trials.

Professor Laporte found:

- In the HPS (Heart Protection Study), 32,145 patients with the inclusion criteria participated in a run in phase, but 11,609 (36%) were excluded because of lack of effect on cholesterol, increase in liver enzymes, increase in CPK, or increase of creatinine, or also because "the patient had little probability of complying with the treatment during 5 years".
- In the MEGA trial (Management of Elevated Cholesterol in the Primary Prevention Group of Adult Japanese), 15,210

patients entered a four-week run in phase, but 7,201 (48%) were excluded for similar reasons, and only 8,009 finally participated in the trial.

- In the JUPITER trial (Justification for the Use of Statins in Prevention: an Intervention Trial Evaluating Rosuvastatin), 89,890 were initially screened, but 78% were excluded for unclear reasons, and only 19,323 were considered for randomisation. Then, an additional 1,521 were excluded during a run in phase because of poor treatment adherence, and only 17,802 patients (19.8%) were finally randomised.

Professor Laporte concluded that in view of these massive exclusions, the data from these trials may be considerably flawed and lacked validity, and that no conclusions could be drawn from the results of the trials.

Paper 486:
Statins do not prevent cardiovascular and all-cause deaths

Vos E et al Point: Why statins have failed to reduce mortality in just about anybody. *Journal of Clinical Lipidology* 2013 May-Jun;7(3):222-4

A team based at McGill University reviewed the scientific evidence regarding statins and death rates.

- In JUPITER (Justification for the Use of Statins in Primary Prevention: An Intervention Trial Evaluating Rosuvastatin trial), a trial involving 17,802 participants randomised to rosuvastatin or placebo found for all participants the cardiovascular mortality was not reduced.
- All published trials with placebo controls conclusively establish that statins do not reduce mortality in women.
- There are no mortality figures suggesting a positive effect for people taking statins for more than five or six years.
- In the PROSPER (PROspective Study of Pravastatin in the Elderly at Risk) study, in patients older than 70 years of age, there appeared to be arising increased rate of cancer, which may indicate that longer intervals of statin therapy may have other costs in the elderly.
- For both genders, the lack of all-cause mortality benefit is also illustrated by all published studies using atorvastatin vs.

placebo, including the summary of 49 in-house studies including 14,236 individual patients.

- The secondary prevention study SPARCL (Stroke Prevention by Aggressive Reduction in Cholesterol Levels) ended with five more deaths on high dose atorvastatin than on placebo.
- To date, there are no placebo-controlled studies showing a mortality benefit when patients used lovastatin, fluvastatin, cerivastatin, or pitavastatin.
- No mortality benefit from statins has ever been shown in patients older than 70 years of age.
- No mortality benefit from statins has ever been shown in patients with heart failure.
- No mortality benefit from statins has ever been shown in patients with kidney failure.
- Patients believing consciously or subliminally that "their cholesterol is under control" because they take a statin may postpone embarking on lifestyle changes, such as stopping smoking and abandoning eating habits that produce obesity and diabetes.
- There is evidence that statins themselves promote diabetes, a life-long health risk.

The first author of the paper, Eddie Vos advises: "*Because the lack of circulating statins is not the cause of atherosclerosis and their benefit on mortality is highly questionable, we should concentrate on lifestyle changes. Exercise, no smoking, and a healthy diet are well demonstrated in population studies to reduce the high mortality seen in so many economically developed countries*".

He concludes that statins: "*do not prevent cardiovascular and all-cause deaths*".

Paper 487:
Statin major adverse effects have been under-reported and the way in which they withheld from the public, and even concealed, is a scientific farce

Sultan S The Ugly Side of Statins. Systemic Appraisal of the Contemporary Un-Known Unknowns. *Open Journal of Endocrine and Metabolic Diseases*, Vol. 3 No. 3, 2013, pp. 179-185

Dr Sherif Sultan, leading Vascular and Endovascular surgeon from the Galway Clinic in Ireland, undertook a comprehensive review of the scientific literature for articles relating to cardiovascular primary prevention and statin side effects.

His review found:

- There is a categorical lack of clinical evidence to support the use of statin therapy in primary prevention.
- Not only is there a dearth of evidence for primary cardiovascular protection, there is ample evidence to show that statins actually augment cardiovascular risk in women, patients with diabetes mellitus and in the young.
- Statins are associated with triple the risk of coronary artery and aortic artery calcification.
- There is increased risk of diabetes mellitus, cataract formation, and erectile dysfunction in young statin users.
- There is a significant increase in the risk of cancer and neurodegenerative disorders in the elderly plus an enhanced risk of a myriad of infectious diseases.
- A review of the use of statins found evidence of selective reporting of outcomes and failure to report adverse events.

Dr Sultan concluded: *"These finding on statin major adverse effects had been under-reported and the way in which they withheld from the public, and even concealed, is a scientific farce".*

Paper 488:
Cardiologist questions the benefits of statins

Vos E et al Questioning the benefits of statins. *Canadian Medical Association Journal* November 8, 2005; 173 (10)

One of the authors of the paper, Dr Colin Rose, is a cardiologist at McGill University.

He notes that:

- Statins have failed to deliver in reducing all cause mortality.
- There are no statin trials with even the slightest hint of a mortality benefit in women.
- In patients over 70 years old evidence shows no mortality benefit of statin therapy.
- In the ALLHAT study says it best: "Trials (primarily in middle-aged men) demonstrating a reduction in (coronary artery

disease) from cholesterol lowering have not demonstrated a net reduction in all-cause mortality". What is the point of decreasing the number of "events" without decreasing overall mortality, when the harm caused by the side effects of statin therapy is factored in?

Paper 489: Bad medicine: statins

Spence D Bad medicine: statins. *British Medical Journal* 2013 May 31;346:f3566

This article in the *British Medical Journal,* regarding statin drugs, is by Dr Des Spence, a general practitioner from Glasgow in the UK.

- Public health "wisdom" dictates that statins are offered to all middle aged people to prevent vascular disease.
- There is no longer a "normal" concentration of cholesterol in the blood, so is treating everyone over a specific age good medicine?
- The cardiovascular disease model is a paradigm based on risk factors, all now morphed into "diseases" –cholesterol, glucose, and the elasticity of arteries based on assessment using a Victorian hearing aid. However, the evidence that supports this model is far from conclusive.
- Medicine believes in this model, worshipping at the educational cathedrals of the pharmaceutical industry.
- The effects of statins need to be quantified. In low risk patients older than 60 and taking standard statin treatments, the number needed to treat per year to prevent one cardiovascular event is 450, and the number needed to treat per year to prevent one vascular death ranges from 1250 to 5000. So, almost none of these patients will actually benefit directly despite taking statins for the rest of their lives.
- What about the long-term side effects?
- 60 million statins a year, are prescribed in the UK, yet we can't prove that statins work in the real world.
- Scepticism is futile. Guidelines will be issued to expand statin use, and these orders dutifully followed. Patients trust doctors and will go along with this advice, eroding societies' wellbeing and fanning health anxiety.

- Soon the natural extension of this logic will see a clamour for statins in ever younger age groups and for more aggressive treatment.
- Is "statins for all" bad medicine? Time will tell.

Paper 490: Professor says science ceases to exist when no one else than those who have conflicts of interest are allowed to see the data on statins adverse effects

Gotzsche PC Muscular adverse effects are common with statins. *British Medical Journal* 2014 Jun 11;348:g3724

Professor Peter Gotzsche from the Nordic Cochrane Centre in Copenhagen makes the following comments regarding statins muscular effects.

- The 2011 Cochrane review of statins for the primary prevention of cardiovascular disease, reported a risk ratio of 1.03 for muscle pain, i.e. 3% more patients developed muscle pain on drug than on placebo.
- However, industry-funded randomised trials are notoriously unreliable when it comes to the harms of drugs.
- A publicly-funded randomised trial from 2012 that studied the impact of statins on energy and exertional fatigue got results that could be interpreted as 20% of the men and 40% of the women experiencing a worsening in either energy or exertional fatigue.
- I therefore wonder why Rory Collins has pressured the BMJ in a most unacademic fashion for having published a paper that reported a similar incidence of harms based on a cohort study.
- He has even called for a retraction of the paper, just like drug companies have often done when a paper appeared that could threaten their sales.
- Collins and his colleagues publish meta-analyses based on company data to which no one else has access because of the confidentiality clauses Collins and colleagues have accepted.
    - o Collins is co-director of the Clinical Trial Service Unit (CTSU) at Oxford University. He is also head of the Cholesterol Treatment Trialists (CTT) Collaboration.

- o The Cholesterol Treatment Trialists (CTT) Collaboration is a division of the Clinical Trial Service Unit (CTSU).
- o The Cholesterol Treatment Trialists (CTT) Collaboration push for aggressive treatment of cholesterol to low levels.
- o The Clinical Trial Service Unit (CTSU) have received £268 million pounds in funding over the years from pharmaceutical companies such as; Astra Zeneca (rosuvastatin), Merck (lovastatin, simvastatin), Novartis (fluvastatin) and Pfizer (atorvastatin).
- o To clarify, Collins heads an organisation that holds data on statin side effects, which he won't share with doctors and patients who would like to know about these statin side effects. Collins has received millions in funding from companies that produce statins. Collins organisation pushes for aggressive treatment of cholesterol to low levels.

Professor Gotzsche concludes: *"I believe science ceases to exist when no one else than those who have conflicts of interest are allowed to see the data"*.

Paper 491:
Open letter raises concerns about NICE guidance on statins

Wise J Open letter raises concerns about NICE guidance on statins. *British Medical Journal* 2014 Jun 11;348:g3937

The National Institute for Health and Care Excellence (NICE) provides national guidance and advice on health and social care in the UK.

A group of leading doctors have written an open letter to David Haslam, chairman of NICE, and to the health secretary, Jeremy Hunt, raising serious concerns about the latest draft guidance on statins.

The draft guidance from NICE, published in February 2014, recommended lowering the threshold for treatment with statins to include people who had a 10% or higher 10 year risk of developing cardiovascular disease.

The letter dated 10th June. 2014 was as follows:

Concerns about the latest NICE draft guidance on statins

Introduction:

We are concerned about your draft guidance on CV risk for discussion and debate. We would ask for a delay until our concerns are addressed. Whilst we agree with much of the guidance, our concerns focus on six key areas: medicalisation of healthy individuals, true levels of adverse events, hidden data, industry bias, loss of professional confidence, and conflicts of interest.

The draft guidance recommends offering statin treatment for the primary prevention of CVD to people who have a 10% or greater ten-year risk of developing CVD.

1. Medicalisation of five million healthy individuals

Firstly, we believe that the benefits in a low risk population do not justify putting approximately five million more people on drugs that will then have to be taken lifelong.

The important questions for clinicians and for patients include: (1) does treatment of elevated cholesterol levels with statins in otherwise healthy persons decrease mortality or prevent other serious outcomes? (2) What are the adverse effects associated with statin treatment in healthy persons? (3) Do the potential benefits outweigh the potential risks? Recent papers have suggested that statin therapy should not be recommended for men with elevated cholesterol who are otherwise healthy.[2]

Furthermore, atorvastatin 20mg is also recommended as the first-line treatment. This appears counterintuitive, as atorvastatin has never been demonstrated to reduce mortality for primary prevention in any clinical study.

2. Conflicting levels of adverse events

In emphasising the cost per Quality Adjusted Life Year (QALY), NICE is clearly making a major assumption that the key issue is mortality reduction, and that statins lead to very few adverse effects. We would question this very strongly.

The levels of adverse events reported in the statin trials contain worrying anomalies. For example, in the West of Scotland Coronary Prevention Study (WOSCOPS, the first primary prevention study done), the cumulative incidence of myalgia was 0.06% in the statin arm, and 0.06% in the placebo arm.

However, the METEOR study found an incidence of myalgia of 12.7% in the rosuvastatin arm, and 12.1% in the placebo arm. Whilst it can be understood that a different formulation of statin could cause a different rate of myalgia, it is difficult to see how the placebo could, in one study, cause a rate of myalgia of 0.06%, and

12.1% in another. This is a 200-fold difference in a trial lasting less than half as long.

Furthermore, the rate of adverse effects in the statin and placebo arms of all the trials has been almost identical. Exact comparison between trials is not possible, due to lack of complete data, and various measures of adverse effects are used, in different ways. However, here is a short selection of major statins studies.

AFCAPS/TEXCAPS: Total adverse effects lovastatin 13.6%: Placebo 13.8%

4S: Total adverse effect simvastatin 6%: Placebo 6%

CARDS: Total adverse effects atorvastatin 25%: Placebo 24%

HPS: Discontinuation rates simvastatin 4.5%: Placebo 5.1%

METEOR: Total adverse effects rosuvastatin 83.3%: Placebo 80.4%

LIPID: Total adverse effects 3.2% pravastatin: Placebo 2.7%

JUPITER: Discontinuation rate of drug 25% rosuvastatin 25% placebo. Serious Adverse events 15% rosuvastatin 15.5% placebo

WOSCOPS: Total adverse effects. Pravastatin 7.8%: Placebo 7.0%

Curiously, the adverse effect rate of the statin, it is always very similar to that of placebo. However, placebo adverse effect rates range from 2.7% to 80.4%, a 30-fold difference.

3. Hidden data

Without access to the raw data, it is difficult to understand how statin related adverse events, and placebo related adverse events can mirror each other so precisely, whilst the absolute rates can vary 30-fold (almost 3,000%). These data most certainly require analysis by a third party with appropriate expertise.

A further serious concern is that the data driving NICE guidance on statins comes almost entirely from pharmaceutical company funded studies. Furthermore, these data are not available for review by independent researchers, only those who work for the Oxford Cholesterol Treatment Trialists Collaboration (CTT).

The CTT has commercial agreements with pharmaceutical companies which apparently means that they cannot release data to any other researchers who request to see it. Which, in turn, means that the latest reviews of the data by NICE and also by the Cochrane group are totally reliant on the CTT 2012 meta-analysis analysis of this concealed data?

4. Industry bias

The overdependence on industry data raises concerns about possible biases. Extensive evidence shows that industry funded trials systematically produce more favourable outcomes than non-industry sponsored ones.

Notably, only one major non-industry funded study on statins has been done. ALLHAT-LLP. The main findings were summarised: *'Although pravastatin has been shown in multiple large clinical trials to reduce CHD morbidity and mortality,* **NO** *benefit was demonstrated in ALLHAT-LLT, the largest clinical event trial of pravastatin published to date.*'

True levels of adverse events.

We are also concerned that the rate of adverse effects in post-marketing studies is, in most cases, far higher than that found in the premarketing studies. In part this is due to the fact that the clinical trial populations studied in premarketing trials are highly selected. Furthermore, industry sponsored trials include prerandomisation run-in periods where those who fail to tolerate statins are excluded. RCT patients may therefore not represent the population that will actually take the drugs in the real world. RCTs may thus grossly underestimate adverse effects such as myopathy or cognitive impairment, and fail to detect drug interactions e.g. amlodipine and statins.

Important findings from some other non-industry sponsored studies.

A double-blind randomised controlled trial that compared 1,016 low risk patients receiving simvastatin 20 mg or pravastatin 40 mg with placebo showed that both drugs had a significant adverse effect on energy/fatigue exercise score with 40% of women reporting reduced energy or fatigue with exertion. Reducing exercise capacity in a healthy group when physical inactivity is a major contributor to the development of cardiovascular disease is extremely counterproductive.

A large observational study involving 153,840 postmenopausal women aged between 50 and 80 years enrolled in the Women's Health Initiative study found that statins were associated with a 48% increased risk of developing diabetes.

Potential psychiatric symptoms including depression, memory loss, confusion, and aggressive reactions have also been associated with statin use.

Erectile dysfunction, to take another significant adverse effect, is not mentioned in the statin trials. Yet, when it was specifically looked for, around 20% of men appeared to be affected.

5. Loss of professional confidence

We are also concerned that GPs feel that this guidance is a 'step too far'. It is instructive to note that a survey of 511GPs carried out by Pulse magazine revealed that '*....almost six out of ten (57%) oppose the plan to lower the current 10-year risk threshold for primary prevention, while only 25% support it. Furthermore, 55% would not personally take a statin or recommend a family member does so based on a 10% 10-year risk score.*'

More recently the General Practitioners Committee (GPC), which negotiates on behalf of GPs in the UK passed the following resolution: '*In light of the Cochrane review of the effectiveness of antiviral influenza treatments, the GPC will request that NICE refrain from recommending a reduction to the current treatment threshold for primary prevention of cardiovascular disease with statin therapy unless this is supported by evidence derived from complete public disclosure of all clinical trials' data*'.

Asking GPs to meet targets that they feel uncomfortable with risks a damaging split within the profession, and a loss of confidence among the public, who are likely to recognise increasingly that GPs are being asked to prescribe statins despite feeling it is inappropriate.

6. Conflicts of Interest (real and perceived)

We are also seriously concerned that eight members of NICE's panel of 12 experts for its latest guidance have direct financial ties to the pharmaceutical companies that manufacture statins. Furthermore, some members of the guideline panel are also involved in next generation, more expensive, cholesterol lowering drugs, which are not yet on the market. If cholesterol lowering becomes established in low risk people, the indications for these new cholesterol lowering drugs, such as the ApoB Antisence drugs and PCSK9 inhibitors, will probably expand as well. We feel that parties with industry conflicts should not be participants in generating recommendations regarding drug use that will influence medical care across the population.

We fear that the CTSU could be perceived as having a major conflict of interest in the area of cardiovascular disease prevention/ lipid modification, which has an impact on the Unit's perceived objectivity. We strongly urge that other researchers, for example, the Cochrane Stroke Group and Cochrane Heart Group, should be able to scrutinize and assess all the data that the CTT has utilised over the years to produce their extremely influential studies.

CTT is a part of the Clinical Trials Service Unit (CTSU) in Oxford, which has carried out many very large studies on statins, and other lipid modification agents with pharmaceutical company support, and has received hundreds of millions in funding over the years. To consider just one such study (REVEAL). REVEAL is being funded by Merck Sharp & Dohme, which developed anacetrapib. A grant of £96 million towards the cost of this multi-million dollar study has been provided to the University of Oxford.

We are concerned that financial conflicts of interest and major commercial bias may have corrupted the database on statins, resulting in an underestimate of the incidence of statin side-effects. Unless all of the data are made available it is impossible to establish a cost per QALY, as there may be DALYs [disability adjusted life years] not accurately accounted for.

We call for all of the data from the clinical trials to be made available to credible researchers, for example, the Cochrane Stroke and Heart Groups. We believe that there is a need for a more robust post-marketing analysis of suspected adverse effects from statins prescribed in a community setting.

To conclude, we urge you to withdraw the current guidance on statins for people at low risk of cardiovascular disease until all the data are made available. The potential consequences of not doing so are worrying: harm to many patients over many years, and the loss of public and professional faith in NICE as an independent assessor. Public interests need always to be put before other interests, particularly Pharma.

Yours Sincerely

Sir Richard Thompson, President of the Royal College of Physicians

Professor Clare Gerada, Past Chair of the Royal College of General Practitioners and Chair of NHS Clinical Transformation Board

Professor David Haslam, General Practitioner and Chair of the National Obesity Forum

Dr J S Bamrah, Consultant Psychiatrist and Medical Director of Manchester Mental Health and Social Care Trust

Dr Malcolm Kendrick, General Practitioner and Member of the British Medical Association's General Practitioners sub- Committee

Dr Aseem Malhotra, London Cardiologist

Dr Simon Poole, General Practitioner

David Newman, Assistant Professor of Emergency Medicine and Director of Clinical Research, Mount Sinai School of Medicine, New York

Professor Simon Capewell, Professor of Clinical Epidemiology, University of Liverpool

Of course, the letter was ignored by NICE.

The NICE guidelines were introduced in July 2014.

(The panel that developed the NICE guidelines comprised of 12 members. See Appendix 3 for the conflicts of interest the panel members have with pharmaceutical companies that manufacture cholesterol lowering drugs.)

Paper 492:
Doctors raises concerns about conflicts of interest in proposed new statin guidelines

Spence D NICE is busted. *British Medical Journal* 2014 Jun 13; 348/bmj.g3937/rr/702032

Dr Des Spence comments on the new UK statin proposals by National Institute for Health and Care Excellence (NICE).

- Concerns about conflicts of interest (COI) in NICE guideline groups have been raised in the recent statin proposals. But this is the norm not the exception for authors of NICE guidelines who are often steeped in COI, for example, hypertension, diabetes and depression. These of course are chronic incurable common conditions that is the financial life blood of the Pharma Industry balance sheets.
- Regrettably institutions like NICE dismiss these COIs, claiming that as long as these are declared, they do not impact on the advice given. This of course is a nonsense and those looking from outside are bemused that experts with COI are allowed to be involved in such important guidance.
- Experts on the take from Pharma companies believe that medication "works", so have a closed therapeutic mindset, never questioning the current paradigm of medical care.

Medications are always the solution to all problems medical or social.

- Indeed there other conflicts of interests that are non financial. Academics have their own careers to carve out, empires to build and pet theories to disseminate. Being on NICE gives credence and status. So even expert academics without links to Big Pharma are by no means truly impartial. So we have the known knowns of academic bias; the known unknowns of academic bias but also unknown unknowns, the ones we don't know we don't know!
- The road to medical truth is barricaded by squat-set-balaclava- -bowtied thuggish experts touting professorships and heavy biases! And we don't really need experts, for most medical research at its core is so basic that having O level statistics would make you over qualified.

Dr Spence concludes: "*NICE is over complicated, flat-footed, bureaucratic, opaque and addled by conflicts of interest, financial and otherwise. Big Pharma and vested specialist interests lurk malevolently in the shadows of many a guideline. Yet these guidelines directly affect our families' medical care, everywhere and everyday. Is NICE fit for purpose? We need to tear it down and start again with a system that actively prohibits all conflicts of interest and is less reliant on a select few experts*".

Paper 493: Editor of the British Medical Journal finds that statin manufacturers exaggerate the benefits of statins and hide the harmful side-effects

Godlee F et al Statins for all over 50? No. *British Medical Journal* 2013;347:f6412

Dr Fiona Godlee, editor of the *British Medical Journal*, discusses whether statins should be prescribed to everyone over the age of 50.

- A detailed critique by John Abramson and colleagues' of the Cholesterol Treatment Trialists Collaboration meta-analysis found that an analysis of the data finds no evidence of a reduction in all cause mortality or in the total number of serious events.
- They also highlight the failure of the trials included in the Cholesterol Treatment Trialists Collaboration analysis to

adequately report important harms of statin treatment, including myopathy and diabetes.

- They conclude that broadening the use of statins to low risk individuals "*will unnecessarily increase the incidence of adverse events without providing overall health benefits.*"
- There is a concern underlying their critique that will be familiar to *BMJ* readers. It is that all of the trials included in the Cholesterol Treatment Trialists Collaboration meta-analysis were funded by the manufacturer of the statin being studied.
- They list the various ways in which these trials might have exaggerated the benefits of statins and minimised the harms, and they summarise what low risk patients need to know. Top of the list is the benefit of lifestyle change, something that the dominance of industry sponsored clinical trials too often obscures.
- None of this does much to bolster confidence in the published literature. Nor am I reassured by discussions at two recent meetings co-hosted by the European Federation of Pharmaceutical Industry Associations (EFPIA). Drug company AbbVie is suing the European Medicines Agency to stop summary reports of its clinical trials becoming publicly available. AbbVie's lawyer made clear that the company considers even the data on adverse events to be commercially confidential.
- Despite industry's claims to be in favour of greater transparency, EFPIA and its American counterpart PhRMA are supporting Abbvie. The *BMJ* and BMA have joined forces to intervene on behalf of the European Medicines Agency.

Dr Godlee concludes: "*As for a way forward, I can't improve on the list of solutions proposed by Richard Lehman*"... "*All phase 3 trials to be designed and conducted independently of manufacturers, using the best available comparator. Research priorities to be determined by patients (James Lind Alliance). Value-based pricing. All data available from all trials, with meta-data: IPD [individual patient data] level for qualified independent centres. Big increase in comparative effectiveness research, much more research into non-pharmacological treatments.*"

Paper 494:
Healthy men should not take statins

Redberg RF et al Healthy men should not take statins.
Journal of the American Medical Association
2012 Apr 11;307(14):1491-2

Dr Rita Redberg, Editor of the *Archives of Internal Medicine* asks the following important questions for clinicians (and for patients):

Does treatment of elevated cholesterol levels with statins in otherwise healthy persons decrease mortality or prevent other serious outcomes?

What are the adverse effects associated with statin treatment in healthy persons?

Do the potential benefits outweigh the potential risks?

The answers to these questions suggest that statin therapy should not be recommended for men with elevated cholesterol who are otherwise healthy.

Does treatment of elevated cholesterol levels with statins in otherwise healthy persons decrease mortality or prevent other serious outcomes?

- Data from a meta-analysis of 11 trials including 65,229 persons with 244 000 person-years of follow-up in healthy but high-risk men and women showed no reduction in mortality associated with treatment with statins.
- A 2011 Cochrane review of treatment with statins among persons without documented coronary disease came to similar conclusions. The Cochrane review also observed that all but one of the clinical trials providing evidence on this issue were sponsored by the pharmaceutical industry.
- It is well established that industry-sponsored trials are more likely than non-industry-sponsored trials to report favourable results for drug treatment because of biased reporting, biased interpretation, or both of trial results.

What are the adverse effects associated with statin treatment in healthy persons?

- All treatments designed to prevent disease – such as death from coronary disease – can also result in adverse effects.

Data from observational studies show much higher rates for statin-associated myopathy and other adverse events in actual use than the 1% to 5% rate reported in clinical trials.

- This underestimation of adverse events occurs because the trials excluded up to 30% of patients with many common comorbidities, such as those with a history of muscular pains, as well as renal or hepatic insufficiency.
- Many randomized trials also excluded patients who had adverse effects of treatment during an open-label run-in period. For example, in the Treat to New Targets trial, after initial exclusions based on comorbidities, an additional 35% of eligible patients, or 16% of patients, were excluded during an eight-week, open-label, run-in phase because of adverse events, ischemic events, or participants' lipid levels while taking the drug not meeting entry criteria.
- Additionally, the results of randomized trials of statin treatment likely underestimate common symptoms such as myalgia, fatigue, and other minor muscle complaints because these studies often only collect data on more quantifiable adverse effects such as rhabdomyolysis.
- Numerous anecdotal reports as well as a small trial have suggested that statin therapy causes cognitive impairment.
- One population-based cohort study in Great Britain of more than two million statin users found that statin use was associated with increased risks of moderate or serious liver dysfunction, acute renal failure, moderate or serious myopathy, and cataract.
- The risk of diabetes with statin use has been seen in randomized clinical trials such as JUPITER, which found a 3% risk of developing diabetes in the rosuvastatin group, significantly higher than in the placebo group.
- In observational data from the Women's Health Initiative, there was an unadjusted 71% increased risk and 48% adjusted increased risk of diabetes in healthy women taking statins.

Do the potential benefits outweigh the potential risks?

- Based on all current evidence, a healthy man with elevated cholesterol will not live any longer if he takes statins. For every

100 patients with elevated cholesterol levels who take statins for five years, a myocardial infarction will be prevented in one or two patients.

- Preventing a heart attack is a meaningful outcome. However, by taking statins, one or more patients will develop diabetes and 20% or more will experience disabling symptoms, including muscle weakness, fatigue, and memory loss.

Dr Redberg concluded: *"Recent data on increased risk of diabetes, cognitive dysfunction, and muscle pain associated with statins suggest that there is risk with no evidence of benefit. Advising healthy patients to take a drug that does not offer the possibility to feel better or live longer and has significant adverse effects with potential decrement in quality of life is not in their interest"*.

Paper 495: Women should not be prescribed statins as they fail to provide any overall health benefit

Kendrick M Should women be offered cholesterol lowering drugs to prevent cardiovascular disease? No. *British Medical Journal* 2007 May 12; 334(7601): 983

Dr Malcolm Kendrick, a General Practioner from the UK, believes there is little or no evidence of health benefits for women taking statins.

He makes the following observations:

- To date, none of the large trials of secondary prevention with statins has shown a reduction in overall mortality in women.
- The primary prevention trials have shown neither an overall mortality benefit, nor even a reduction in cardiovascular end points in women.
- Statins carry a substantial burden of side effects.
- Mass medicalisation is a dangerous road with many psychological and societal consequences.
- In the Scandinavian simvastatin survival study, three more women died taking statins than the women who took the placebo.
- In the studies of primary prevention, neither total mortality nor serious adverse events have been reduced.

- A meta-analysis published in the *Lancet* found that statins even failed to reduce coronary heart disease events in women.
- Another meta-analysis of statins in primary prevention suggested that overall mortality may actually be increased by 1% over ten years (in both men and women).
- Data from 124,814 women in 19 studies and trials found that cholesterol levels had no impact on total death rates and heart disease.
- Studies have suggested that side effects from statins may be much more common than is recognised.
- One study found that 80% of athletes could not tolerate statins.
- Research by Golomb and McGraw found that doctors often dismiss most (probable) statin related events. Patients who met the criteria for definite or probable adverse events reported that their doctors tended to dismiss symptoms, deny specific statins adverse events, and failed to appreciate the effect of the adverse reaction on their quality of life.
- More evidence comes from the US Food and Drug Administration adverse event reporting system. Between November 1997 and May 2004 simvastatin was reported as a direct cause of 49,350 adverse events and 416 deaths. Adverse events are greatly under-reported, so the actual figures are likely to be much higher.
- Of further concern, as statins are increasingly prescribed to younger women, is the potential for birth defects, with severe neurological abnormalities reported. Spending millions on a treatment that has no proved benefit and may cause serious harm goes against the rationale of evidence based prescribing.

As no trials have shown that stains reduce death rates or heart disease in women, Dr Kendrick asks: "*This raises the important question whether women should be prescribed statins at all*".

After reviewing the evidence, Dr Kendrick answers: "*I believe that the answer is clearly no. Not only do statins fail to provide any overall health benefit in women, they represent a massive financial drain on health services. This money could be diverted to treatments of proved value*".

Paper 496:
The medical profession is running a massive statin drug trial on fat children and don't actually know what long-term effects statins will have on children

Radcliffe M We are running a massive drug trial on fat children. *Nursing Times* 2008 Jul 22-28;104(29):56

This article by Mark Radcliffe, a Senior Lecturer in the School of Nursing, University of Brighton, notes that American paediatricians are currently recommending wider cholesterol screening for overweight children and more aggressive use of cholesterol-lowering drugs, starting as early as the age of eight.

- Radcliffe comments: "*We don't actually know what effect statins will have on children. There is no research base yet and we are only going to find out by prescribing them and monitoring the long-term effects. So what we have is a potentially massive drug trial, on fat kids*".

He asks the very pertinent question: "*I wonder how history will judge that?*"

Paper 497:
Doctor finds that statins do not help diabetics and official guidelines regarding statin use should be re-examined and reformulated by experts independent from the pharmaceutical industry

de Lorgeril M et al Is the use of cholesterol-lowering drugs for the prevention of cardiovascular complications in type 2 diabetics evidence-based? A systematic review. *Reviews on Recent Clinical Trials* 2012 May;7(2):150-7

Dr Michel de Lorgeril is internationally known for his work on cardiovascular disease. In this paper, he systematically reviewed the results of high-quality double-blind trials testing whether cholesterol-lowering drugs (statins and fibrates) reduce mortality and cardiovascular complications specifically in type two diabetics.

The review of the scientific literature found four trials, three statin and one fibrate.

- Statin trials:
  - o The Collaborative Atorvastatin Diabetes Study (CARDS) trial was discontinued two years before the anticipated

end and in the absence of significant effect on both overall and cardiovascular mortality, suggesting that the trial should not have been prematurely stopped.

- o The Deutsche Diabetes Dialyse Studie (4D) trial showed no significant effect on heart attack, stroke or cardiovascular and overall death rates.
- o The Atorvastatin Study for Prevention of Coronary Heart Disease Endpoints in Non-Insulin-Dependent Diabetes Mellitus (ASPEN) trial showed no significant effect in nonfatal heart attacks, nonfatal stroke, coronary artery bypass surgery, resuscitated cardiac arrest, worsening or unstable angina requiring hospitalization or cardiovascular and overall death rates.

- Fibrate trial: The Fenofibrate Intervention and Event Lowering in Diabetes (FIELD) trial showed no significant effect on coronary heart disease death, non-fatal heart attack or death rates.

Dr de Lorgeril concluded: *"This review does not support the use of cholesterol-lowering drugs (such as statin and fibrate) to reduce mortality and cardiovascular complications in type two diabetics. Official guidelines should be re-examined and reformulated by experts independent from the pharmaceutical industry"*.

Paper 498:
Cardiologist asks for a full reappraisal of the cholesterol theory

de Lorgeril M et al Recent cholesterol-lowering drug trials: New data, new questions. *Journal of Lipid Nutrition* Vol. 19 (2010), No. 1 pp.65-92

The French cardiologist Dr Michel de Lorgeril again analysed the outcome of recent cholesterol-lowering drugs trials.

He found:

- The cholesterol-lowering drug trials published in 2008-2009, were either negative (ENHANCE, SEAS, GISSI-HF, AURORA) or obviously biased and therefore not credible (JUPITER).
- It is also noteworthy that most cholesterol-lowering drug trials published between 2005 (the year of the Vioxx affair and of enforcement of new clinical trial regulations) and 2007 were also negative or ambiguous (CORONA, ASPEN, 4D, PREVEND IT, IDEAL, and ILLUMINATE).

- Taken together, these trials strongly suggest that the results of previous, highly positive trials with statins – particularly in the secondary prevention of coronary heart disease – published between 1994 and 2004 and that were used to issue guidelines for medical practitioners, should be carefully re examined by experts independent from the pharmaceutical industry.
- The positive results from trials published between 1994 and 2004 were before the Vioxx affair and of enforcement of new clinical trial regulations. (Vioxx was a drug that was supposed to greatly relieve the pains of arthritis sufferers, the problem was that it caused heart attacks and strokes and three-fold increase in death rates. The company that manufactured the drug (Merck) tried to hide these side effects by manipulating data. Eventually the drug was withdrawn and now, in an attempt to prevent pharmaceutical companies hiding or manipulating evidence, the US Food and Drug Administration require that all pharmaceutical companies file any and all trial results to a federal registry within one year of the completion of the trial.)

With all the negative results of the recent statin trials, Dr de Lorgeril asks: *"Is it not time for a full reappraisal of the cholesterol theory?"*

Paper 499: Results from JUPITER statin trial raise troubling questions concerning the role of commercial sponsors

de Lorgeril M et al Cholesterol Lowering, Cardiovascular Diseases, and the Rosuvastatin-JUPITER Controversy. A Critical Reappraisal. *Archives of Internal Medicine* 2010;170(12):1032-1036

In this paper, Dr de Lorgeril notes that the results of cholesterol-lowering drug trials show no evidence that statin drugs lower the disease rates or death rates of people with or without coronary heart disease with one exception, and that is the JUPITER (Justification for the Use of Statins in Primary Prevention) trial. JUPITER reports a substantial decrease in the risk of cardiovascular diseases among patients without coronary heart disease and with normal or low cholesterol levels.

The results of the JUPITER study were met with a massive media fanfare proclaiming the benefits of statin drugs. This enthusiastic recommendation has no doubt persuaded many people with normal cholesterol levels to start long-term statin treatment.

The JUPITER trial tested the effects of rosuvastatin in patients without heart disease and with normal or low cholesterol levels but relatively high levels of C-reactive protein, a marker of inflammation. The study spanned 1,315 sites in 26 countries and included 17,802 people who were assigned either 20 mg/d of rosuvastatin or placebo.

Three recent trials with rosuvastatin (with the acronyms CORONA, GISSI-HF and AURORA) had been conducted, and all had failed to provide evidence that rosuvastatin therapy reduces heart disease complications.

The JUPITER trial was prematurely terminated on the grounds that it had generated evidence that the statin treatment had definitely reduced heart disease rates.

However, the evidence shows otherwise:

- If you include people who had fatal and nonfatal heart attack and stroke – the trial was stopped after only 240 incidents.
- There was no difference in the incidence of serious adverse events (total hospitalizations, prolongations of hospitalizations, cancer, and permanent disability) between the two groups.
- There was hardly any difference in death rates when the trial was ended, and the trend was showing that the statin groups death rate was increasing compared to the placebo group.

An "unequivocal reduction in cardiovascular mortality" was announced in March 2008 as the main justification for the premature trial termination.

However, the actual facts again beg to differ:

- Fatal heart attacks were nine in the statin group and six in the placebo group.
- Stroke death was three in the statin group compared to six taking the placebo.

So there were 12 cardiovascular deaths in each group. Hardly an "unequivocal reduction in cardiovascular mortality" as the JUPITER study authors concluded.

So why was the trial stopped early?

As stated earlier, JUPITER was hailed in the media as a ringing endorsement for us all to start statin therapy. This was achieved by the authors of the study only highlighting some results of the trial and completely ignoring other, less favourable data. It also raises the suspicion that if the trial had continued then the results would have shown statins in an even more unfavourable light.

Rosuvastatin (sold under the brand name crestor) is marketed and distributed by AstraZeneca Pharmaceuticals.

The JUPITER trial involved multiple conflicts of interest:

- o It was conducted by Astra Zeneca with their obvious commercial interests.
- o Nine of 14 authors of the JUPITER article have financial ties to the Astra Zeneca.
- o The principal investigator has a personal conflict of interest as a co-holder of the patent for the C-reactive protein test.
- o AstraZeneca's own investigators controlled and managed the raw data which increases the chance of bias appearing in the data.

Dr de Lorgeril's findings reveal:

- The results of the JUPITER trial are clinically inconsistent and therefore should not influence medical practice or clinical guidelines.
- The results of the JUPITER trial show that commercially sponsored clinical trials are at risk of poor quality and bias.
- The failure of the JUPITER trial to demonstrate a protective effect of rosuvastatin confirms the results of more than 12 other cholesterol-lowering trials published in recent years, which all provided no evidence of protection against heart disease by cholesterol lowering.
- These failed trials strongly suggest that the presumed preventive effects of cholesterol-lowering drugs have been considerably exaggerated.

Dr de Lorgeril concludes: "*The results of the trial do not support the use of statin treatment for primary prevention of cardiovascular diseases and raise troubling questions concerning the role of commercial sponsors. Clearly the time has come for a critical reappraisal of cholesterol-lowering and statin treatments for the prevention of coronary heart disease complications. The emphasis on pharmaceuticals for the prevention of coronary heart disease diverts individual and public health attention away from the proven efficacy of adopting a healthy lifestyle".*

Paper 500:
Doctor says there is no evidence that statins are safe

Nehrlich HH Statins – Safe? *Canadian Medical Association Journal* May 6: 2008

Dr Herbert Nehrlich, a doctor from Australia, discusses the effects of statin drugs.

- Statins reduce the body's production of mevalonate through the suppression of a liver enzyme called hydroxymethylglutaryl (HMG) coenzyme A reductase.
- This enzyme is crucial in enabling the body to synthesize such substances as cholesterol, coenzyme Q-10 etc., substances that are essential for every living cell.
- So, if you reduce the supply of mevalonate, the liver can no longer keep up production of sufficient cholesterol and has to slow the shipping of cholesterol from the depot (liver) to the various areas in need of it via the bloodstream. Hence, blood cholesterol will be lower in lab tests.
- Mevalonate is not just important in this respect but is heavily involved in muscle metabolism as well as in the production of thromboxane. Thromboxane, of course, is the agent responsible for the important stage in healing called clotting and originates in the platelets of our blood.
- Mitochondria are energy factories that MUST have coenzyme Q-10, the very substance that is in short supply when people undergo statin treatment.
- The dismal success record of statin treatment, combined with their sometimes atrocious side effects (identified and hidden) makes the prescription of statins in humans an assault with unknown and likely dire consequences.
- People tend to die with low cholesterol blood levels.
- May I ask for the studies that have shown that lowering cholesterol is reasonable and thus good practice? Statins are

safe? Let us look at the PROSPER Trial and the all cause mortality. It is not improved by statins.

- I prefer to see cholesterol as an extremely vital substance, essential for good health and indispensable when it comes to repair and maintenance of the body.
- Statins are now Big Pharma's golden goose and the price of gold is rising.
- If we think of rhabdomyolysis, of transient global amnesia and of the propensity of statins to initiate cancer in many animals, if we consider the truly dismal success of statin treatment then we can skip looking at the plausibility of using these drugs altogether.
- Statins are mayhem to Coenzyme Q-10 and it follows that statins may thus weaken the heart. They may cause cancer in humans.

Dr Nehrlich concludes: "*There is no evidence that statins are safe*".

The papers in this chapter were authored by doctors, professors, cardiologists, vascular surgeons, the president of the Royal College of Physicians, and the editors of two peer-reviewed scientific journals *The British Medical Journal* and *The Archives of Internal Medicine.*

These papers present the viewpoint that statins provide no benefit but have many toxic side effects.

- Statin use may lead to low cholesterol and many health problems.
- Advertising by statin manufacturers promotes risky use of statins.
- Health legislation and payment incentives in the UK and USA make it virtually compulsory for doctors to prescribe statins.
- Doctors under-report the side effects of statins because they don't know of them, or they don't believe when the patients complain of adverse effects.
- Statins increase the risk of diabetes and don't prevent cardiovascular disease.
- Men, women, children and the elderly should not take statins.
- Statins trials are at risk of bias because they are generally funded by statin manufacturers.

- Statin manufacturers exaggerate the benefits, but hide the harmful side effects of the drugs.
- There are conflicts of interest in the people that recommend cholesterol lowering guidelines.
- A full re-appraisal of the cholesterol theory should be initiated and the cholesterol lowering guidelines should be re-assessed by experts independent from the pharmaceutical industry.
- There is no proof that statins work in the real world and no evidence that statins are safe.

Chapter 21

Summary of the evidence

- The scientific evidence has revealed that statins do not save lives. The data from some studies show that statins increase the death rate in those who are healthy, those who have "high" cholesterol and patients with a diverse range of conditions and diseases.
- Since the advent of statin drugs there has been an epidemic of heart failure. This may be because statins weaken the heart by depleting levels of the essential nutrient, coenzyme Q10.
- The risk of brain hemorrhage is also increased in people using statins.
- Diabetes risk is exacerbated by statin use. Statins increase insulin levels, insulin resistance and blood glucose levels, all of which increase the likelihood of diabetes.
- Long-term use of statins has been shown to increase cancer rates, possibly by inhibiting the production of selenoproteins.
- Muscle pain and muscle damage is a common occurrence in people prescribed statins. Many studies reveal that at least a quarter of statins users suffer muscle problems.
- A serious muscle disease, rhabdomyolysis, is a statin side effect that can lead to kidney failure, liver disease, pancreatitis and multiorgan failure.
- Statins interfere with liver function. Some people will suffer immediate liver damage, whilst in others the damage will manifest and worsen over time.
- Studies have shown that statin users have a 40% increased risk of pancreatitis.
- Long-term statins users have a 27-fold increase in neuropathy, a disease in which statins damage the peripheral nerves especially in the outer extremities of the body.

- The medical literature reveals that statins may trigger or aggravate autoimmune diseases such as lupus, an can also promote a variety of skin abnormalities.
- Statins can also stimulate asthma, cause lung disease and reduce the capacity of people to exercise. 80% of athletes don't tolerate statins and older people's ability to walk is diminished.
- Brain function is slowed down when taking statins. Statins have been shown to increase the risk of neurodegenerative diseases such as Alzheimer's, dementia, Parkinson's, multiple sclerosis and amyotrophic lateral sclerosis.
- Increase in irritability, anger, aggression and violence are associated with statins, as is an elevated danger of depression and suicidal thoughts.
- Cataracts, macular degeneration, double vision and eye fatigue are abnormalities linked to statins.
- Statins increase impotence in men and birth defects in babies.
- A whole host of many other diseases, conditions and injuries may also be caused or worsened by statins.
- A large percentage of people report having adverse effects when taking statin drugs. Data from one trial revealed that nearly all the participants suffered from side effects.
- Statins poison us by their effects of blocking the mevalonate pathway. They inhibit the production of vital and essential molecules and compounds such as cholesterol, coenzyme Q10, dolichols, selenoproteins, isopentenyl adenine, prenylated proteins, heme A and some vitamins, minerals and antioxidants.
- By inhibiting the above molecules and compounds, statins promote and worsen an almost infinite number of ailments.
- Vested financial interests have been the driving force in the clamour of official advice to ever lower cholesterol level targets, and ever increase the number of people eligible for statin drugs.
- Statins generate $34 billion in annual sales. Data from 192 countries from the World Health Organisation shows that people with lower cholesterol have higher overall death rates and even higher death rates from cardiovascular causes.
- Eminent doctors and professors have commented on the increased risk of health problems associated with statin use:
    - Legislation and advertising has resulted in a massive over prescription of statin drugs.

- o Doctors and scientific researchers receive $billions over the years in payments from statin manufacturers.
- o Statin manufacturers fund most of their drug trials.
- o Statin drug trials are flawed and designed to show positive results for the drug.
- o Data suggests statins and dangerous for all sections of society such as men, women, children, the elderly and the unborn fetus.

I shall leave you with the thoughts of Dr Michel de Lorgeril, the internationally renowned cardiologist:

"*We'll come to the inevitable conclusion in the end that these drugs are unnecessary and toxic, they must be removed from the market*".

Appendix 1

Glossary

3-hydroxy-3-methylglutaryl-coenzyme (HMG-CoA) reductase inhibitors
Statins full name.

Abdominal aortic aneurysm
Dilation (ballooning) of part of the aorta that is within the abdomen.

Acipimox
Reduces the amount of certain lipids in the blood.

Acute coronary syndrome
Term given by doctors for various heart conditions, including heart attack and unstable angina.

Acute generalised exanthematous pustulosis
Skin eruption characterised by superficial pustules.

Adenoma
A type of non-cancerous tumour that may have the potential to become cancerous.

Alanine (amino)transaminase
Transaminase enzyme. Elevated levels may be an indicator of liver damage.

Alkaline phosphatase
Protein found in all body tissues. Tissues with higher amounts include the liver, bile ducts, and bone.

Amitriptyline
Antidepressant, also prescribed to relieve pain and aid sleep.

Amylase
Enzyme that helps digest carbohydrates.

Amyotrophic lateral sclerosis
Progressive neurodegenerative disease that affects nerve cells in the brain and the spinal cord.

Aneurysm
Bulge in a blood vessel that's caused by a weakness in the blood vessel wall.

Angina
Chest pain caused by the blood flow to the heart muscles being restricted.

Angioplasty
Technique of mechanically widening narrowed or obstructed arteries.

Anicteric hepatitis
Hepatitis without jaundice.

Antinuclear antibodies
Found in patients whose immune system is predisposed to cause inflammation against their own body tissues.

Anti-neutrophil cytoplasmic antibodies (ANCAs)
Group of autoantibodies associated with a number of autoimmune disorders particularly with systemic vasculitis, so called ANCA-associated vasculitides.

Antioxidants
Substances that may prevent or delay some types of cell damage.

Antisynthetase syndrome
Autoimmune disease affecting the muscles, lungs and joints.

Aortic stenosis
Obstruction of blood flow across the aortic valve.

Arthritis
Condition that causes pain and inflammation in a joint.

Arthropathy
Collective term for any disease of the joints.

Aspartate (amino)transaminase
Transaminase enzyme. Elevated levels may be an indicator of liver damage.

Asthenia
Loss or lack of bodily strength.

Asthma
Inflammation of the airways.

AstraZeneca
British-Swedish multinational pharmaceutical company that markets rosuvastatin. It is the world's seventh-largest pharmaceutical company.

Atherosclerosis
Build up of plague inside the arteries.

Atorvastatin
Type of statin marketed by Pfizer under the trade name lipitor.

Atrial fibrillation
Heart condition that causes an irregular and often abnormally fast heart rate.

Atrium
Two blood collection chambers of the heart. The atrium is a chamber in which blood enters the heart, as opposed to the ventricle, where it is pushed out of the organ.

Autoimmune disease
Occurs when the body's immune system attacks and destroys healthy body tissue by mistake.

Bacille Calmette–Guérin vaccine
Provides immunity or protection against tuberculosis. It is also used to treat bladder tumors or bladder cancer.

Balloon angioplasty
Angioplasty.

Balloon occlusion test
A test to see whether one artery can be temporarily or permanently blocked without significantly affecting the level of blood in your brain. The procedure utilizes an X-ray and a special dye to create detailed images of your arteries and a small balloon, which when inflated will temporarily block your artery.

Basal cell carcinoma
Type of skin cancer.

Benign prostatic hyperplasia
Increase in size of the prostate gland without malignancy present and it is so common as to be normal with advancing age.

Bile Acid Sequestrants
Medications that lower LDL cholesterol levels.

Bilirubin
Yellowish pigment found in bile, a fluid made by the liver.

Biochemical recurrence
A rise in the blood level of prostate-specific antigen (PSA) in prostate cancer patients after treatment with surgery or radiation.

Blunt trauma
Injury caused by a blunt object or collision with a blunt surface, as in a vehicle accident or fall from a building.

Bristol-Myers Squibb
Large American pharmaceutical company that markets pravastatin.

Calcific aortic stenosis
Where calcium deposits narrow the aortic valve of the heart and decrease blood flow from the heart.

Canadian Cardiovascular Society Angina Grading
Commonly used for the classification of severity of angina

Cancer
Condition where cells in a specific part of the body grow and reproduce uncontrollably.

Carcinoma
Cancer that begins in the skin or in tissues that line or cover body organs.

Cardiac insufficiency
Medical term that refers to a type of heart failure in which the heart is not able to pump enough blood throughout the body.

Cardiologist
Doctor with special training and skill in finding, treating and preventing diseases of the heart and blood vessels.

Cardiometabolic
Concerning both heart disease and metabolic disorders such as diabetes.

Cardiopulmonary bypass
Technique that temporarily takes over the function of the heart and lungs during surgery, maintaining the circulation of blood and the oxygen content of the body.

Cardiovascular diseases
A class of diseases that involve the heart or blood vessels, such as heart disease, heart failure and stroke.

Cardiovascular event
Any incident that may cause damage to the heart muscle. E.g. arrhythmias, heart valve disease, enlarged heart, carotid or coronary artery disease and chest pain.

Carotid Intima-Media Thickness Test
Measures the thickness of the inner two layers of the carotid artery – the intima and media.

Celecoxib
Drug prescribed to prevent cancer.

Cholestasis (cholestatic hepatitis, cholestatic jaundice)
Can occur when the normal flow of bile from the liver to the small intestine is interrupted by either a blockage in the duct system or a side effect of medications.

Cholesterol
A waxy substance found in your body that is needed to produce hormones, vitamin D and bile. Cholesterol is also important for protecting nerves and for the structure of cells.

Cholestyramine
Drug used for reducing cholesterol levels.

Coenzyme Q10 (CoQ10)
Substance that's found naturally in the body and helps convert food into energy. CoQ10 is found in almost every cell in the body, and it is a powerful antioxidant.

Cohort
Group of subjects who have shared a particular event together during a particular time span.

Colestipol
Bile acid sequestrant used to lower blood cholesterol.

Collagen
Major constituent of bone and provides the bone with strength and flexibility.

Collateral blood vessels
Small capillary-like branches of an artery that form over time in response to narrowed coronary arteries. The collaterals "bypass" the area of narrowing and help to restore blood flow.

Colorectal
Relating to or affecting the colon and rectum.

Compartment syndrome
Painful and potentially serious condition caused by bleeding or swelling within an enclosed bundle of muscles (a muscle "compartment").

Congestive heart failure
Condition in which the body's tissues aren't receiving enough blood and oxygen due to the heart's reduced pumping action.

Coronary artery bypass graft
Surgical procedure performed to relieve angina and reduce the risk of death from coronary artery disease.

Coronary artery bypass surgery
See coronary artery bypass graft.

Coronary artery calcification
Build up of calcium deposits in the coronary arteries.

Coronary artery calcium scan
Test that looks for specks of calcium in the walls of the coronary (heart) arteries. The amount of calcium detected in the coronary arteries is converted to a calcium score. A high coronary artery calcium score is an independent predictor of coronary heart disease events.

Coronary artery disease
Coronary heart disease.

Coronary heart disease
The narrowing or blockage of the coronary arteries.

Coronary revascularisation procedures
Coronary artery bypass graft and coronary angioplasty with and without stenting. Procedures used to restore adequate blood flow to blocked coronary arteries.

Cortical stroke
Occurs when the blood supply to the outside, or cortex, of the brain is reduced or blocked, which results in brain damage.

Cortico-subcortical region of the brain
Outer layers and the area beneath the outer layers of the brain.

C-reactive protein
Produced by the liver. The level of C-reactive protein rises when there is inflammation throughout the body.

Creatine kinase (see creatine phosphokinase)

Creatine phosphokinase
Enzyme found mainly in the heart, brain, and skeletal muscle. (High levels are considered a marker of muscle damage.)

Creatinine
Formed by the metabolism of creatine, that is found in muscle tissue and blood and normally excreted in the urine as a metabolic waste.

Crestor
Trade name of rosuvastatin.

Deep vein thrombosis
Blood clot in a vein. Blood clots in veins most often occur in the legs but can occur elsewhere in the body, including the arms.

Delirium
Severe confusion and disorientation.

Dermatologist
Medical expert that is concerned with the diagnosis and treatment of diseases of the skin, hair and nails.

Dermatomyositis
Muscle disease that involves inflammation and a skin rash.

Diabetes
Disease in which there are high blood sugar levels over a prolonged period. Untreated, diabetes can cause many complications which include heart disease, stroke, kidney failure, foot ulcers and damage to the eyes.

Diastolic
Referring to the time when the heart is in a period of relaxation and dilatation (expansion). In a blood pressure reading, the diastolic pressure is typically the second number recorded. For example, with a blood pressure of 120/80 ("120 over 80"), the diastolic pressure is 80. By "80" is meant 80 mm Hg (millimetres of mercury).

Dolichols
Compounds that play an important role in cell vitality, immune system health and in helping the body build proteins and other important compounds.

Double-blind study
A study in which neither the subject nor the investigator nor the research team interacting with the subject or data during the trial knows what treatment a subject is receiving (e.g. active or placebo).

Dysglycemia
Defined as diabetes and/or impaired fasting glucose.

Dysphagia
Medical term for swallowing difficulties.

Echocardiogram
A test that uses sound waves to create pictures of the heart. The picture is more detailed than a standard X-ray image.

Ejection fraction
Measurement of the percentage of blood leaving the heart each time it contracts.

Elective cardiac surgery
Planned, non-emergency surgical procedure on the heart or major blood vessels.

Electromyography (EMG)
Diagnostic procedure to assess the health of muscles and the nerve cells that control them (motor neurons).

Endocrinology
Branch of medicine that deals with the diagnosis and treatment of diseases related to hormones.

Endothelial cells
Thin layer of cells that line the interior surface of blood vessels and lymphatic vessels.

Eosinophilic fasciitis
Disease in which muscle tissue under the skin, called fascia, becomes swollen and thick.

Epidemiologic Study
The study of health in populations to understand the causes and patterns of health and illness.

Erectile dysfunction
Inability to get and maintain an erection.

Erythrocyte sedimentation rate
Test that indirectly measures the degree of inflammation present in the body.

Ezetimibe
A drug that lowers cholesterol levels by decreasing cholesterol absorption in the small intestine.

F-actin cytoskeleton
Part of the cells scaffolding or skeleton.

Fasciotomy
Surgical procedure that cuts away the fascia to relieve tension or pressure.

Fasting blood sugar levels
A measurement of blood glucose after you have not eaten for at least eight hours. It is often the first test done to check for prediabetes and diabetes.

Fenofibrate
Type of fibrate. Used to reduce cholesterol levels.

Fibrates
Fibric acid derivative agents that are used to lower plasma lipids, particularly triglyceride levels.

Fluvastatin
Type of statin marketed by Novartis under the trade name lescol.

Focal myositis
Inflammatory pseudotumor of skeletal muscle.

Gamma-glutamyltransferase (gamma-glutamyl transpeptidase)
See γ glutamyl transferase.

Gastroenterology
Branch of medicine focused on the digestive system and its disorders.

Gemfibrozil
Generic name for an oral drug used to lower lipid levels. It belongs to a group of drugs known as fibrates.

Gilbert's syndrome
Hereditary cause of raised bilirubin and may lead to bouts of jaundice.

Gleason score
The Gleason score provides an effective measurement that helps determine how severe the level of prostate cancer. Scores from two to four are very low on the cancer aggression scale. Scores from five to six are mildly aggressive. A score of seven indicates that the cancer is moderately aggressive. Scores from eight to ten indicate that the cancer is highly aggressive.

Glucose
Common carbohydrate. Also called dextrose. In the human bloodstream it is called blood sugar.

Glutamic oxaloacetic transaminase
See aspartate (amino)transaminase.

Glycated haemoglobin (HbA1c)
Develops when haemoglobin, a protein within red blood cells that carries oxygen throughout your body, joins with glucose in the blood,

becoming 'glycated'. By measuring glycated haemoglobin, clinicians are able to get an overall picture of what our average blood sugar levels have been over a period of weeks/months. For people with diabetes this is important as the higher the HbA1c, the greater the risk of developing diabetes-related complications.

Glycemia
Refers to the concentration of sugar or glucose in the blood.

Glycaemic control
Medical term referring to the typical levels of blood sugar (glucose) in a person with diabetes. Many of the long-term complications of diabetes result from many years of elevated levels of glucose in the blood.

Guillain–Barré syndrome
Disorder affecting the peripheral nervous system.

Haematocrit (packed cell volume (PCV) or erythrocyte volume fraction (EVF))
Blood test that measures the percentage of the volume of whole blood that is made up of red blood cells. This measurement depends on the number of red blood cells and the size of red blood cells.

Haemofiltration
Kidney replacement therapy similar to haemodialysis.

Haemodialysis
The filtering of circulating blood through an apparatus to remove waste products.

HbA1c
Term for glycated haemoglobin.

Heart failure
Condition in which the heart can't pump enough blood to meet the body's needs.

Heme A
Important component in the system of mitochondrial energy production.

Hemodynamics
The study of blood flow or the circulation.

Hepatic toxicity
Implies chemical-driven liver damage.

Hepatology
Branch of medicine that incorporates the study of liver, gallbladder, biliary tree, and pancreas as well as management of their disorders.

High density lipoprotein (HDL cholesterol)
HDL particles can pick up cholesterol from other tissues and transport it back to the liver for re-processing and/or disposal as bile salts.

HMG CoA reductase inhibitors
Full name of statins.

HOmeostasis Model Assessment (HOMA-IR)
Method used to quantify insulin resistance and beta-cell function. Low HOMA values indicate high insulin sensitivity, whereas high HOMA values indicate insulin resistance.

Hypercholesterolemia
Alleged, "high" levels of cholesterol in the blood.

Hyperlipidemia
"High" lipid levels.

Hypertension
High blood pressure.

Hyperthyroidism
Increase in activity of the thyroid gland.

Hypertriglyceridemia
Condition in which triglyceride levels are elevated.

Hypoesthetic
An abnormally low sensitivity to stimuli.

Hypothyroidism (under active thyroid)
Disorder in which the thyroid gland does not produce enough thyroid hormone.

ICU
Intensive care unit.

Immunotherapy
Treatment of disease by inducing, enhancing, or suppressing an immune response.

Impaired fasting glucose (prediabetes)
Refers to a condition in which the fasting blood glucose level is consistently elevated above what is considered normal levels; however, it is not high enough to be diagnosed as diabetes.

Impaired glucose tolerance
Where blood glucose is raised beyond the normal range but it is not so high to have diabetes.

Inegy
Combination of ezetimibe and simvastatin. Marketed by Merck.

Insulin
A hormone produced by beta cells in the pancreas. With each meal, beta cells release insulin to help the body use or store the glucose it gets from food.

Insulin resistance
A condition in which the body produces insulin but does not use it effectively. When people have insulin resistance, glucose builds up in the blood instead of being absorbed by the cells, leading to type two diabetes or prediabetes.

Insulin sensitivity
Describes how sensitive the body is to the effects of insulin. Someone said to be insulin sensitive will require smaller amounts of insulin to lower blood glucose levels than someone who has low sensitivity. Low insulin sensitivity can lead to a variety of health problems. The body will try to compensate for having a low sensitivity to insulin by

producing more insulin. However, a high level of circulating insulin (hyperinsulinemia) is associated with damage to blood vessels, high blood pressure, heart disease and heart failure, diabetes, obesity, osteoporosis and even cancer.

Internist
Doctor that specializes in the diagnosis and medical (nonsurgical) treatment of adults.

Interstitial lung disease
Name for a large group of diseases that inflame or scar the lungs.

Intra-aortic balloon pump
The intra-aortic balloon pump, also called the balloon pump, is a machine that helps the heart pump blood throughout the body. It consists of two parts: a balloon inserted into the aorta, one of the large arteries through which blood passes from the heart to the rest of the body; and a machine outside the body. The intra-aortic balloon pump is used when the heart cannot pump enough blood on its own.

Intracerebral
Within the brain.

Intracranial
Within the skull.

Intraoperative
Occurring, carried out, or encountered in the course of surgery.

Intravenous thrombolysis
The use of thrombolytic drugs to break down and dissolve blood clots.

Invasive ductal carcinoma
Refers to cancer that has broken through the wall of the milk duct and begun to invade the tissues of the breast.

Invasive lobular carcinoma
This means that the cancer started in the cells that line the lobules of the breast and has spread into the surrounding breast tissue.

Ischemic stroke
Occurs when an artery to the brain is blocked.

Isoprenoids
Compounds that play widely varying roles in the physical and chemical processes of plants and animals.

Kennedy's disease
Motor neuron disease that affects males.

Kidney disease (renal failure)
Condition where the kidneys do not work effectively.

Kowa Pharmaceuticals America
Global pharmaceutical organisation that markets pitavastatin.

Lactate dehydrogenase
Enzyme that catalyzes the conversion of lactate to pyruvate.

Large fibre neuropathy
Characterized by numbness, tingling, weakness and loss of deep tendon reflexes.

Lescol
Trade name of fluvastatin.

Lipase
Enzyme produced by the pancreas to help digest dietary fats.

Lipids
Group of naturally occurring molecules that include fats, waxes, sterols, fat-soluble vitamins (such as vitamins A, D, E, and K), monoglycerides, diglycerides, triglycerides, phospholipids, and others.

Lipitor
Trade name of atorvastatin.

Lipoprotein
Combination of a lipid (fat) surrounded by a protein. Carries nutrients around the body.

Livalo
Trade name of pitavastatin.

Liver disease (hepatic disease)
Damage or disease of the liver.

Liver enzymes (elevated)
Elevated liver enzymes may indicate inflammation or damage to cells in the liver.

Liver enzyme tests
Group of blood tests that detect inflammation and damage to the liver.

Liver function tests
See liver enzyme tests

Lovastatin
Type of statin marketed by Merck under the trade name mevacor.

Low density lipoprotein (LDL cholesterol)
LDL delivers important nutrients such as cholesterol, phospholipids, vitamins E, K1, K2, carotenoids, alpha lipoic acid and coenzyme Q10 to the cells and tissues of the body.

L-Thyroxine
Synthetic form of the human hormone thyroxine.

Lung disease
Refers to many disorders affecting the lungs, such as asthma, infections like influenza, pneumonia and tuberculosis, lung cancer, and many other breathing problems.

Lupus
Can cause various symptoms, the most common being joint pains, skin rashes and tiredness. Problems with kidneys and other organs can occur in severe cases.

Lymphangioleiomyomatosis
Rare progressive cystic lung disease.

Lymphoid malignancies
Cancer of the lymphatic system. Includes lymphoma and myeloma.

Lymphoma
Cancer that starts in the lymph glands or other organs of the lymphatic system.

Magnetic resonance imaging
Medical imaging technique used to visualize internal structures of the body in detail and can create more detailed images of the human body than possible with X-rays.

Major histocompatibility complex-I
Cell surface molecule that interacts with white blood cells to destroy diseased cells.

McArdle's disease
Enzyme deficiency (myophosphorylase) which renders patients unable to release glucose from glycogen in muscle.

Melanoma
The most lethal form of skin cancer

Merck
American pharmaceutical company that markets lovastatin and simvastatin. One of the largest pharmaceutical companies in the world.

Meralgia paresthetica
Numbness or pain in the outer thigh not caused by injury to the thigh, but by injury to a nerve that extends from the thigh to the spinal column.

Merkel cell carcinoma
Rare type of skin cancer. It develops in Merkel cells which are in the top layer of the skin.

Meta-analysis
Systematic method that takes data from a number of independent studies and integrates them using statistical analysis.

Metabolic acidosis
Occurs when the body produces too much acid, or when the kidneys are not removing enough acid from the body.

Mevacor
Trade name of lovastatin.

Mevalonate Pathway
The Mevalonate pathway is an important metabolic pathway which plays a key role in multiple cellular processes by synthesizing sterol isoprenoids, such as cholesterol, and non-sterol isoprenoids, such as dolichol, heme-A, isopentenyl tRNA and ubiquinone.

Microalbuminuria
This is when excess amounts of a protein called albumin pass through the kidneys and into the urine. This can be a sign of underlying conditions such as kidney disease or cardiovascular disease.

Microbleeds
Pinpoint drops of blood that leak from blood vessels in the brain that may increase the risk of stroke and cognitive dysfunction.

Microhaemorrhages
See microbleeds.

Mitochondria
Are often referred to as the powerhouses of the cells. They generate the energy that our cells need to do their jobs.

Mitochondrial myopathy
Disease caused by damage to the mitochondria.

Modified Rankin scale
Measures the degree of disability in people that have suffered a stroke and runs from 0-6 where 0 is perfect health without symptoms and 6 is death.

Mononeuritis multiplex
Damage to one or more peripheral nerves.

Mononeuropathy
Type of neuropathy that only affects a single nerve.

Multiorgan failure
Failure of several interdependent organ systems.

Multiple myeloma
Type of bone marrow cancer.

Musculoskeletal
The musculoskeletal system is made up of the body's bones (the skeleton), muscles, cartilage, tendons, ligaments, joints, and other connective tissue that supports and binds tissues and organs together.

Myalgia
Muscle pain.

Myeloma (multiple myeloma)
Cancer arising from plasma cells, a type of white blood cell which is made in the bone marrow.

Myocardial infarction
Heart attack.

Myoglobin
Protein in heart and skeletal muscles.

Myopathy
Disease of the muscles.

Myositis
Inflammation of the muscles.

Myotonic dystrophy
Progressive muscle wasting and weakness.

Naproxen
Nonsteroidal anti-inflammatory (NSAID) drug.

National cholesterol Education Program
US government program set up to persuade the medical profession and the public to lower cholesterol levels.

Necrotizing myopathy
Disorder in which the muscle fibres suffer destruction.

Neoplasm
A tumour; any new and abnormal growth, specifically one in which cell multiplication is uncontrolled and progressive. Neoplasms may be benign or malignant.

Nervous system
Consists of the brain, spinal cord, sensory organs, and all of the nerves that connect these organs with the rest of the body.

Neuroleptic malignant syndrome
Life-threatening neurological disorder most often caused by an adverse reaction to neuroleptic or antipsychotic drugs.

Neurology
Branch of medicine concerned with the study and treatment of disorders of the nervous system. (Brain, spinal cord, and nerves.)

Neuromuscular
Relating to nerves and muscles.

Neuropathy
See peripheral neuropathy.

New York Heart Association Functional Classification
Provides a simple way of classifying the extent of heart failure. It places patients in one of four categories based on how much they are limited during physical activity. Class I is mild cardiac disease, whilst class IV is very severe cardiac disease.

Niacin
Sometimes prescribed to lower "high" cholesterol.

Niacinamide
Type of vitamin B3. Decreases LDL cholesterol.

Non-insulin-dependent diabetes mellitus
Type two diabetes.

Non-melanoma skin cancer
Group of cancers that slowly develop in the upper layers of the skin.

Novartis
Swiss multinational pharmaceutical that markets fluvastatin. Ranked number one in sales among the world-wide industry in 2013.

NSAIDs (nonsteroidal anti-inflammatory drugs)
Among the most common pain relief medicines in the world.

Oliguria
Defined as passing a reduced urine volume. It is a clinical characteristic of acute kidney injury

Osteoblasts
Cells that helps to build bone.

Osteoclasts
Type of cell that destroys bone.

Otolaryngologists
Physicians trained in the medical and surgical management and treatment of patients with diseases and disorders of the ear, nose, throat, and related structures of the head and neck.

Pancreatitis
Inflammation in the pancreas. Symptoms include: nausea/sickness ; abdominal pain below the ribs, often spreading to the back; poor digestion, resulting in pale stools and weight loss.

Parallel study
Type of clinical study where two groups of treatments, A and B, are given so that one group receives only A while another group receives only B.

PCSK9 (proprotein convertase subtilisin/kexin type 9) inhibitor
Inhibits the PCSK9 enzyme to lower cholesterol.

Percutaneous coronary intervention
Term for angioplasty.

Pericarditis
Swelling of the pericardium, which is the fluid-filled sac surrounding the heart.

Perioperative
The period of time extending from when the patient goes into the hospital, clinic, or doctor's office for surgery until the time the patient is discharged home.

Peripheral neuropathy
Damage to your peripheral nerves, often causes weakness, numbness and pain, usually in your hands and feet.

Pfizer
American multinational pharmaceutical corporation that markets atorvastatin. It is one of the world's largest pharmaceutical companies.

Pharmacoepidemiology
The study of the utilization and effects of drugs in large numbers of patients.

Pitavastatin
Type of statin marketed by Kowa Pharmaceuticals America under the trade name livalo.

Placebo
Placebo-controlled studies are a way of testing a medical therapy in which, in addition to a group of subjects that receives the treatment to be evaluated, a separate control group receives a sham "placebo" treatment which is specifically designed to have no real effect.

Plasma
The liquid portion of blood – a protein-salt solution in which red and white blood cells and platelets are suspended. Plasma, which is 92% water, constitutes 55% of blood volume.

Polycystic ovary syndrome
Condition where a woman's hormones are out of balance. It can cause period problems, reduced fertility, excess hair growth, and acne.

Polymyalgia rheumatica
Condition that causes pain, stiffness and inflammation in the muscles around the shoulders, neck and hips.

Polymyositis
Chronic inflammation of many muscles.

Polyneuropathy
Damage or disease affecting peripheral nerves.

Polyp
An abnormal growth of tissue projecting from a mucous membrane.

Pravachol
Trade name of pravastatin.

Pravastatin
Type of statin marketed by Bristol-Myers Squibb under the trade name pravachol.

Prediabetes
See impaired fasting glucose.

Prospective study
A study in which the subjects are first identified and then followed forward as time passes.

Pulmonary embolism
Blockage in the artery that transports blood to the lungs (pulmonary artery). It is usually caused by a blood clot.

Radical cystectomy
The removal of the entire bladder, nearby lymph nodes, part of the urethra, and nearby organs that may contain cancer cells.

Radical prostatectomy
Operation to remove the prostate gland and some of the tissue around it. It is done to remove prostate cancer.

Radical retropubic prostatectomy
Surgical procedure in which the prostate gland is removed through an incision in the abdomen. It is most often used to treat individuals who have early prostate cancer.

Renal
Kidneys.

Renal cell carcinoma
The most common type of kidney cancer.

Resins
Bind to bile acids in the intestine and prevent them from being reabsorbed into the blood. The liver then produces more bile to replace the bile that has been lost. Because the body needs cholesterol to make bile, the liver uses up the cholesterol in the blood, which reduces the amount of LDL cholesterol circulating in the blood.

Restenosis
Recurrence of stenosis, a narrowing of a blood vessel, leading to restricted blood flow.

Retrospective study
A study that looks backward in time, usually using medical records and interviews with patients.

Rhabdomyolysis
Condition in which damaged skeletal muscle tissue breaks down and is released into the bloodstream which may lead to kidney failure.

Rippling muscle disease
Characterized by painful muscle stiffness involving skeletal muscle contractions which produces a visible rippling effect.

Rosuvastatin
Type of statin marketed by AstraZeneca under the trade name Crestor.

Simvastatin
Type of statin marketed by Merck under the trade name zocor.

Single blind study
Study or clinical trial in which the researchers but not the subjects know which subjects are receiving the active medication or treatment and which are not.

Sleep apnea
Disorder in which you have one or more pauses in breathing or shallow breaths while you sleep. As a result, the quality of your sleep is poor, which makes you tired during the day.

Small fibre neuropathy
Condition characterized by severe pain attacks that typically begin in the feet or hands.

Statins
A class of drugs used to lower cholesterol levels. They have many adverse side effects.

Stent thrombosis
This is when a previously placed stent in a heart artery (coronary artery) suddenly becomes blocked by a blood clot. This can result in a heart attack or even death.

Strain imaging
Echocardiographic tool that evaluates the function of the heart muscle using cardiac ultrasound.

Stroke
The sudden death of brain cells in a localised area due to inadequate blood flow.

Subarachnoid
Refers to the space in the brain between the arachnoid and the pia mater.

Thiazolidinediones
Medications used in the treatment of type 2 diabetes.

Thrombolysis
Pharmacological treatment to dissolve dangerous clots in blood vessels, improve blood flow, and prevent damage to tissues and organs. Is often used as an emergency treatment to dissolve blood clots that form in arteries feeding the heart and brain.

Thrombocytopenia
Medical term for a low blood platelet count.

Thromboembolism
Formation in a blood vessel of a clot (thrombus) that breaks loose and is carried by the blood stream to plug another vessel. The clot may plug a vessel in the lungs (pulmonary embolism), brain (stroke), gastrointestinal tract, kidneys, or leg.

Thyroid stimulating hormone
High levels indicate hypothyroidism.

Thyroxine (T4)
Thyroid hormone.

Tissue Doppler imaging
Echocardiographic tool that assesses heart function.

Transaminases (alanine transaminase (ALT) and aspartate transaminase (AST)
Elevated levels may be an indicator of liver damage.

Transient global amnesia
Syndrome where there is a temporary but almost total disruption of short-term memory with a range of problems accessing older memories.

Transient ischemic attack
'Mini stroke' is caused by a temporary disruption in the blood supply to part of the brain.

Transurethral resection of the bladder
Surgical procedure that is used both to diagnose bladder cancer and to remove cancerous tissue from the bladder.

Triiodothyronine (T3)
Thyroid hormone.

Ubiquinone
Co-enzyme Q10.

Under active thyroid (hypothyroidism)
Disorder in which the thyroid gland does not produce enough thyroid hormone.

Urinary tract infection (acute cystitis or bladder infection)
Infection that affects part of the urinary tract.

Urology (genitourinary surgery)
Branch of medicine that focuses on the surgical and medical diseases of the male and female urinary tract system and the male reproductive organs.

Vascular surgery
Refers to diseases affecting the vascular system including diseases of arteries, veins and lymphatic vessels.

Vasculitis
Inflammation of the blood vessels.

Vasospasm
Refers to a condition in which a blood vessel's spasm leads to a narrowing of the blood vessels resulting from contraction of the muscular wall of the vessels. This can lead to tissue to a restriction in blood supply to tissues causing tissue death.

Ventricle
Chamber of the heart, having thick muscular walls, that receives blood from the atrium and pumps it to the arteries.

Vytorin
Combination of ezetimibe and simvastatin. Marketed by Merck.

World Health Organization
Agency of the United Nations that is concerned with international public health.

γ glutamyl transferase
Enzyme found in cell membranes of many tissues mainly in the liver, kidney, and pancreas.

Zocor
Trade name of simvastatin.

Appendix 2

Further resources

Websites:

www.thincs.org
The International Network of Cholesterol Skeptics (or THINCS) is a group of scientists, physicians, and other academicians from around the world who dispute the widely accepted saturated fat/cholesterol causes heart disease hypothesis. THINCS was founded in January 2003.

www.drmalcolmkendrick.org
Website of the Scottish doctor Malcolm Kendrick. Dr Kendrick says the blog is his best effort at providing some balance to the increasingly strident healthcare lobby that seems intent on scaring everyone about almost everything.

www.spacedoc.com
Dr Duane Graveline, MD and others have submitted over 250 articles on Cholesterol, Statin Drugs and their Side Effects.

www.dietsandscience.com
I've run this website since 2010. I've written easy to read reviews on over 1,400 diet, lifestyle & health studies from research centres, universities and peer-reviewed journals.

Books:

Ignore the Awkward: How the Cholesterol Myths Are Kept Alive by Dr Uffe Ravnskov
Fat and Cholesterol are Good For You by Dr Uffe Ravnskov
The Great Cholesterol Con by Dr Malcolm Kendrick

Doctoring Data: How to sort out medical advice from medical nonsense by Dr Malcolm Kendrick
Statin Damage Crisis by Dr Duane Graveline
The Dark Side of Statins by Dr Duane Graveline
Cholesterol and Saturated Fat Prevent Heart Disease by David Evans
Low Cholesterol Leads To An Early Death by David Evans
The Great Cholesterol Con by Anthony Colpo
Nutrition and Physical Degeneration by Weston A Price

DVD:

Statin Nation by Justin Smith
Informative information on the harm, often irreversible, caused by the wholesale prescribing of statin drugs.

Appendix 3

NICE conflict of interest

The National Institute for Health and Care Excellence (NICE) provides national guidance and advice on health and social care in the UK.

The following is a list of the NICE panel (Guideline Development Group) that developed the latest cholesterol guidelines for the UK. Many have direct financial ties to the pharmaceutical companies that manufacture statins, and some are involved in the next generation, more expensive, cholesterol lowering drugs, which are not yet on the market such as the ApoB Antisence drugs and PCSK9 inhibitors.

Dr Anthony Wierzbicki (Chair)

- Received funding for clinical trials from Sanofi – Aventis, Amgen, Pfizer, Genzyme, Merck Sharp & Dohme and Pfizer.

Dr Rajai Ahmad

- Received speaker fees from Bayer and Boehringer Ingelheim for providing educational presentations and from Bayer for participation in advisory board.
- Paid by Merck Sharp & Dohme to participate on symposium on commissioning in cardiovascular disease.

Ms Lindsay Banks

- Editor, 'NICE Bites' – a monthly bulletin for healthcare professionals involved in prescribing. The aim of the publication is to provide healthcare professionals with a clear and succinct summary of key prescribing points taken from NICE guidance.

Ms Liz Clark

- Has been involved in some NICE guidelines and activities.

Dr Martin Duerden

- Has written a number of articles and editorials on subject of Lipid modification.
- Has reviewed the North Wales Lipid lowering guideline.

Mrs Eleanor Grey

- No declared interest.

Dr Michael Khan

- Paid fees for been member of advisory boards at Genzyme and Amgen.
- Supported by AstraZeneca and Pfizer.
- Funding for clinical trial by Amgen.
- Salaried position as Chief Medical Officer and director of Silence Therapeutics Ltd.
- Member of advisory board for Amgen.
- Gave a talk sponsored by an educational grant by AstraZeneca.
- Has shares in and is a director of Pharmalogos Ltd (owned by his wife).
- Has sat on paid advisory boards for Genzyme/Sanofi and Novartis.
- Advisor to Oxford Pharmascience on behalf of his wife's company.
- Host and local organiser of Heart UK 2014.

Mrs Emma McGowan

- Sponsored by the Pharmaceutical company Astra Zeneca.
- Received personal payment from Merck Sharp Dohm for speaking at a meeting for nurses.
- Received personal payment from Astra Zeneca UK for attending the Heart UK Annual conference.
- Study coordinator for an Amgen study.
- Involved in the making of a video on behalf of Astrazeneca and Heart UK.

Dr Robert Dermot Neely

- Participated in advisory boards including Roche Pharma, Genzyme and Aegerion.
- Trustee and board member of the Heart UK.

- Member of Newcastle FATS guideline group on cholesterol lowering treatment.
- Sponsored by Merck to attend European Arteriosclerosis society.
- Received an honorarium from Sanofi UK & Ireland to participate in the UK Lipid Strategic Advisory Board.
- Gave an educational lecture at the HEART UK North West Lipid Forum. The meeting was supported by Sanofi UK & Ireland.
- Employed by Newcastle upon Tyne Hospitals NHS Foundation Trust as a Consultant and Clinical Lead for Clinical Biochemistry Department, a contracted provider of lipid profiles and other blood tests to primary and secondary care organisations which generate income for the Trust.
- He is also Clinical Lead for the Lipid and Metabolic Clinic in the same Trust, which accepts patient referrals for investigation and management of lipid disorders, which generate income for the Trust.
- Received an honorarium from Amgen for a short presentation.
- Participated in JBS3 on behalf of Heart UK.
- Involved in the production of lipid lowering guideline produced for the North East (FATS).

Dr Nadeem Qureshi

- Has received research grants. Published a paper underpinning NICE guidelines.
- Involved in developing NICE guidelines. Gave a talk at Heart UK.

Dr Alan Rees

- Member of advisory boards for Merck Sharp & Dohme, Pfizer and Genzyme.
- Received sponsorship to attend international meetings.
- Ex-chair of heart UK.
- Involved in trials for new drugs from Genzyme/Sanofi and Novartis.
- Chaired a medical meeting on Diabetes, sponsored by AstraZeneca.
- Sponsored by Merck Sharp & Dohme for giving lectures.
- Attended an Association of the British Pharmaceutical Industry dinner as guest of Abbott Healthcare.

- Gave a lecture on the forthcoming JBS3 Guidelines at a meeting sponsored by Merck Sharp & Dohme.
- Member of Sanofi Pharmaceutical Advisory Board.
- Received a speaker fee for giving a talk at a symposium sponsored by Bristol Myers Squibb and AstraZeneca on Diabetic Services.
- Received an honorarium for attending an Advisory Board for Aegerion.
- Member of JBS-3 guidelines development.
- Paid member of an Advisory Board for Novartis and to Amgen.
- Speaking at a forthcoming meeting on diabetes which is sponsored by AstraZeneca.
- Principle investigator to 2 trials involving monoclonal antibody to PCSK9 and an antisense oligonucleotide to Apo B.
- Trustee of Heart UK.

Dr David Wald

- Director of Polypill Ltd.
- His father, Nicholas Wald is also a Director of Polypill Ltd.
- Prinicipal Investigator of a Trial examining the effect of text message reminders on adherence to preventive cardiac treatment (including statins) which is partly funded by an education grant from Astra Zeneca.
- Has published and given lectures on the efficacy of cholesterol and blood pressure reduction in the general population in the prevention of cardiovascular disease.

List of pharmaceutical companies and the drugs they market.

Abbott: Niaspan, increases HDL cholesterol.

Aegerion: Lomitapide (trade nam Juxtapid), inhibits microsomal triglyceride transfer protein and inhibits the synthesis of chylomicrons and very low-density lipoprotein.

Amgen: Evolocumab, a monoclonal antibody PCSK9 inhibitor.

Astra Zeneca: Rosuvastatin (crestor) statin.

Bayer: Adempas (riociguat) For the treatment of Chronic Thromboembolic Pulmonary Hypertension and Pulmonary Arterial Hypertension.

Bayer: Cerivastatin (baycol, lipobay) statin.

Boehringer Ingelheim: Pradaxa (dabigatran etexilate mesylate) is a competitive, direct thrombin inhibitor. Used for risk reduction of stroke and embolism due to atrial fibrillation.

Bristol Myers Squibb: Pravastatin (pravachol) statin.

Genzyme: Mipomersen (trade name Kynamro) is a cholesterol-reducing drug. It is an antisense therapeutic that turns off the gene for apolipoprotein B.

Genzyme/Sanofi: Sanofi bought Genzyme for over $20 Billion in 2011.

Heart UK: Charity that advocates cholesterol lowering.

Joint British Societies 3 guidelines group (JSB3): Group that advocates pharmacological therapy to prevent heart disease.

Merck: Anacetrapib, CETP inhibitor is a member of a class of drugs that inhibit cholesterylester transfer protein (CETP), that may 'improve' cholesterol levels.

Merck Sharp & Dohme: Ezetimibe reduces the amount of cholesterol which is absorbed from the intestine.

Merck Sharp & Dohme: Simvastatin (zocor) statin.

Newcastle FATS guideline group: A group that develops strategy for the use of cholesterol lowering drugs in Newcastle, North Tyneside and Northumberland.

Novartis: Diacylglycerol O-acyltransferase 1 (DGAT1) inhibitor. Lowers triglycerides.

Novartis: Fluvastatin (lescol) statin.

Novartis: LCZ696 heart failure drug.

Oxford Pharmascience: Reformulate statin drugs.

Pfizer: Atorvastatin (lipitor) statin.

Pfizer: Bococizumab is a monoclonal antibody PCSK9 inhibitor.

Pharmalogos Ltd: Have provided educational/training activity in FH on behalf of Astra-Zeneca. The company may also provide consultancy/advisory services in these areas in the future.

Polypill Ltd: Developing a combination pill (including a statin) for the prevention of cardiovascular disease.

Roche Pharma: Dalcetrapib, increases HDL cholesterol.

Sanofi – Aventis: Alirocumab (trade name praluent) monoclonal antibody PCSK9 inhibitor.

Silence Therapeutics Ltd: Company are interested in preclinical studies of novel targets for homozygous FH, including ApoB.

The above reveals how an intimate beneficial financial tangled web is woven between pharmaceutical companies, government advisory bodies, doctors, scientists, charities and non-elected repesentitives that recommend national and local health policy.

Index

(Refers to paper numbers)

CPSIA information can be obtained
at www.ICGtesting.com
Printed in the USA
BVHW042034090822
644147BV00001B/3

9 781781 483909